Health Politics:

Power, Populism and Health

Other Books by Mike Magee, MD

All Available Boats
The Book of Choices
Positive Leadership
The Best Medicine
The New Face of Aging
Positive Doctors in America

To order, call (866) 543-5140

Health Politics:
Power, Populism and Health

Mike Magee, MD

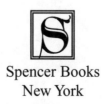

Spencer Books
New York

Published in the United States by Spencer Books.

Published simultaneously in Canada.

Spencer Books
3 Stoneleigh Plaza, Suite 5D
Bronxville, NY 10708

To order, call (866) 543-5140
www.spencerbooks.com

ISBN 1-8897-93-17-5

Text design: Jeanette Koon
Cover design: Ana Schedler

Manufactured in Canada

Foreword

No one who works close to the health care delivery system can be in that position long without realizing that the system is broken. The urge to fix it is what this book is all about. There has certainly been no shortage of suggestions for improving the system, but the doomsday prophets, academics, and policy makers alike do little to raise our expectation for the future. Instead, they leave the impression that perhaps our problems may be too big to address fundamentally. Few, it seems, believe in their own abilities, in this era of enormous challenges and intense change.

The issues are complex and have largely been the province of this country's thought elites. But as our unbelievable access to information has increased, especially over the past decade, a new cohort has joined in the debate — the public. Consumers come at our daunting health care issues from a different knowledge base than even the preceding generation: with instant communication, public discussion, and an increasingly well-developed ability to discern hype and spin from truth.

Top this off with the technology of the Internet and the public has produced a generation of remarkably savvy individuals who understand their own bodies, the challenges of maintaining health, the benefits of preventive medicine and their power to influence outcomes. The right to be heard is so deeply ingrained in them that it has even affected the way medicine is now practiced.

The baby boomers have essentially written the agenda of America for the past 30 years. I have long looked forward to the day when they would encounter the problems of the health care system — particularly Medicare — because their previous performance indicated they would not put up with the things that their parents accepted as norms. That day has arrived.

Led by the boomers, consumers are increasingly empowered by knowledge and an understanding of the process of health care policy making. They clamor for action and results, and they expect our leaders — whether in government, academia, or the private sector — to step forward into their arena with new ideas.

Within that arena is a sensitive voice of honesty and innovation in the person of Mike Magee, MD, the author of this book. He rightly calls the emergence of empowered consumers a "populist uprising in health care," and he comes to the debate with thoughts they — and policy makers — need to hear. Dr. Magee has been speaking and writing for many years, testing his ideas with the public; and now many of these ideas appear here as essays.

Health Politics: Power, Populism and Health isolates Dr. Magee's many specific concerns against the key trends that are shaping our health care future and gives the reader a health care context in which to judge health care issues, such as the demography of aging; the need for, rise of, and exhaustion of family caregivers; the dual burden of disease — both acute and chronic; and the role played by the two-edged sword of the Internet, which engenders consumer activism and power.

The issues touched upon in this book loom large and complicated. How will we deal with the impending crush of chronic disease globally? As we prolong lives by the increased knowledge of, say, cardiology, so that other acute diseases become chronic, have we given any thought to the public health impact of having people live longer but sicker and unable to care for themselves? What will we do about the uninsured? Immigrants account for the largest cohorts of uninsured (26 percent), and they represented 86 percent of the growth of the uninsured between 1998 and 2003. How will we care for them? With obesity listed as the number two cause of death by lifestyle decisions in the United States, do we really have a plan for managing these social risks? With 500 million tobacco-related deaths predicted by statisticians within the next 25 years, has anyone really taken in the enormity of those figures and adequately calculated the role of avarice and greed that contributes to the death of these people? Can any of the above be tackled legislatively without true malpractice and health insurance reform?

I raise these questions at a particularly appropriate time in history. I have been lecturing, debating, and holding seminars on health care reform in this country since the days when the elder Bush was president. Through those years there were always activists fighting for the "Canadian System" or extolling the virtues of any "Single Payer" system, when at the same time, what we used to call socialized medicine was failing in many places on the planet.

On June 9, 2005, the Supreme Court of Canada took unusual action and essentially labeled the health system (as it then worked) as dangerous, and it struck down portions of the law that make current health care in Canada, at the very best, uncertain. Not many predicted this outcome. Statistics indicate that approximately 1.2 million Canadians lack a family doctor and are looking for one. Without the health care provided in the United States for many Canadians, the situation would be even worse than it is.

The Prime Minister of the United Kingdom, Tony Blair, won re-election in 2005 partly on promises made for radical changes in the National Health Service. In spite of all this, the United States in recent months has seen Vermont, California, and Maine vote for some type of single payer system.

The point is: We are divided nationally, and nations are divided globally. The answers some may have thought obvious in recent years are not so obvious anymore. New answers are needed, new thinking, new hope. And it all must be geared toward practical, workable, long-term solutions.

Connecting the divide between an abstract health policy argument and its very real impact on the lives of individuals and families is just one of Mike Magee's many talents, and it is evident throughout this book. His observations about our health care system offer just what we need at the moment — objective thinking, a sense of urgency, hope for the future, a batch of fresh ideas, and an end to the crass political infighting that seeks the victory of one political party over the other in any skirmish rather than serving the needs of the American people.

Dr. Magee primarily intended this book as a classroom resource, to spur debate on college campuses while coalescing academic disciplines; I believe it is just as relevant, but perhaps more important, to policy makers and private sector leaders.

Health Politics: Power, Populism and Health illuminates the growing disconnect between those who shape policy and those who are affected by it — and our leaders must acknowledge this gap before they are overwhelmed by it.

I cannot believe that this disconnect will lead to anything other than a continuation of the current uprising by enlightened consumers seeking a populist health policy.

It may be that history will show that the public eventually won the day because it sickened of the tinkering at the edges that characterized politics and health in the last three decades and in a sense empowered policy makers to work for the greater good with the assurance of enormous public support.

Hopefully, *Health Politics: Power, Populism and Health* will help history play out accordingly. In the meantime, Mike Magee's book is an invaluable resource for anyone who cares about our health care future.

C. Everett Koop, MD, ScD
Surgeon General 1981-1989
McInerny Professor of Surgery
Senior Scholar, C. Everett Koop Institute at Dartmouth

"Medicine is a social science. And politics is simply medicine on a large scale."

— Rudolf Virchow
Pioneer in public health
1821-1902

Preface

The Social Science of Health: A New Value Proposition

Over the past five years, the World Health Organization and other groups have actively engaged the question, "What is health?" A large part of this thought process has involved defining what health is not. It is not the health care system or a bureaucratic delivery mechanism. It is not the reactive elimination of disease. It is not a simple commodity to be weighed against all other commodities in society. It is different from these things, and more than these things.

Health is universal and common to the people of the world, independent of geography, race, income, gender and culture. Health is an active state of well-being that encompasses mind, body and spirit. It is the capacity to reach one's full human potential, and, on a larger scale, a nation's leading edge of development.

Dr. Gro Brundtland, former director general of the World Health Organization, wrote in the World Health Report 2000 that "The objective of good health is twofold — goodness and fairness; goodness being the best attainable average level; and fairness, the smallest feasible differences among individuals and groups."[1]

Now, five years later, this notion that health is a preferred state of being, rather than a set of disconnected functions or services, is increasingly being embraced.

With this in mind, it becomes impossible to ignore a significant modern truism. Health is profoundly political. Why is this the case? For multiple reasons: Health is a collection of resources unequally distributed in society. Health's "social determinants," such as housing, income and employment, are critical to the accomplishment of individual, family, and community well-being and are themselves politically determined. Health is recognized by many throughout the world as a fundamental right, yet it is irreparably intertwined with our social, economic and political systems. And growth in health, health care, and health systems requires political debate and political consensus.[2]

For these reasons and more, it is entirely reasonable to acknowledge and attempt to structure in a purposeful manner the social science of health. To do so requires mention of some of the major forces shaping health worldwide. These include aging demographics, the growth of home-based caregivers, the dual burden of disease, the Internet, and consumer empowerment and activism.

In the United States, nearly 50 percent of all 60-year-olds have a parent alive, and by 2050 there will be 1 million people over age 100.[3] This means the three-generation family has been supplanted by the four- and five-generation family. Twenty-five percent of American homes have an elder caregiver in place, and 85 percent of them are volunteer family members. The vast majority of these caregivers are third-generation women, managing parents and grandparents on the one hand and children and grandchildren on the other.[4,5] In the United States, their focus is predominantly on chronic diseases, seven of which cause 90 percent of the disability in senior populations.[6]

In the developing world, the health focus remains primarily on infectious diseases, nutrition, and maternal and fetal issues, which are challenging the human and financial resources of these countries. But urbanization and the influx of tobacco and unhealthy foods are accelerating the onset of chronic diseases and creating a dual burden of disease.[7]

As for the last trend that's shaping health, consumer empowerment is being fueled by the Internet and supported by physicians, nurses and other caregivers. This has led to emancipation and engagement of an increasingly activist-oriented public.[8] We desire education, behavioral modification, home-based care solutions, inclusion in the health care team, and financial incentives to reward wellness.[9]

As these trends play out and the definition of health continues to evolve, we will see the seat of political power in health continue to shift. It will move away from paternalism toward partnership. It will move away from individual care models to team approaches. And it will move away from intervention toward prevention. It will embrace evidence-based clinical care but incorporate educational and social missions as well. It will move away from hospitals and outpatient care sites toward home settings. And it will move away from thought elites toward patients and their care teams.

Despite this shifting environment, there is a growing political disconnect between those who make health policy and those most affected by health policy. While the former continue to reinforce silos and the status quo, the latter seek broad, fundamental and comprehensive reform. Such reform might include expansion of insurance coverage, realignment of financial incentives toward prevention, increased reimbursement of physicians and nurses for team coordination that includes home health managers, support for early diagnosis and screening, and expansion of education and behavioral modification for individuals and families.

Due to its profound impact on the future of individuals, families, communities, and societies, the social science of health deserves broad debate, active public participation, and focused scholarly pursuit. We must harness the best scholars in medical sociology, political sociology and political psychology, health economics, public health, medicine, nursing, pastoral care and bereavement, to create interdisciplinary social health leadership curricula and degrees that are equipped to manage the rapidly evolving health environment, and to more effectively challenge outdated thinking, outdated systems, and outdated approaches to health.

Health Politics: Power, Populism and Health is a collection of 76 individual essays that explore the complex health issues of the day. They have been loosely organized into nine general categories, but by no means fully address these themes in a comprehensive or coordinated way. Rather, the essays provide an entry point to a focused topic, key questions, and a rich array of electronic resources, accessible online at www.HealthPolitics.com. The resources provided are designed to support discussion, interaction and debate. If this text advances public involvement and engagement around today's most pressing health issues, it will have served its purpose.

REFERENCES

1. World Health Organization. World Health Report 2000 – Health Systems: Improving Performance. Available at: http://www.who.int/whr/2000/en/index.html. Accessed June 8, 2005.
2. Bambra C, Fox D, Scott-Samuel A. Towards a politics of health. *Health Promotion International*. 2005;20:187-193.
3. Alliance for Aging Research. *Medical Never-Never Land: Ten Reasons Why America is Not Ready for the Coming Age Boom*. Available at: http://www.agingresearch.org/brochures/nevernever/nevernever.pdf. Accessed June 8, 2005.
4. Census 2000 Brief. The 65 years and over population: 2000. Available at: http://www.census.gov/prod/2001pubs/c2kbr01-10.pdf. Accessed June 8, 2005.
5. Magee M. Aging — New Environments for Mature Living. Health Politics. Available at: http://www.healthpolitics.com/program_info.asp?p=prog_10. Accessed June 8, 2005.
6. Yach D, Hawkes C, Gould CL, Hofman KJ. The global burden of chronic diseases. *JAMA*. 2004;291:2612-2622.
7. Action on smoking and health. Tobacco global trends. Available at: http://www.ash.org.uk/html/international/html/globaltrends.html. Accessed June 8, 2005.
8. Magee M. Relationship-Based Health Care in the United States, United Kingdom, Canada, Germany, South Africa and Japan. World Medical Association Annual Meeting in Helsinki, Finland. Sept. 11, 2003.
9. Nash D. *Connecting with the New Health Care Consumer*. New York: McGraw Hill;2001.

Acknowledgments

Health Politics, the web-based health policy program that I host, recently celebrated a milestone by publishing its 100th weekly show since it was launched two years ago.

Health Politics would not be possible without the help of a number of talented individuals and organizations whose shared experience in health care has provided a tremendous asset. Their insights and collective experience in health care has helped me think in new ways about the issues. To mention individually the wide range of physicians, nurses, health professionals, caregivers, and patients who have been remarkably generous with their friendship, knowledge and wisdom would require many pages and risk important omissions. Please know that you have been on my mind each and every day, and that I listen carefully to you, appreciate you, and respect you.

As a group, participants over the past seven years in the Pfizer Medical Humanities Initiative programming deserve my thanks as partners who have been willing to make policy "house calls" to our program; to inform our thinking and help us better shape our shared health care environment. For your extraordinary contributions, openness and for the trust established between us, I extend my sincere gratitude.

It is also important to acknowledge the extraordinary efforts of our Health Politics partners and associates who have provided feedback, or contributed to our content, aided our distribution and who share credit for our growth. They include Alpha Epsilon Delta, American Academy of Family Physicians, American College of Physicians, American College of Nurse Practitioners, American College of Surgeons, American Federation for Aging

Research, American Gastroenterological Association, American Geriatrics Society, American Medical Association Alliance, American Medical Association Foundation, American Medical Women's Association, American Osteopathic Association, American Society on Aging, Association of American Medical Colleges, Bone and Joint Decade, California Academy of Family Physicians Foundation, Center for Aging Services Technologies, Columbia University Global Health Initiative, International College of Surgeons, Department of Surgery at Johns Hopkins, Medical Group Management Association, National Alliance for Caregiving, the National Eating Disorders Association, National Women's Health Resource Center, United Nations Department of Economic and Social Affairs (DESA), UCLA Healthcare Collaborative and the World Medical Association.

A special thanks to Paul Larson, Leslie Green and Jeanette Koon for their daily contributions to the success of this program; and to Karen Carey, Eneida Clarke, Kate Frohlinger, Kaveri Nair, Jim Tosone and Zach Sikes for making time from their otherwise busy schedules to contribute to our success.

Finally, my thanks to Trish, Mike, Sue, Mitchell, Marc, Kathleen, Meredith, Dave, Anabella and Fiona, and to our extended families, who have daily reinforced in me that caring individuals, families, communities and societies are built upon compassion, understanding and partnership; and that life and death must be embraced. I will always appreciate your love, guidance and support.

Mike Magee, MD
New York
2005

How to Use This Book

Health Politics: Power, Populism and Health has been written and designed as a classroom resource. Seventy-six essays have been grouped into nine categories, with fully sourced references at the end of each essay. Each chapter includes a section titled "Teaching Tools," which organizes the material for academic use. The classroom tools include:

• Policy Premises: The key policy issues driving each essay, boiled down and stated succinctly in bullet form to frame class discussions.

• Review: Five to ten study-and-review questions related to chapter content.

• Online Resources: Web-based resources, ranging from scholarly studies to government websites, offering related information and analysis for research purposes.

• Health Politics Online: Links to supporting material for each of the essays, found at the website www.HealthPolitics.com. Supporting material includes videos and downloadable Power Point slides.

How to Use the Health Politics CD

The CD included with this book includes all of the materials located in the "Online Resources" section of each chapter. Note: All of the web links listed in each chapter are included as "live" links on the CD — which allows users to easily access these resources. Just insert the CD in your computer, find the chapter you need, and click on any of the links to visit a website or a down-loadable source.

How to Use HealthPolitics.com in the Classroom

All essays in this book are based on similar essays previously published at the website www.HealthPolitics.com. The website includes a video presentation of each essay by Dr. Magee, accompanied by a synchronized set of Power Point slides. These free videos may be assigned to students or viewed in class.

Videos and slides at the HealthPolitics.com website are archived and easily accessible, and they include a wide range of background and support materials for research purposes.

About the Pfizer Medical Humanities Initiative

Health Politics is supported by the Pfizer Medical Humanities Initiative, an education and research project founded in1997 and supported by Pfizer Inc. In addition to worldwide studies of health care, leadership and the patient-physician relationship, the initiative funds numerous scholarship and grant programs for physicians, medical students and patient groups.

To the caregivers,
who give so much of themselves every day.

Table of Contents

Health Politics:
Power, Populism and Health

CHAPTER 1

Placing Health in Context

"Remarkable gains in health, rapid economic growth and unprecedented scientific advances — all legacies of the 20th century — could lead to a new era of human progress. The world enters the 21st century with hope, but also with uncertainty."

— GRO BRUNDTLAND
Former Director General
World Health Organization

CHAPTER 1.1

Globalization

DEFINING THE BURDEN OF DISEASE

"Remarkable gains in health, rapid economic growth and unprecedented scientific advances — all legacies of the 20th century — could lead to a new era of human progress. The world enters the 21st century with hope, but also with uncertainty." So wrote Gro Brundtland, director general of the World Health Organization in her World Health Report in 1999.[1] Today, both hope and uncertainty seem on the rise, with good reason for both.

The Global Burden of Disease study, published in *Science* in 1996, looked at the effect of disease not only on "lifespan" but also on "health span" for the first time.[2] It did so by moving beyond mortality rates and creating a new measure called DALY, which stands for Disability Adjusted Life Year, and expresses one year of life lost to premature death and years lived with a disability of specified severity and duration; one year of life lost to poor health.

Lifespan equals the number of years living, while health span equals the number of years of healthy living. These are two enormously different measures. We increasingly appreciate that disease and disability can significantly limit an individual's productivity and happiness, and radically alter individual, family and community well being. For example, malnutrition is responsible for approximately 12 percent of total deaths worldwide, radically altering global lifespan, but affects health span to an even greater degree, contributing nearly 16 percent of the world's total disability.[2]

The DALY measure for the first time provided a comparative tool to analyze and prioritize our most pressing health challenges worldwide, regionally, and nationally. The study, extending over multiple years and led by epidemiologist Alan Lopez of the WHO and Harvard professor Christopher Murray, is clearly just the beginning of a new way of thinking strategically about health as the leading edge of development.

Let's start at the beginning. There are some 6 billion people in the world and hundreds of millions experience disease or injury each year. Taken as a whole, the combined pain, suffering, loss of productivity and unrealized hopes and dreams are our world's burden of disease.

The Global Burden of Disease study, begun in 1992, involved 100 collaborators in more than 20 countries. It attempted to quantify disease and injury burden of more than 100 conditions and make projections out 30 years for 500 consequences or results of these conditions. In the analysis, more than 50,000 estimates were made.[2,3] In the process, opinions were replaced by facts and it became clear that disease burden involved more than premature death. It also involved living life marred by chronic, debilitating and incapacitating disease.

Out of this enormous groundbreaking effort came an avalanche of data. Table 1.1-1 shows the top ten disease entities that have or will alter health span in 1990 and 2020, ranked from high to low by the percentage of total years of healthy living that our global population loses as a result of specific disease or disability.

Table 1.1-1. Top Ten Disease Entities in 1990 and 2020

1990	% DALY	2020	% DALY
1. Respiratory infections	8.2	1. Ischemic heart disease	5.9
2. Diarrheal disease	7.2	2. Major depression	5.7
3. Perinatal illnesses	6.7	3. Auto accidents	5.1
4. Major depression	3.7	4. Cerebrovascular disease	4.4
5. Ischemic heart disease	3.4	5. Chronic obstructive	4.1
6. Cerebrovascular disease	2.8	pulmonary disease	
		6. Respiratory infections	3.1
7. Tuberculosis	2.8	7. Tuberculosis	3.1
8. Measles	2.6	8. War	3.0
9. Auto accidents	2.5	9. Diarrheal disease	2.7
10. Congenital birth defects	2.4	10. HIV	2.6

Source: Murray CJL, Lopez AD. Science 1996; 274:741

Topping off the list in 1990 are respiratory diseases, diarrheal diseases, perinatal illnesses, depression and ischemic heart disease. As you can see, by 2020, the rankings have changed, and heart disease worldwide has achieved top billing, followed by depression, auto accidents, cerebrovascular disease and chronic obstructive pulmonary disease or emphysema.[2]

Even this high-level review reveals some surprises.

First, on the whole, while communicable infectious diseases are still overwhelming in underdeveloped countries, they will gradually be overtaken by non-communicable chronic diseases as the leading cause of world death and disability, especially in developed countries. Predictive models suggest that by 2020, 73 percent of the world's disease burden will result from chronic disease, 15 percent from infectious diseases and 12 percent from trauma.[4]

Secondly, the worldwide burden of mental illness was exceedingly high. 3.7 percent of the total global burden of disease was attributed to major depression alone.[1]

Third, violence, war and injuries accounted for 12 percent of deaths worldwide. But shockingly, in the United States, for people under 20, it accounted for 41 percent of deaths with 14 percent homicides and 7 percent suicides.[5]

Fourth, alcohol-related problems were the leading cause of male disability and the tenth leading cause of female disability in developed nations.[4] Tobacco use was predicted to cause more disease and disability than any other single cause, and to a greater extent in underdeveloped nations by the year 2020.[2,4]

Chronic diseases are already the major cause of limited health span and DALYs in the developed world. Looking at sources of total DALYs in developed countries, 18.6 percent are the result of cardiovascular disease, 15.4 percent from mental illness, 15 percent from cancer, 4.8 percent from all respiratory diseases, and 4.7 percent from alcohol.[2]

What does this data tell us then about the relationship between economic development and health? It tells us to be aware of DALYs' "downward spiral." As we concentrate resources on combating the disability related to communicable diseases in developing countries, and harness economic resources to advance standard of living and movement toward more developed economies, we must be prepared to address the significant threat to health of chronic disease, which is literally right around the corner.

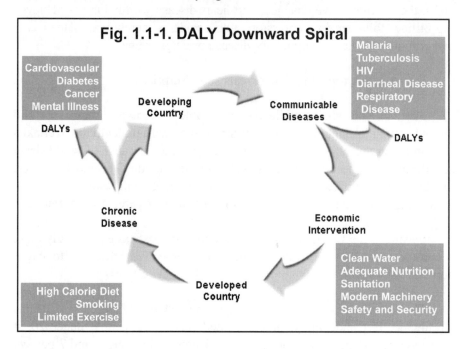

Fig. 1.1-1. DALY Downward Spiral

Economic development on the most basic level addresses fundamental health needs including clean water, adequate nutrition, sanitation, work-saving machines and safety. However, development carries with it the hazard of high calorie diets, smoking, sedentary lifestyles and vehicular trauma, which gradually shift the risk of disease from infectious agents to chronic conditions including cancer and cardiovascular disease. Dr. K. Srinath Reddy, Professor of Cardiology at the All India Institute of Medical Sciences, recently noted, "This study compels us to focus downstream on health and economic consequences of the disease burden, as well as upstream on the risk factors and determinants."[6]

What are the specific factors most affecting the burden of disease, and where are these factors most prevalent?

INFLUENCING FACTORS

Thanks to the Global Burden of Disease study, reported in 1996, and the creation of a new health measure, the DALY, or the disability adjusted life year — one DALY equals one year lost to poor health — we've begun to think more clearly about the health of our planet's 6 billion human inhabitants.

Aristotle said, "Men do not think they know a thing until they have grasped the why of it." Dr. A.D. Lopez, lead author of the Global Burden of Disease study, echoed those sentiments when he said, "The purpose of the research into the global burden of disease was not only to measure and describe the health of the world, but also, and more important in many ways, to explain why these events and phenomena have occurred."[6]

The global burden of disease is a product of complex and interwoven demographic, economic, social, political, religious and environmental factors. Probably the strongest factor yielding the greatest impact on global health span is the aging of the world's population.[7] There are currently approximately 184 million global citizens over the age of 65. This number is projected to increase to 678 million by the year 2030. This will make four- and five-generation families, with all their complexity and competing resource needs, the norm worldwide. It will also mean that chronic disease will dominate as sources of DALYs. This is already the case in the developed world where cardiovascular disease accounts for 18.6 percent of lost health, mental illness results in 15.4 percent of lost health and cancer delivers 15 percent of lost health.[5] But by 2020, global percentages of total lost health span in both developed and underdeveloped nations will be dominated by chronic disease. Global lost health from cardiovascular disease, as a percentage of total lost health, will rise from 11.1 percent to 14.7 percent. Losses from cancer will rise from 5.1 percent to 9.9 percent, and losses from neuropsychiatric disorders will rise from 10.5 percent to 14.7 percent.[8]

The reality of aging is causing health policy experts to go back to the drawing board and consider the relationship between lifespan and health span. Stated in another way, when examining the application of health resources, experts have often focused on the first 15 years of life and the last 15 years. But today, with the five-generation global family increasingly the norm, we have begun to appreciate that the health gains achieved in the first 15 years must be consolidated and leveraged to the benefit of the next 15 years, and so on up the ladder of life. Early and continuous investment delivers long-term gains.

If aging is an undeniable reality, then so is urbanization. Rapid urbanization, with dense populations, unsafe water, poor sanitation and poverty, is a perfect breeding ground for disease. In 1950 only one-third of the global population resided in urban settings. By 2000 this number had risen to 45 percent. And by 2020, 60 percent of the world's population is projected to be urban.[7] As people migrate, they may leave behind diseases endemic to their region only to inherit new ones. For example, where once they grew their own food, city dwellers must now purchase food, often high in salt, dietary fats and sugar. With these changes come higher levels of obesity, diabetes and heart disease. Smoking, high fat diets and poor exercise habits all accompany industrialization and urbanization. Where developed nations have had the resources to at least challenge these harmful changes in behavior, the developing nations may neither have the time nor the means to cope.

Finally, economic factors clearly impact the global burden of disease. Nils Daulaire, president of the Global Health Council, has noted that, "Poor people are often sick because they are poor, and sometimes poor people are poor because they are sick." The economic impact of just infectious diseases is overwhelming. It is estimated that developing nations have an annual per capita loss of income of 2 percent as a result of infectious diseases. This in effect eliminates the potential of an individual to double his income over a 35-year period.[9] And the gap between rich and poor is growing. In 1900, the per capita income gap between the richest 20 percent and the poorest 20 percent was 25 to one. In 2000, that gap was 67 to one.[9]

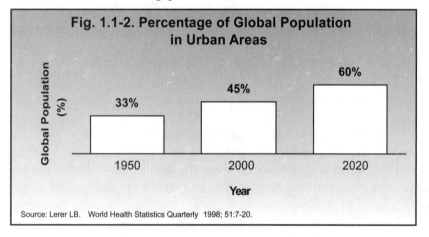

Fig. 1.1-2. Percentage of Global Population in Urban Areas

Source: Lerer LB.   World Health Statistics Quarterly 1998; 51:7-20.

Yet, when resources are focused, there is a glimmer of hope. Gro Brundtland, director general of the WHO, said in 1999, "The most sustainable investment we can make in healthy populations is to take proper care of our children's health."[9] In the latest analysis of the global burden of disease, lead researcher Dr. Lopez noted that mortality in children under age 5 declined from 13.5 million deaths per year to about 10.5 million deaths per year over an eight year period. That's a 22 percent improvement. Experts believe that increases in availability of basic health services are a part of this success story. But Dr. Lopez feels that the secret to success is another factor: "Education of the mother is perhaps the most significant parental factor in determining child survival."[10]

So the factors are many. But one thing is clear, needs must be matched by resources. Currently 85 percent to 90 percent of global health expenditures occur in developed nations, which harbor only 10 percent to 15 percent of the global burden of disease. In contrast, developing nations are left to cope with 85 percent to 90 percent of the disease burden utilizing only 10 percent to 15 percent of the world's resources.[10]

Is it possible to use the burden of disease data and the power of the DALY to direct resources toward greatest need?

FROM RESEARCH TO ACTION

The 1996 Global Burden of Disease study, using 100 collaborators from more than 20 countries worldwide, was the first comprehensive attempt to measure the world's current and future health needs.[5] The creation of a unit of measure — the DALY, the equivalent of one year of active living lost to poor health — provided a method of comparing and prioritizing the many competing health needs of the world's population.

We've considered definitions and findings, environmental contributors and individual risk factors. Now, we'll consider how best to use those findings to influence action.

Dr. Lopez, one of the lead authors of the study, has said, "Development of health care policy is not about predictions or wish lists for the future. Rather, it is a process that aims to challenge assumptions and encourage fresh thinking to better understand the future."[11]

In accessing global health, we are no longer starting from scratch. We now have a common language and set of tools. Nils Daulaire has said, "In the past we were comparing apples and oranges and grapes. Although there are imperfections in the data that require ongoing research and refinement, at least there is now a common language."[11]

Turning words into action, however, requires knowledge of what works and how much it costs. Both are required to substantially alter the burden of disease. In developing countries, resources are required to create infrastructure for clean water, sanitation, adequate nutrition and medical supplies. Equally necessary are strategies that successfully accomplish vaccination, maternal education and safe-sex education. In developed countries, the resources to educate, diagnose, and treat — long term — a population currently overwhelmed by diabetes, heart disease, cancer and depression; and more importantly, to develop educational and motivational tools that successfully promote healthy diets, exercise, early screening, and treatment compliance, are all required.

In short, there is the need to finance and execute programs that address acute threats and promote healthy behaviors. What do we know works? First, facts, in the form of statistics and hard data, that are accurate, up-to-date and compelling. Second, stories — true stories — that put a human face on data. Third, political pressure, the ability to mobilize a constituency around a concrete goal and objective, with a target time for completion. And fourth, a "knight in shining armor," a compelling and effective spokesperson. Witness the impact of Christopher Reeve or Michael J. Fox on research into neurodegenerative diseases, or C. Everett Koop's influence on HIV prevention and cigarette smoking.

Prioritization is critical to success. In health, one must be extraordinarily pragmatic, focusing on what is possible now, rather than on a long-term and currently unrealistic goal. How does one select achievable goals? Here are three hints. First, choose small achievable goals that will impact large numbers of people, rather than large goals that affect only a few people. Second, find what people value, what they are willing to take action on to protect or correct, and build your campaign around those values. Third, invest in patient education, especially maternal education, as well as preventive screening and early intervention.

In the past, there were sharp demarcations between the health challenges of developing and developed countries. But today, with mass migration, high-speed travel, global trade, the Internet and progressive urbanization, we must be prepared to address the double burden of disease in all geographies. Certainly the burden of infectious diseases, malnourishment, and maternal-fetal ill health will continue to dominate the public health horizon in developing countries. But these issues will find visibility in pockets of poverty and limited health access in our most developed nations, as well. Similarly, the rapid conversion to poor diet and physical inactivity that accompanies rising standards of living and leads to outbreaks of heart disease, diabetes and cancer, will increasingly find a foothold in underdeveloped countries as multinational franchises market and spread these behaviors. The global health movement must be prepared to wage its campaign for health on two fronts simultaneously around the world. Tobacco and the health of infants are two areas worthy of special focus, considering the long-term health implications of failure in these arenas.

A.C. Achutti of the World Heart Federation recently sounded a cautionary alarm when he said, "Unfortunately, much of the ground work for the burden of disease in 2020 has already been laid in infants born in poverty or at low birth weights, who are then malnourished or unprotected from infection as children. We need to end this continuum."[11]

So perhaps that is a good place to conclude this discussion of the Global Burden of Disease, with the notion that poor health is a downward spiral, a negative continuum that requires aggressive coordinated action to assure course reversal. It is clear that a challenge of this magnitude requires cross-sector health platforms and cooperative partnerships.[12] What might each sector contribute? Government can provide consistent high-health objectives, presidential leadership and multinational agreements. Academics can provide ongoing research, evolving diagnostic and treatment strategies, and outcome measurements. Nongovernmental organizations, or NGOs, can provide health services on the ground, real-time surveillance, and expertise in internet organization. And industry can provide financial and human resources, political contacts and multinational infrastructure.

We all have something to bring to the table. The Global Burden of Disease study seems to be calling out, prodding us, reminding us, "The time is right. The time is now." John Seffrin, CEO of the American Cancer Society, summed it up nicely with these words: "The burden of disease is the great oppressor, perhaps the single greatest cause of loss of personal freedom. Now, more than any other time in human history, we can influence this great oppressor with our actions. We have it within our power to improve the health of people on the earth."[11]

REFERENCES

1. Kalfoglou AI, Boenning DA, et al. IOM: Summary of the Symposium on Public Confidence and Involvement in Clinical Research: Clinical Research Roundtable. Washington, DC: *National Academy of Sciences*; Sep 2000.
2. Lichter, A. Bench, Bedside, and Beyond: Clinical Research at the Crossroads. *The Pfizer Journal*. Vol 6:3, 2002. p. 10-12.
3. Getz K. Patient experiences in industry-sponsored clinical trials. In: Kalfoglou AI, Boenning DA, et al. IOM: Summary of the Symposium on Public Confidence and Involvement in Clinical Research: Clinical Research Roundtable. Washington, DC: *National Academy of Sciences*; Sep 2000.
4. Nationwide survey reveals public support of clinical research studies on the rise [news release]. Denver, CO: Harris Interactive; Jun 27, 2001.
5. Murray CJL, Lopez AD. Evidence-based health policy-lessons from the Global Burden of Disease Study. *Science*. 1996; 274:740-743.
6. Murray CJL, Lopez AD. The utility of DALYs for public health policy and research: a reply [point of view]. Bull World Health Org. 1997; 75:377-381.
7. Lerer LB, Lopez AD, KjellstromT, Yach D. Health for all: analyzing health status and determinants. World Health Stat Q. 1998;51:7-20.
8. Murray CJL, Lopez AD. Alternative projections of mortality and disability by cause. 1990-2020: Global Burden of Disease Study. *Lancet*. 1997;349:1498-1504.
9. Daulaire, N. Understanding the Burden of Disease: A Global Perspective. *The Pfizer Journal*. 1:1, 2000. p.23-24.
10. Lopez AD. Understanding the Burden of Disease. A Global Perspective. *The Pfizer Journal*. 1:1, 2000, p. 24-25.
11. Understanding the Burden of Disease: A Global Perspective. *The Pfizer Journal*. www.thepfizerjournal.com. Volume 1:1, 2000. Accessed May 2003.
12. Magee, M. Qualities of enduring cross-sector partnerships in public health. *The American Journal of Surgery*. 185(2003) 26-29.

TEACHING TOOLS

Policy Premises

1. The global burden of disease is a product of complex and inter-woven demographic, economic, social, political, religious and environmental factors.
2. The strongest demographic driving the global burden of disease is the aging of the world's population.
3. Rapid urbanization with dense populations, unsafe water, poor sanitation and poverty is a perfect breeding ground for disease.
4. Globalization — the sharing of people, communications, capital, images, ideas and values across borders — is creating tactical alliances and potential new solutions to many complex health challenges.
5. Poverty is a breeding ground for compromised lifespan and health span.
6. Global needs must be matched with resources.
7. In assessing global health, we are no longer starting from scratch. We have a common language and set of tools.
8. To turn words into action you must know what works and how much it costs.
9. Prioritization must be extraordinarily pragmatic, focusing on what is possible now, rather than on a long-term and currently unrealis-tic goal.
10. Address the double burden of disease, which coexists in develop-ing countries and in pockets of poverty in developed countries.
11. Control of tobacco and the health of infants are priorities every-where because of their extensive long-term downward spiraling illness continuum.
12. Success requires cross-sector platforms and long-term cooperative partnerships.

Review

1. What is a DALY?
2. How do medical researchers use DALYs?
3. What is the difference between lifespan and health span?

4. What are five of the top ten diseases that will alter health span in the year 2020?

5. What is the relationship between economic development and health?

6. What factor has the greatest impact on global health span?

7. How many people worldwide are over the age of 65?

8. What impact does global urbanization have on health span?

9. During the past century, to what extent did the gap between the world's wealthiest and poorest people widen?

10. What is the most sustainable investment we can make in improving worldwide health?

11. What is required to substantially alter the burden of disease in developing countries?

12. What four things work to finance and execute programs that address acute threats and promote healthy behaviors?

13. How can achievable goals be selected to address health issues?

14. How have factors such as mass migration, high-speed travel, global trade, the Internet and widespread urbanization altered the relationship between the health challenges of developed and developing nations?

15. Addressing the Global Burden of Disease requires cross-sector health platforms and cooperative partnerships. What can NGOs and industry contribute to this effort?

Online Resources

 Access online resources with this book's CD.

Burden of Disease Unit
http://www.hsph.harvard.edu/organizations/bdu/

**New Vaccines Could Balance Global Burden of Disease —
Programs Often Depend as Much on Political Will as Scientific
Capacity**
http://www.researchmatters.harvard.edu/story.php?article_id=206

Burden of Disease Project
http://www3.who.int/whosis/menu.cfm?path=evidence,burden&lan
guage=english

Health Politics Online

For Original Health Politics Programs and Slides:

Global Burden of Disease: Part 1 – Defining the Problem
http://www.healthpolitics.com/program_info.asp?p=prog_01
Slide Briefing
http://www.healthpolitics.com/media/prog_01/brief_prog_01.pdf

Global Burden of Disease: Part 2 – Influencing Factors
http://www.healthpolitics.com/program_info.asp?p=prog_02
Slide Briefing
http://www.healthpolitics.com/media/prog_02/brief_prog_02.pdf

Global Burden of Disease: Part 4 – From Research to Action
http://www.healthpolitics.com/program_info.asp?p=prog_04
Slide Briefing
http://www.healthpolitics.com/media/prog_04/brief_prog_04.pdf

CHAPTER 1.2

Aging

THE SCOPE OF THE CHALLENGE

In his book "The Virtues of Aging," former President Jimmy Carter said, "You are old when regrets take the place of dreams."[1] His title is especially fitting today, since aging is making real advances in quantity and quality of years.

Clearly, we have entered an era of new longevity. One need only look at the trend lines to see that the senior block is growing in leaps and bounds. There are now approximately 184 million global citizens over the age of 65. This number is projected to increase to 678 million by the year 2030.[2] In 2000, there were some 35 million Americans over the age of 65 (see Fig. 1.2-1). This number will more than double to 79 million by 2050.[2] And the oldest old, those over 85 years of age, are growing as well, from 4 million in 2000 to a projected 18 million in 2050 (See Fig. 1.2-2).[3]

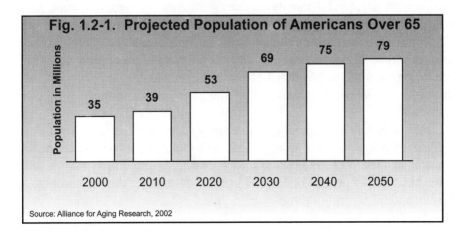

Fig. 1.2-1. Projected Population of Americans Over 65

Year	Population in Millions
2000	35
2010	39
2020	53
2030	69
2040	75
2050	79

Source: Alliance for Aging Research, 2002

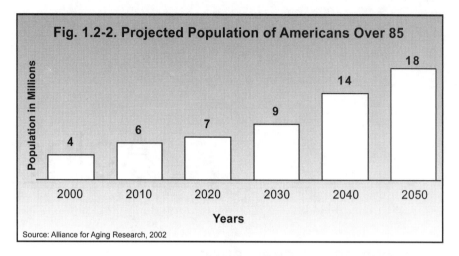

Fig. 1.2-2. Projected Population of Americans Over 85

Source: Alliance for Aging Research, 2002

The numbers alone imply a fundamental shift in the American family. Nearly 50 percent of all current 60-year-olds have at least one parent alive. This means that the four-generation American family has arrived. By the year 2050, there will be an estimated 1 million Americans over the age of 100, making the five-generation American family commonplace.[3]

Even today, we can see the impact of these demographics on our day-to-day lives. Despite the fact that we've seen a 15 percent drop in the presence of chronic disability and institutionalization in our older population, largely as a result of improvements in medical care, technology, and lifestyle behavior, we still have a long way to go.[4]

One need not look far for evidence that American families are having trouble keeping up with changing demographics. Home care of dependent, frail seniors falls predominantly on third-generation women, who struggle to manage up and down the generation divide. Family and friends provide 80 percent of long-term care.[5] The inability to adequately address chronic disease ensures organ damage and disability. This cycle has created the "The Sandwich Generation," which finds itself squeezed between children and grandchildren on the right, and parents and grandparents on the left.

While clearly the demographics of aging seem overwhelming, reinforced by "boomers," who begin to hit 65 in 2011, there are forces deflecting the impact. In fact, poor health is not as prevalent in the elderly as we once thought. A full 75 percent of 65- to 74-year-olds consider themselves in good health, and 67 percent of those over 75 give themselves similar grades.[6]

Dr. Gene Cohen, director of the Center of Aging, Health and Humanities at George Washington University, said, "The better health, higher level of education, and larger number of individuals with ample financial assets among today's older population — compared with earlier aging cohorts — speak to the greater collective role that those age 65 and older can play in assisting contemporary society."[7]

It's a race then: advancing age and traditional chronic, disease-instigated disability against advancing health and systems to support individual vitality and independence. Science and prevention must keep one step ahead of the demographic changes. A starting point is a clear understanding of the leading causes of death and disability in seniors.

The top five causes of mortality for those over 65 are heart disease, cancer, stroke, emphysema and pneumonia. The top five sources of disability are arthritis, high blood pressure, heart disease, hearing impairments and cataracts.[8] The risk factors most likely to interfere with successful aging include smoking, alcohol abuse, depression, lack of exercise and incontinence.[9,10,11] Addressing these behavioral issues can postpone the onset of disability by at least five years.[12]

Maintaining the functional capacity of aging Americans is critical to the long-term financing of health care. The direct health care costs for a chronically disabled senior are seven times greater than for a healthy senior.[12] The cost of care for a senior with dementia is 70 percent higher than a senior without mental impairment.[13] And none of this considers the indirect cost on family caregivers. A recent study of family caregivers of Alzheimer's patients found the average caregiver missed 23 days of work per year.[14]

So the challenge is clear: There must be a concerted effort on two fronts if the advance of health is to keep step with the advance of longevity. The first front is health maintenance. Currently, the average 75-year-old in America has three chronic conditions and takes 4.5 medications.[3] Early diagnosis, effective treatment and healthy behaviors must continue to lower these numbers.

The second front is prevention. There's a great deal that can be done to better manage the changes and disabilities that are associated with aging. One simple example is hip fractures — mainly the result of poor supervision and unsafe environments for seniors — which are growing at an alarming rate and projected to hit a half-million per year by 2050, with half of the injured never regaining independence.[3] Good management could positively impact those numbers.

PREVENTING ILLNESS, MAINTAINING HEALTH

We have clearly entered a new era of longevity in the United States and world-wide. This reality has political, social, economic and health consequences that are fluid and not yet fully determined.

What we do know is that we will live longer and that four- and five-gen-eration American families will be the norm. We also know that, because of the arrival of the "boomers," beginning in 2011, the projected increase in numbers of seniors and their future lifespans in America over the next 50 years will be unprecedented.[6] The projected increase in years for men and even more so for women is extraordinary, and this is in addition to an already added 28 years of life expectancy for Americans since the turn of the 20th century.[15]

Absent effective preventive measures and improved health management, senior health care costs will financially cripple our health care system. Currently, Americans over 65 represent 13 percent of all hospital care, and 50 percent of all physician work hours.[4] But there are positive signs on the hori-zon. First, seniors' disability rates are declining in the United States. Since 1980 there has been a nearly 15 percent decrease in the prevalence of chronic disability and institutionalization among people 65 and older.[12] A drop in dis-ability translates directly into cost savings since it is seven times more expen-sive to care for a disabled senior versus a healthy one.[3]

A second reason for optimism is that boomers are healthier than their par-ents. Earlier diagnosis and treatment of chronic diseases, behavioral changes in diet and exercise, and the health consumer empowerment movement have each played a role.[3] And the third sign of positive change is that both science and technology are progressing and contributing to a better understanding of diseases and the execution of methods to both diagnose and treat them.

If that is the good news, what are the concerns? One major concern is that our country is poorly prepared from a health-professional manpower stand-point to properly manage the complexity of aging. The average 75-year-old today has multiple chronic diseases and is on several medicines, yet fewer than one percent of all doctors, nurses, pharmacists and physical therapists have had advanced geriatric training.[4] How does this disconnect play out? Let's take just one case in point, the underdiagnosis of depression in the elderly — an easy miss if you've not been alerted by your training to look for it, and if you've been raised in the age of, "Mom's slowing down is just part of her getting old."

Depression is often misdiagnosed as cognitive impairment, in spite of the fact that there are many good reasons to be depressed: retirement, widowhood, bereavement and isolation.[4] But the cause of depression can be much more subtle. For example, having a hearing impairment is frequently associated with depression. More aggressive approaches to hearing loss would be very beneficial. Hearing loss affects quality of life and interpersonal relationships, and is a significant safety issue.[16] And if other diseases cause depression in the elderly, the reverse is true as well. Depression increases the risk of disability from all other causes in the elderly by 67 percent.[16] Training in geriatrics sensitizes clinicians to these various interactions.

A second concern is treatment strategies. Where should we begin? A logical starting point is with cognitive impairment. There are some four million American seniors currently suffering from Alzheimer's disease and dementia, with numbers expected to reach 14 million by 2040 (see Fig. 1.2-3). The numbers increase with age. While 2 percent may have the disease at age 65, 16 percent are affected by 85.[17] The costs are staggering, estimated currently at $100 billion per year, making it the third most expensive disease in the United States.[18] Nearly 50 percent of all nursing home patients are cognitively impaired.[4] The scientific focus on neurodegenerative diseases in both public and private sectors is enormous, and reflects both the seriousness of the problem and the potential positive impact that would accompany a solution.

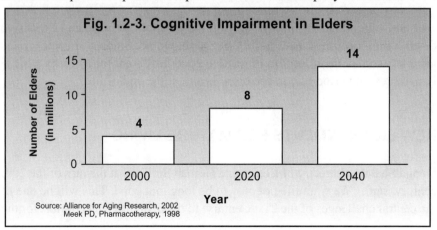

Fig. 1.2-3. Cognitive Impairment in Elders

Source: Alliance for Aging Research, 2002
Meek PD, Pharmacotherapy, 1998

Where else is there significant pay dirt? Incontinence affects 13 million Americans, including half of all nursing patients, at a cost of nearly $12 billion per year.[19] Experts suggest that we also target other conditions that lead to institutionalization. Major activity limitations are a common cause of nursing home admissions. The most common cause is arthritis, affecting 50 percent of people over 65, and an estimated 60 million people by 2020.[20] Hip fractures are a second source of immobility, projected to occur 420,000 times in the year 2020, nearly all fall related, and resulting in a loss of independence in nearly 30 percent of those affected. Fully 80 percent occur in women, who are at special risk because of osteoporosis.[4]

In addition to the obvious benefits of medical treatment and the creation of safe environments, the expansion of exercise and muscle strengthening could make a real difference in the incidence of falls and fractures. At present, even minimal exercise is totally absent in one-third of those over 65, and weight training is nearly nonexistent.[21]

Finally, a focus on medications, their interactions, assistance in their accurate and regular administration, and regular evaluation would lead to further improvement.

Dollars spent on both geriatric training and the prevention of those conditions most likely to cause disability and institutionalization are an extraordinarily wise investment. Adding a single month of independence and health to America's senior population would save $5 billion. A 10 percent decrease in hospitalization and institutionalization would accrue $50 billion in savings per year.[3]

But is good health simply delaying the inevitable, a long and expensive deterioration occurring later in life? Surprisingly, no. Studies of centenarians have shown that their decades of relative good health are followed by a highly compressed period of compromised health at the end of life.[22]

NEW ENVIRONMENTS FOR MATURE LIVING

Donna Shalala, secretary of Health and Human Services at the turn of the 20th century, said: "We want life not only to be long, but good. This will be one of the central challenges of the 21st Century: to make dignity and comfort for the elderly as much a part of our national consciousness as education and safety are for our children."[23]

We are in a scientific and social service race against the very real challenges of aging demographics. We have outlined the need for a two-pronged strategy. The first arm is enlightened prevention and health maintenance, intended to help elders maintain vitality and independence for as long as possible, by aggressively addressing those conditions that lead to disability and institutionalization.

The second arm, which is complementary to the first, is the creation of new environments that actively manage the changes and disabilities that come with advanced age. Long-term care is part of the natural fabric of life. It is fundamentally different than acute care in that it integrates health services and supports for daily living. The explosive growth of the long-term care industry simply reflects the numbers, with a projected doubling of the over-65s and tripling of the over-85s in the next 50 years.[24, 25] During this period, the number of people requiring long-term care is projected to grow from less than 10 million to 24 million.[26] But one should not confuse our future vision of long-term care with older images of restrictive nursing homes.

Even with excellent health maintenance and prevention, most of us will need to confront the issue of long-term care. Fully 43 percent of those over 65 will require some long-term care services in their lifetime, including 52 percent of all women and 33 percent of all men.[27] What's more, 51 percent of all Americans believe that it is likely that in their lifetime they will be responsible for the care of an elderly family member.[28]

What is it that causes individuals to require this support? The need for long-term care is measured by the limitation in capacity to perform certain basic functions or activities called "Activities of Daily Living," or ADLs. ADLs include bathing, dressing, getting in and out of bed, eating, toileting, and moving about. There are other activities, called "Instrumental Activities of Daily Living," or IADLs, such as getting out, driving, preparing meals, shopping, maintaining a home, using a phone, managing finances and taking medications, which are critical and require help if absent, though not on the level of absent ADLs.

About 97 percent of nursing home patients have ADL limitations.[26] By age 85, the need for help is not at all unusual. As shown in Table 1.2-1, some 35 percent need assistance with walking, 31 percent with bathing, 22 percent with getting in and out of bed, 17 percent with dressing, 14 percent with toileting, and 4 percent with eating.

Table 1.2-1. Percentage of Elders Over 85 With ADL Difficulty

Activities of Daily Living (ADL)	Percentage of Difficulty
Walking	35%
Bathing	31%
In/Out Bed	22%
Dressing	17%
Toileting	14%
Eating	4%

Source: US Bureau of Census, 1996

Most of those requiring long-term care prefer to "age in place," in their own home and community, in familiar settings. And most do just that. In fact, the use of nursing homes is declining in all categories of aging, with numbers of nursing home patients over 85 declining by nearly 10 percent between 1985 and 1995.[29] Instead, what we see is nearly 90 percent of seniors living in their own homes, independently or with informal care that's almost always provided by family or close friends. This compares with 4.5 percent who are living at home with professional care and 4.6 percent residing in nursing homes (See Fig. 1.2-4).[30]

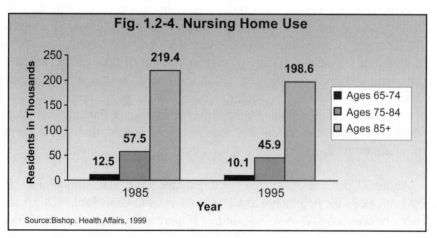

Fig. 1.2-4. Nursing Home Use

Source:Bishop. Health Affairs, 1999

The primary challenge for providing long-term care support for fourth and fifth generation Americans is falling predominantly on third generation female family members. As Jim Firman, president of the National Council on Aging has noted, "We mistakenly define long-term care problems as medical concerns rather than disability concerns. The care needs of most frail older people are primarily supportive: for example, help them move from here to there, help them eat and dress, and help them keep track of their medicine."[31]

If family members provide the muscle of home care, they also provide a significant portion of the dollars. For 40 percent of Americans, long-term care is the most costly purchase ever made.[32] As shown in Fig. 1.2-5, more than 32 percent of the total costs of long-term care in 1999 came directly from patients, while the government shouldered approximately 56 percent of the bill — 38 percent in Medicaid and 18 percent in Medicare. Only 5.5 percent was covered by private insurance.[33]

As family members critically assess the financial consequences of these difficult decisions, costs are being assigned to each option. The ability to live independently at home is less expensive than institutionalization. But, as Gail Hunt, executive director of The National Alliance for Caregiving, says, "There's a reason for that. The quality of life at home is better, yes, but only the federal government saves money. And that's because family caregivers are the unpaid extensions of the health care system." In 1992 it was roughly five times more expensive to be elderly and dependent in a nursing home versus independent in one's own home.[34] The nursing home charge then averaged $29,000 per year. Today, the cost approaches $60,000 per year.[34, 35]

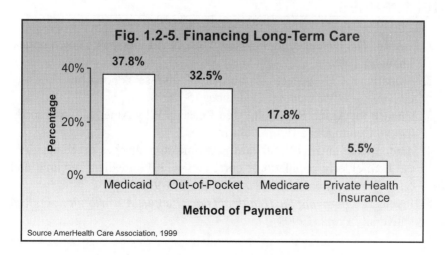

Fig. 1.2-5. Financing Long-Term Care

Source AmerHealth Care Association, 1999

The race against the aging juggernaut, then, is about science, about independence, and about "aging in place." Long-term care is rapidly evolving with a primary focus on dignity, personal autonomy, and support for caregivers.

What are the major trends in long-term care? First, less institutionalized care. Nursing homes are being reserved for the most severely impaired. Second, more reliance on home care and community-based alternatives. Day care options, blended services, "assisted living," and care for the caregiver programs all signal a shift in emphasis that presages a shift in finances. Third, these environments will feature more choices, greater use of supportive new life-assist technologies, a greater emphasis on prevention, and the opportunity for shared learning and community-based strategic planning.

If one were to plan, what might emerge as the best environment for mature living? It would be a place that supports dignity and privacy, a place that balances personal autonomy with safety, a place that leverages technology to enhance personal security and safety, a place that provides stimulation and social interaction, and a place that assures easy access to affordable services.

There is a great deal of work to be done to get ahead of the aging curve. But we should be optimistic for two reasons. The solution relies on the goodness of America's individuals, families and communities on the one hand, and on the power of innovation imbedded in America's scientific and medical enterprise on the other.

REFERENCES

1. Carter J. *The Virtues of Aging*. New York, NY: Library of Contemporary Thought; 1998.
2. Brundtland GH. Speech on burden of disease concept at Hopitaux Universitaires de Geneve; December 15, 1998.
3. Alliance for Aging Research. "Ten Reasons Why America is not ready for the Coming Age Boom." Spring 2002.
4. Manton KG, Corder LS, Stallard E. Monitoring changes in the health of the U.S. elderly populations: correlates with biomedical research and clinical innovations. *FASEB J.* 1997;11:923-930.
5. Havens B. *Improving the Health of Older People. A World View*, Oxford University Press. 1990.

6. Hobbs FB, Damon BL, eds. 65+ in the United States. Washington, DC: US Bureau of the Census; 1996.
7. Biomedical innovations, Baby Boomers and Aging. *The Pfizer Journal.* 3:1, 1999. p.5-6.
8. National Center for Health Statistics. 2000.
9. Valliant GE, Meyer SE, Mukamal K, Soldz S. Are social supports in late midlife a cause or result of successful physical aging? *Psychol Med.* 1998; 28:1159-1168. Journal article is not available online without subscription to Psychological Medicine.
10. Strawbridge WJ, Cohen RD, Shema SJ, Kaplan GA. Successful dying: predictors and associated activities. *Am J Epideiol.*1996;144:135-141.
11. Vita AJ, Terry RB, Hubert HB, Fries JF. Aging, health risks, and cumulative disability. *N Engl J Med.* 1998;338:1035-1041.
12. Pardes H, Manton KG, Lander ES, Tolley HD, Ullian AD, Palmer H. Effects of medical research on health care and the economy. *Science.* 1999;283:36-37. Article not available without subscription fee or partial registration.
13. Alzheimer's Association. 1998 National public policy program to conquer Alzheimer's disease. Washington, DC: Alzheimer's Association; 1998.
14. Koppel R. Alzheimer's cost to U.S. business. Washington, DC: Alzheimer's Association; September 1998.
15. Hodes RJ, Cahan V, Pruzan M. The National Institute on Aging at its twentieth anniversary: achievements and promise of research on aging. *J Am. Ger Soc.* 1996;44:204-206.
16. Penninx BW, Leveille S, Ferrucci L, et al. Exploring the effect of depression on physical disability: longitudinal evidence from the established populations for epidemiologic studies of the elderly. *Am J Public Health.* 1999; 89:1346-1352.
17. Kane RA, Kane RL, Ladd RC. *The Heart of Long-Term Care.* New York, NY: Oxford University Press. 1998.
18. Meek PD. McKeithan K, Schumock GT. Economic considerations in Alzheimer's disease. *Pharmacotherapy.* 1998;18:79-82.
19. Freiman M, Brown E. Special care units in nursing homes — selected characteristics, 1996. Rockville, Md: Agency for Health Care Policy and Research; 1999. MEPS Research Findings #6. *ACHPR* Publication No. 99-0017; January 1999.
20. American Association of Retired Persons (AARP). Fitness: do you make physical activity an integral part of your daily routine? AARP Webplace. Available at:
http://www.aarp.org/confacts/health/fitness.html. Accessed

September 13, 1999.

21. Fantl JA, Newman DK, Colling J, et al. Urinary incontinence in adults: acute and chronic management. Clinical Practice Guideline Number 2 (1996 Update). Rockville, MD: agency for Health Care Policy and Research; 1996. *AHCPR* Publication No. 97-0682.

22. Perls TT. Centarians prove the compression of morbidity hypothesis, but what about the rest of us who are genetically less fortunate. *Med Hypotheses*. 1997;49:405-407.

23. Shalala D. The United States Special Committee on Aging. Long Term Care for the 21st Century: A Common Sense Proposal to Support Family Caregivers. Testimony before the United States Special Committee on Aging: March 23, 1999. Available at: http://www.senate.gov/~aging/hr29.htm. Accessed October 4, 1999.

24. Administration Association for Homes and Services for the Aging (AAHSA). Nursing homes [fact sheet]. Available at: http://www.aahsa.org/public/nursbkg.htm. Accessed June 16, 1999.

25. The Growing Population of Persons Age 65 and Over: 1990 to 2050. Source: Cheeseman J. Population projections of the United States by Age, Sex, Race, and Hispanic Origin: 1995 to 2050. Current Population Reports. Washington DC: US Department of Commerce, Economics and Statistics Administration, US Bureau of the Census; February 1996. Publication No. P25-1130;12.

26. 1994 Green Book. Overview of Entitlement Programs. Committee on Ways and Means, US House of Representatives. Washington DC; July 15, 1994. [Appendix B: Health Status, Insurance, Expenditures of the Elderly, and Background]. Available at: http://bappend.txt at aspe.os.dhhs.gov. Accessed August 24, 1999.

27. Kemper P, Murtaugh CM. Lifetime use of nursing home care. *N Eng J Med*. 1991;324:595-600.

28. National Partnership for Women and Families. When you become a parent to your parents: finding the balance [press release]. August 10, 1999. Available at: http://www.nationalpartnership.org/news/pressreleases/1999/081099.htm. Accessed October 4, 1999.

29. Nursing Home Use Declining. Source: Bishop CE. Where are the missing elders? The decline in nursing home use, 1985 and 1995. *Health Aff*. 1999;18:146-155.

30. Long-Term Care Use by the Elderly. Source: Van Nostrand JF, Clark RF, Romoren TI. Nursing home care in five nations. Ageing Int. 1993:1-5.

31. New environments for mature living. *The Pfizer Journal*. Volume 3. Number 3. 1999.

32. American Health Care Association (AHCA). Survey finds boomers headed for financial disaster in golden years [press release.] Washington,DC:AHCA;1999.Available at: http://www.ahca.org/brief/nr990407.htm. Accessed September 27, 1999.

33. Who Pays for Long-Term Care? Source: American Association of Homes and Services for the Aging (AAHSA). Long-Term Care Financing [Backgrounder]. Washington, DC: AAHSA; 1999. Available at: http://www.aahsa.org/public/ltfinbkg.htm. Accessed September 1, 1999.

34. Expenditures for Healthcare. Source: Agency for Health Care Policy and Research. AHCPR Research on long-term care. Available at: http://www.ahcpr.gov/research/longtrm1.htm. Accessed August 30, 1999.

35. Reschovsky JD. The roles of Medicaid and economic factors in the demand for nursing home care. *HSR: Health Services Research.* 1998;33:787-813.

TEACHING TOOLS

Policy Premises

1. We have entered an era of new longevity.
2. The four- and five-generation American family is becoming the norm.
3. Home care of dependent, frail seniors falls predominantly on the third generation, which balances the needs of the first and second generations with those of fourth and fifth generations.
4. Science and prevention must keep one step ahead of the demographic change. Major causes of death and disability are preventable and treatable.
5. Maintaining functional capacity of aging Americans is critical to long-term financing of health care.
6. Successful aging will require a concerted effort on two major fronts.
7. The projected increase in numbers of seniors and their future lifespan in America over the next 50 years is unprecedented.
8. Absent effective preventive measures and improved health management, senior health care costs will financially cripple our health care system. But there are positive signs on the horizon.
9. Care for seniors is high in complexity and low in access to geriatrically trained health professionals.
10. Cognitive impairment fundamentally undermines vitality and independence and carries with it huge cost implications.
11. Targeting conditions that lead to institutionalization makes good sense.
12. Dollars spent on prevention and aging research are extraordinarily wise investments.
13. Increased demand for long-term care is being driven by aging demographics. The long-term care industry is one of America's fastest growing industries.
14. The need for long-term care reflects an inability to manage ADLs, or "activities of daily living."
15. Most elderly requiring long-term care prefer to "age in place," receiving informal care from family and friends at home.
16. The four- and five- generation American family is the primary source of home-based long-term care.

17. The costs of long-term care are considerable and fall primarily on the shoulders of family and government.
18. Long-term care is rapidly evolving with a primary focus on dignity, personal autonomy, and support for caregivers.

Review

1. How many global citizens are over the age of 65?
2. What is "The Sandwich Generation?"
3. Fifty percent of all current 60-year-olds have at least one parent alive. How does this impact the American family?
4. What percentage of 65- to 74-year-olds consider themselves to be in good health?
5. What are the top five causes of mortality for those over 65?
6. What effect do senior health care costs have on our health care system?
7. In terms of health care professionals, how is our country not adequately prepared to care for elderly populations?
8. What are some causes of depression among senior citizens?
9. What medical conditions often result in the elderly being placed in nursing homes?
10. How can frequent exercise help the elderly?
11. Why is there growth in the nursing home and other long-term care industries?
12. Why do so many individuals need care in their elder years?
13. Who provides most of the support for long-term care?
14. What are the major trends in long-term care?
15. What is the best environment for elderly living?

Online Resources

Access online resources with this book's CD.

Costs of Family Caregiving for Elderly with Cancer are Significant, Often Forgotten
http://hrsonline.isr.umich.edu/papers/releases/06-29-01.pdf

Costs of Caring for Elders with Dementia
http://hrsonline.isr.umich.edu/papers/releases/nov2001.pdf

HHS Issues Report Showing Dramatic Improvements in Americans' Health Over Past 50 Years
http://www.cdc.gov/od/oc/media/pressrel/r020912.htm

U.S. Census Bureau Age Data
http://www.census.gov/population/www/socdemo/age.html

A Demographic Revolution
http://www.un.org/esa/socdev/ageing/agewpop1.htm

Depression in Older Persons
http://web.nami.org/helpline/elddepres.htm

As Elderly Population Explodes, Study Published in JAMA Calls for Increase in Geriatric Training Programs in U.S. Medical Schools
http://www.americangeriatrics.org/news/jamarelease111202.shtml

Healthy Aging: Preventing Disease and Improving Quality of Life Among Older Americans
http://www.cdc.gov/nccdphp/aag/aag_aging.htm

Elderly - Mental Health
http://www.hpb.gov.sg/hpb/eld/eld04.asp

Chronic Depression in the Elderly: Approaches for Prevention
http://www.ncbi.nlm.nih.gov/entrez/query.fcgi?cmd=Retrieve&db=PubMed&list_uids=11482744&dopt=Abstract

The Importance of Geriatric Medicine - Berkeley Medical Journal
http://www.ocf.berkeley.edu/~issues/spring94/geriatric.html

Characteristics of Long-Term Care Users
http://www.ahcpr.gov/research/ltcusers/ltcuse1.htm

National Alliance for Caregiving
http://www.caregiving.org/

Annual Report on Nation's Health Spotlights Elderly Americans
http://www.hhs.gov/news/press/1999pres/991013.html

The National Council on Aging
http://www.ncoa.org/index.cfm?bType=ie4

Health Politics Online

For the Original Health Politics Programs and Slides:

Aging: Part 1 – The Scope of the Challenge
http://www.healthpolitics.com/program_info.asp?p=prog_08
Slide Briefing
http://www.healthpolitics.com/media/prog_08/brief_prog_08.pdf

Aging: Part 2 – Preventing Illness, Maintaining Health
http://www.healthpolitics.com/program_info.asp?p=prog_09
Slide Briefing
http://www.healthpolitics.com/media/prog_09/brief_prog_09.pdf

Aging: Part 3 – New Environments for Mature Living
http://www.healthpolitics.com/program_info.asp?p=prog_10
Slide Briefing
http://www.healthpolitics.com/media/prog_10/brief_prog_10.pdf

The Evolving Patient-Physician Relationship

ITS ROLE IN SOCIETY

The patient-physician relationship is at the epicenter of stable, civil, relationship-based societies. A national study, conducted in 1997, found that 90 percent of patients and doctors defined the relationship as having three elements: compassion, understanding, and partnership.[1] While science, technology, and professional competency were viewed as important in ensuring a successful relationship, they were separate from the very human emotions that bind patients to doctors — and doctors to patients.

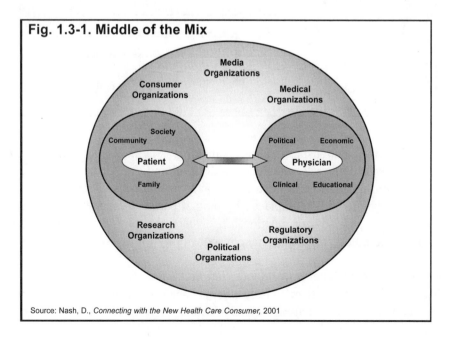

Fig. 1.3-1. Middle of the Mix

Source: Nash, D., *Connecting with the New Health Care Consumer*, 2001

On a broader scale, this relationship is clearly in the "middle of the mix" (See Fig. 1.3-1). Both patients and physicians have important spheres of influence that they bring to the dance. And these spheres move within the orbit of a wide array of consumer, media, medical, regulatory, political and research organizations.[2]

In 2002, studies in six countries on four continents revealed that the citizens of all countries viewed the patient-physician relationship as second in importance to family relationships.[3] As shown in Fig. 1.3-2, in the United States, the patient-physician relationship scored significantly higher than spiritual, financial and co-worker relationships. This finding was repeated in the United Kingdom, Canada, Germany, South Africa and Japan. These high levels of confidence may, in part, reflect the fact that, in all countries studied, strong majorities believe that doctors place the patient's interests above anything else.

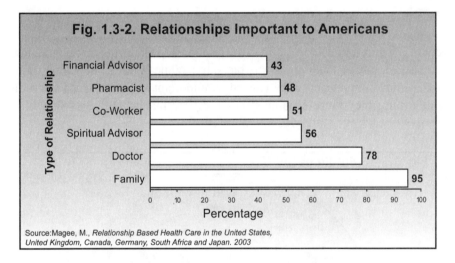

Fig. 1.3-2. Relationships Important to Americans

Source:Magee, M., *Relationship Based Health Care in the United States, United Kingdom, Canada, Germany, South Africa and Japan. 2003*

While the relationship is highly valued, it is certainly not static. In all countries studied, the relationship is rapidly evolving. Authoritarian, paternalistic relationships — where "doctor says" and "patient does" — are now in the minority. They have been replaced by mutual partnerships with 50/50 decision-making, and advisor relationships where the physician serves as a resource and guide, but patients take responsibility for decisions.[3]

What's next? Patients worldwide state that the relationship will move further away from paternalism, to fully embrace one-on-one mutual partnerships, and mutual, service-oriented physician teams. These teams will not only deliver traditional clinical care — for example, with a coordinated group of medical professionals caring for a diabetic patient — but will also include a parallel educational team to support patient empowerment. The patient in these cases has the benefit of access to a nurse educator, dietician, health librarian, web manager, self-help team and consumer activist.

Studies show that patients are realistic and don't expect their physicians to do the educating themselves. But they do expect the physicians to provide oversight to the educational team, to validate their expertise, and to ensure that information is up-to-date and accurate. As educational support is growing, so too is patient confidence in self-management. Between 63 percent and 76 percent of patients in all countries studied, except Japan, are completely or very confident in managing their own health. And in Japan, 57 percent are somewhat confident, moving en masse toward health consumer empowerment (See Table 1.3-1).[3]

Table 1.3-1. Patient Confidence in Self-Management (%)

	U.S.	U.K.	Canada	Germany	South Africa	Japan
Completely	29	18	25	15	24	5
Very	47	48	44	48	48	10
Somewhat	21	29	28	31	23	57
Not Very	2	5	2	4	4	23
Not At All	1	0	1	1	1	5
Not Sure	0	0	0	1	0	0

Source: Magee, M., *Relationship Based Health Care in the United States, United Kingdom, Canada, Germany, South Africa and Japan*, 2003

Empowerment is clearly a function of educational support. While physicians are the patient's primary source of information, this is only one factor in a formula for behavioral change. Physicians are also the most trusted source of information, and the professionals whose recommendations patients are most likely to follow. In all countries studied, the physicians' role in moving patients toward more active self-management is highly noted.[3]

In the United States alone, hundreds of thousands of times each day, on a grassroots level, these very private and highly charged relationships are engaged. The cost to society is not insignificant. But what is the true value? Certainly, the relationships deliver, to a significant portion of society, "nuts and bolts health care" — though irregularly and with a fragile and imperfect safety net. This includes diagnosis, treatment and follow-up care, with greater emphasis still being placed on reactive intervention rather than thoughtful prevention.

But this service alone hardly explains the high reputation of physicians, and the uniform value that is associated with their efforts with patients. The true value extends well beyond "nuts and bolts."

The patient-physician relationship delivers three other important products each and every day.[4] First, it processes the populace's very private fears and worries, channeling most to a positive outcome. In so doing, it effectively vents societal anxiety that might otherwise accumulate to destabilizing effect.

Second, in individualizing care within the context of family, community and culture, the relationship quietly reinforces and affirms the value of individual connectivity to other cornerstone values and to contact points in society.

Third, the relationship quietly and effectively instills hope and confidence in the future, which translates into a willingness to invest money, talent and ideas that shape a society's future.

If the relationship is as highly valued, and the investment made by most countries so significant, why is health care policy so often a source of controversy? Or, stated another way, why is all the money that's expended on health care not viewed as delivering sufficient value?

UNLOCKING THE VALUE

The patient-physician relationship is highly valued by both patients and doctors in the United States and around the world. In importance, it ranks second only to family relationships, dwarfing co-worker relations, spiritual relations and financial relationships. Yet health care delivery systems, their financing, and their organization are highly controversial in most societies, and clearly integral to the success or failure of this relationship.[3]

In a recent study of patient-physician relationships involving six countries, on four continents, large majorities of doctors in all countries agreed with the statement: "The medical system in your country sometimes interferes with your ability to put your patient's interests above everything else." This conflict, felt by physicians, is not as visible to patients, who in large majorities, in the same study, agree strongly or somewhat that "the doctor puts my interests above everything else."[2]

What is the source of this fundamental disconnect between health care system design and its anchoring relationship? The problem in the United States can be traced to two factors: First, a fundamentally flawed understanding of the true value proposition in health care, and second, a lack of understanding of what defines the patient-physician relationship itself.[2]

In nationwide studies, according to patients and their doctors, this relationship consists, fundamentally, of three elements: compassion, understanding and partnership.[5] While science, technology, and competence are recognized as essential and enabling, they are quite separate from the core elements of the relationship, which work in unison to support mutual confidence, trust and respect.[5]

Understanding the relationship is critical if one is to correct what has been a defective value proposition in health care. For almost two decades, value has been defined as quality over cost. Quality refers to measurable and quantifiable, outcomes-measured, protocol-driven, evidence-based quality. Cost is tied to processes and resources. The logic has been that as processes are re-engineered and simplified, costs will decline, outcomes will be more reliable, and safety advanced.[2]

In advancing measurable quality, most agree that progress has been made, at least for those insured Americans. It is clear, as well, that until recently, cost has been better managed. And yet, through this active period of healthcare redesign, heavily centered on a concept of managed care delivered by HMOs, both doctors and patients have not defined the output as valuable.[6]

To understand why, we need only return to the definition of our health system's core relationship. The patient-physician relationship is compassion, understanding and partnership, in both clinical care and educational empowerment. This output fundamentally requires a key ingredient: participation, which was left unaccounted for in the value equation. Had policy experts been basing value redesign decisions on the correct equation, that is, value in health care equals quality over cost plus participation, it is likely we would be further along in our health system evolution, with stronger support from both patients and physicians.[4]

A second core issue, left unaddressed and ignored, is the issue of equity. Gro Brundtland, former head of the World Health Organization, defined care as goodness — that is, the highest quality, outcome-driven care — and fairness, or care delivered equitably across a population. In a first-of-its-kind comparison of worldwide health care systems based on five criteria, the United States ranked a sad 37th, not because of goodness or quality and expertise, but because of fairness or equitable distribution of care and resources to our population. An employer-based health insurance system, with urban and rural pockets of poverty, and an inadequate safety net reliant on the goodwill of doctors, nurses and hospitals, has become frayed and broken. This not only creates a crisis of conscience, but also ensures that our goal of moving from intervention to prevention, from hospital-based to home-based, from paternalism to partnership, from individual approaches to team-based approaches, and from disability to productivity will be a rocky road indeed.

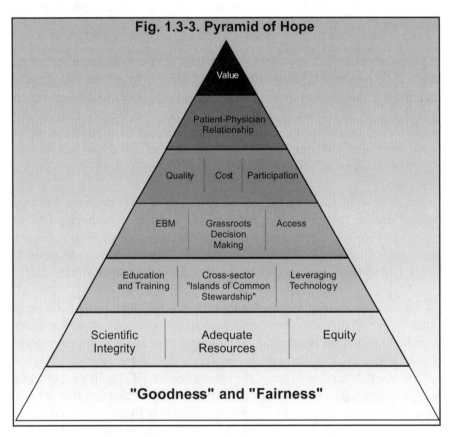

Fig. 1.3-3. Pyramid of Hope

Value

Patient-Physician Relationship

Quality | Cost | Participation

EBM | Grassroots Decision Making | Access

Education and Training | Cross-sector "Islands of Common Stewardship" | Leveraging Technology

Scientific Integrity | Adequate Resources | Equity

"Goodness" and "Fairness"

The solution lies within a pyramid of hope. It is based on a fundamental philosophy of goodness and fairness in health care. Upon this base we build our future with scientific integrity, adequate resources and a commitment to equity. With that basis, areas of concentration naturally evolve, including education and training, cross-sector cooperation on "islands of common stewardship," and wise leveraging of technology. A commitment to evidence-based medicine, to grassroots decision-making, and access — to caregivers and the wide range of diagnostic and therapeutic discoveries — becomes a natural progression, delivering quality, cost and participation. In this environment, the patient-physician relationship will flourish, and at the end of the day citizens and their caregivers will declare the systems and their services valuable.

REFERENCES

1. Magee, M. Enduring Relationships in American Society. New York, NY: Yankelovich Partners, Omnibus Study. 1999.
2. Nash, D. *Connecting with the New Health Care Consumer*: New York, NY: McGraw-Hill; 2001.
3. Magee M. Relationship Based Health Care in the United States, United Kingdom, Canada, Germany, South Africa and Japan. Annual Meeting, World Medical Association. Helsinki, Finland. September 11, 2003
4. Magee, M. *The Best Medicine*. 2003, Spencer Books, New York.
5. Magee, M. The Evolving Patient-Physician Relationship in America: From Paternalism to Partnership. New York, NY. Yankelovich Partners. 1998.
6. Collins KS, Schoen C, Sondman DR. The commonwealth Fund Survey of Physician Experience with Managed Care. Available at: www.omwf.org/health_care/physrvy.html. Accessed August 1998.

TEACHING TOOLS

Policy Premises

1. The patient-physician relationship is at the epicenter of stable civil relationship-based societies.
2. Patients and physicians highly value each other.
3. The patient-physician relationship is rapidly evolving.
4. The patient-physician relationship is moving toward team approaches that support clinical and educational continuums.
5. Patient confidence in self-management is growing; information from physicians is critical.
6. The patient-physician relationship is a wise societal investment.
7. The patient-physician relationship is highly valued by patients and physicians.
8. That said, physicians agree worldwide that health care systems as designed can undermine care.
9. This fundamental disconnect can be traced back to a flawed value equation.
10. A second issue, left largely unaddressed in the U.S., is equity.
11. This has created a "crisis of conscience" in America.
12. The "Pyramid of Hope" must be based on a new value proposition in America.

Review

1. A national study in 1997 found that 90 percent of patients and doctors defined the patient-physician relationship according to what three attributes?
2. In a 2002 study involving six countries, citizens universally viewed the patient-physician relationship as being second in importance to which core interpersonal relationship?
3. Authoritarian relationships — where "doctor says" and "patient does" — have been replaced by what two types of relationships?
4. What are mutual, service-oriented physician teams?
5. What are two factors that cause a disconnect between health care system design and the patient-physician relationship?
6. How do you define the value equation?

7. What key ingredient is missing from the health care value equation?
8. In a comparison of worldwide health care systems, where did the United States rank?
9. What tools are needed to build the future of health care?

Online Resources

Access online resources with this book's CD.

Evolution of the Patient-Physician Relationship
http://www.fda.gov/cder/ddmac/p6magee/tsld002.htm

Patient Perspectives on Spirituality and the Patient-Physician Relationship
http://www.ncbi.nlm.nih.gov/entrez/query.fcgi?cmd=Retrieve&db=PubMed&list_uids=11679036&dopt=Abstract

The Patient-Physician Relationship in the Internet Age: Future Prospects and the Research Agenda
http://www.ncbi.nlm.nih.gov/entrez/query.fcgi?cmd=Retrieve&db=PubMed&list_uids=11720957&dopt=Abstract

The American Academy of Orthopaedic Surgeons Bulletin
http://www.aaos.org/wordhtml/bulletin/aug99/stratp2.htm

Who is Being Difficult? Addressing the Determinants of Difficult Patient-Physician Relationships
http://www.ama-assn.org/ama1/pub/upload/mm/384/apriljdisc2.doc

Simplifying the American Health Care System Implementation
http://www.amga.org/WhoWeAre/AMGAInitiatives/implementation_amgaInitiatives.asp

Restoring the Sanctity of the Patient-Physician Relationship
http://www.pragmatism.org/shook/biomedical_ethics/Module%20One/cooper.htm

Patient-Physician Relationship and Service Utilization:
Preliminary Findings Published in the Journal of Clinical
Psychology
http://www.psychiatrist.com/pcc/pccpdf/v05n01/v05n0104.pdf

Patients Becoming More Empowered, New Study Finds
http://www.wma.net/e/press/2003_15.htm

Health Politics Online

For Original Health Politics Programs and Slides:

The Patient-Physician Relationship: Part I – Its Role in Society
http://www.healthpolitics.com/program_info.asp?p=prog_25
Slide Briefing
http://www.healthpolitics.com/media/prog_25/brief_prog_25.pdf

The Patient-Physician Relationship: Part II – Unlocking the Value
http://www.healthpolitics.com/program_info.asp?p=prog_26
Slide Briefing
http://www.healthpolitics.com/media/prog_26/brief_prog_26.pdf

Home Health Care

ITS RE-EMERGENCE

Some 40 years ago, I recall visiting General Electric's "Carousel of Progress" at the World's Fair in New York. The attraction, now housed at Disney World in Florida, documented the changes in the technology and social structure of the American home over five or six decades, ultimately creating a vision of the future, a case for progress. I think the time has come to build something similar for health care. This "Carousel of Progress" would provide a vision of the past, present and future for something far more important than refrigerators and toasters — our nation's health. At the core of this carousel would be a vision that's just within our reach — something that will change health care as we now know it. I'm talking about the concept of home-centered health, in which technology, advanced information systems and a new, more team-oriented medical approach would make it possible for more health care to take place in the home than we ever imagined possible.

Today, voices are rising once again in the name of health care reform. The various power bases remain much as they were in 1980 — locked in position, facing year-to-year battles for funding support from public and private sources. While they have not changed, the health care world certainly has. We are now immersed in a full-blown health consumer empowerment movement in response to aging demographics, a caregiver revolution, advances in information technology, debates over risks and benefits of various treatments and therapies, and an outpatient office-based delivery system that lacks time and space to advance prevention and wellness.

In the middle of all this noise, quietly below the radar screen, health care is preparing to restructure itself from the inside out. At the end of this silent evolution, we will have a home-centered health care system that will radically realign the current players and power bases. The new system will tilt rewards to those who play prevention, and play it well.[1]

At the center of this home-centered health scenario will be the American family — aging in place, now routinely four and five generations deep, rather than just three. Family caregivers, currently present in 25 percent of American families, are providing most of the care for parents and grandparents.[2] In the next decade, they will embrace the designated role of home health manager and apply their skills up and down the generational divide as designated members of physicians' health care teams.[3]

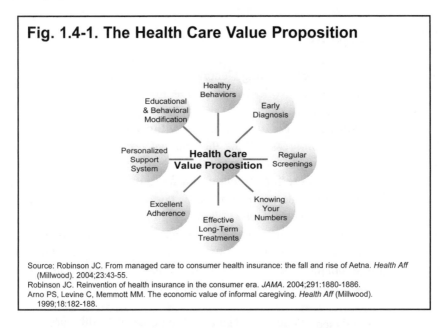

Fig. 1.4-1. The Health Care Value Proposition

Source: Robinson JC. From managed care to consumer health insurance: the fall and rise of Aetna. *Health Aff* (Millwood). 2004;23:43-55.
Robinson JC. Reinvention of health insurance in the consumer era. *JAMA*. 2004;291:1880-1886.
Arno PS, Levine C, Memmott MM. The economic value of informal caregiving. *Health Aff* (Millwood). 1999;18:182-188.

Those teams will carry out both educational and clinical missions. The educational support teams will be coordinated with the physicians' active support, primarily by nurse educators connected 24/7 to virtual networks of family-based home health managers. Through this network, home health managers will receive targeted education, behavioral modification strategies, and financial rewards in the form of reduced insurance premiums for achieving superior outcomes for family members. Physicians, as well, will be tied to performance and fairly reimbursed for team management responsibilities.[4]

The home itself will look quite different — it will generally be more stable, productive, and controlled. Technology, originally directed at seniors with cognitive decline, cancer, and cardiovascular disease who wanted to age in place, will be advancing the health of all ages.[5] The infrastructure for maintaining home-based wellness will include wireless sensors that track movement of people and objects in-home; intelligent software that will analyze data and provide appropriate behavioral clues and guidance; friendly, communicative interfaces through a wide range of devices, such as wristwatches, telephones, and televisions; and Internet connectivity with the rest of the health care team.[6]

This could become our reality, but the pieces must fall into place. According to David Tennenhouse, vice president and director of Intel Research, "The real challenge for research now is to explore the implications and issues associated with having hundreds of networked computers per person. These networked computers will work together to learn our habits and patterns and be proactive in providing us with the information and services we need for a healthier, safer, more productive and enjoyable life."[5]

In the near future, such systems could adjust behavior in physical fitness, nutrition, social activity, and cognitive engagement. They could assist seniors with incontinence, in regular toileting, and assure better adherence to medication regimens. They could provide early diagnostics, streaming data daily to the physician-directed, nurse-led educational team, and adjust daily treatment regimens, substantially decreasing the need for on-site office visits or hospitalization.[5]

Intel is not alone in this vision. Massachusetts Institute of Technology, the University of Michigan, the University of Virginia, and the University of Rochester are just a few of the academic institutions actively engaged.[7,8,9,10] So are General Electric, NASA, the Disney spin-off I.D.E.A.S., Best Buy, and Philips, which all see home health technology as a major growth market.[11,12,13,14,15] They are betting that the technology, privacy and usability barriers can be overcome, and that once health consumers are at financial risk, the logic of prevention will prevail, and a tipping point will have been reached.

Why might they be right? First, there is inadequate funding, time and space to manage an aging, actively disease-ridden population. Second, education, behavioral modification, and preventive screening must be home-based to be successful. Third, the complexity of a four- and five-generation family becomes rapidly unmanageable in the absence of active health planning. Fourth, success in managing home-based health prevention saves time and money, in the short and long term. Fifth, most people don't want to go to a hospital unless they absolutely have to.

Beyond all this, much of our future home-based health workforce is already in place — highly stressed, yet ready, willing, and able. I'm talking about the nation's informal caregivers, present in a quarter of all homes, 34 million strong. Seventy percent of these informal caregivers are women, age 45 to 64 years.[16,17] Ignore for the moment that 20 percent of them have been forced to sacrifice their work status to manage the complexity of caregiving and that nearly half of those managing elder dementia have symptoms of depression from the isolation and constant work load. Sadly, it's clear that what our family caregivers have learned has been hard fought and accomplished with very little help from the system.[18,19]

Now, let us admit these weaknesses and injustices, and recognize that a change in incentives, infrastructure, and goal-directed organization could increase job satisfaction and success for these dedicated workers. You might be wondering, "Who are these caregivers, and what qualifies them to be home health managers?"

A recent survey of 1,005 women, conducted by the National Women's Health Resource Center, begins to answer these questions.[20] Seventy-one percent of the women surveyed said they make health care decisions such as selecting a health care professional and choosing when to go to the doctor for their family. According to Amy Niles, the group's president and chief executive officer, "Our study found that caring for the health of others is perceived to have a major positive impact on women's physical and mental health. Given these findings, it is not surprising that women choose to take on the role of health manager for their family, making the bulk of health care-related decisions."

When women in the study were asked to identify areas that are "very important" to them, 96 percent chose "having a healthy family"; 95 percent chose "being healthy"; and 90 percent said "being close to family." This is all the more remarkable when compared with some of the other results. Only 72 percent of the women said "being financially secure" was "very important"; 66 percent said "having close friends"; and 65 percent said "having a job you enjoy." Only 40 percent said "having enough free time" was "very important" to them.

Women are not only committed to their families' health, they are good at handling and understanding it. Many are consistently ahead of the curve. Fifty-five percent of women are aware that heart disease is the major killer of women; two-thirds are very familiar with their family's medical history; and 95 percent are knowledgeable about diagnosis and treatment of diseases their parents have suffered. It's clear that women are also familiar with and support screening guidelines such as Pap smears, teeth cleanings and cholesterol tests. More than 90 percent have seen their doctors and other care professionals in the past year. Seventy-four percent are most likely to get their information on health issues from their health care professional, and 60 percent have used the Internet for information research.[20]

According to the results of the National Women's Health Resource Center survey, women's views of health are multidimensional and integrated, emphasizing body, mind and spirit. When asked in the study to identify what "being healthy" means, "having a healthy family" ranked No. 1, followed by spiritual well-being, being happy, being physically active, not having chronic disease, and not being overweight. As for issues women consider contributors to unhealthiness, stress, lack of exercise, poor nutrition, and low income all scored high.[20]

Let me suggest for the moment that this workforce will expand as boomers age, and that some men of like mind will join. If we were to move from an informal to a formal home health workforce, what might be done to strengthen the home health managers' performance, longevity and retention? First, have physicians include these managers as part of their health care team. Second, organize, on the local practice level, physician-led, nurse-directed "virtual teams" of home health managers to provide information and address isolation. Third, advocate for health insurance reform to reward home health managers for success in managing their multigenerational family's wellness and prevention. Fourth, support smart technology development to outfit homes for efficiency, safety, education and behavioral modification. Fifth, experiment with best practices that save time, lower stress, and build efficient, reliable care processes.

A home-centered health care system, where information begins at home, connects to physicians and care teams, and circles back home, seems impossible only because the pieces of our system, built long ago for vertical disease intervention, are locked in place by historic silos and outdated business plans. But we're now moving toward a horizontal model of health care, one that flattens the old silos, rearranges and reconstructs the pieces, and connects all the players together in a much more logical way.

As we enter this new millennium, we are experiencing a shifting health care value proposition. Americans are attempting to move from reactive intervention to proactive prevention, and this changes the playing field for everyone — hospitals, doctors' offices, health insurers, and pharmaceutical and medical device companies alike. It implies healthy behaviors, early diagnosis, regular screenings, knowing your numbers, effective long-term treatments with excellent adherence, and a personalized, information- and relationship-rich support system that is equitable and just. It suggests that to be valued in our future health care system, each player, in addition to his or her traditional unique contributions, will also need to be engaged in educational and behavioral modification to claim insider status.[16,21,22]

With these in mind, the health care "Carousel of Progress" has been created. Now, we're circling counter-clockwise and the last set appears. Ten realities have been skillfully integrated into this calm and well-organized vision of a healthy home:

1. A home health manager, previously the informal family caregiver, has been designated for each extended family.

2. Health insurance covers nearly all Americans, and a medical information highway has been constructed primarily around the patient, with caregivers integrated in, rather than the other way around.

3. The majority of prevention, behavioral modification, monitoring and treatment of chronic diseases now takes place at home.

4. Physician-led, nurse-directed virtual health networks of home health managers provide a community-based, 24/7, educational and emotional support team.

5. Health care insurance premiums for families have just gone down due to expert performance of the home health manager, as reflected in outcome measures of family members.

6. Basic diagnostics, including blood work, imaging, vital signs, and therapeutics are performed by the home health manager and transmitted electronically to the physician-led, nurse-directed educational network, which provides feedback, coaching, and treatment options as necessary.

7. Sophisticated behavioral modification tools, age-adjusted for each generation, are present and utilized, funded in part by diagnostic and therapeutic companies who have benefited from expansion of insurance coverage and health markets as early diagnosis and prevention has taken hold.

8. Physician office capacity has grown, as most care does not require a visit. Physician reimbursement has increased in acknowledgement of their roles in managing clinical and educational teams and multigenerational complexity. Nursing school enrollment is up as the critical role as educational director of home health manager networks has become a major magnet for the profession.

9. Family nutrition is carefully planned and executed; activity levels of all five generations are up; weight is down; cognition is up; mental and physical well-being are also up.

10. Hospitals continue to right size — they're more specialized and safer, with better outcomes. And scientific advances have allowed early diagnosis and more effective treatment, making the need for hospitalization increasingly rare.

Is this all a far-fetched scenario? Not really. Many of these elements are well within the reach of an integrated and progressive vision for tomorrow's health.

REFERENCES

1. Cohen JL. Human Population: The Next Half Century. *Science*. November 14, 2003:1172-1175.
2. Alliance for Aging Research. Medical Never-Never Land: Ten Reasons Why America is Not Ready for the Coming Age Boom. 2002.
3. Magee M. *The Best Medicine*. New York:St. Martin's Press;2001.
4. Nash D. *Connecting with the New Health Care Consumer*. New York:McGraw-Hill;2001.
5. Dishman E. Inventing Wellness Systems for Aging in Place. *Computer*. 2004;37:34-41.
6. R.W. Pew and S.B. Van Hemel, eds. *Technology for Adaptive Aging*. Nat'l Research Council, 2003. Cited in Dishman E.

7. Massachusetts Institute of Technology Web site. Available at: http://architecture.mit.edu/house_n/. Accessed April 12, 2005.

8. University of Michigan Web site. Available at: http://www.eecs.umich.edu/~pollackm/. Accessed April 12, 2005.

9. University of Virginia Web site. Available at: http://marc.med.virginia.edu/projects_smarthomemonitor.html. Accessed April 15, 2005.

10. University of Rochester Web site. Available at: http://www.centerfor-futurehealth.org/. Accessed April 12, 2005.

11. General Electric Web site. Available at: http://geglobalresearch.com/01_coretech/homeAssurance.shtml. Accessed April 12, 2005.

12. NASA Web site. Available at: http://science.nasa.gov/headlines/y2004/28oct_nanosensors.htm. Accessed April 12, 2005.

13. I.D.E.A.S., a spin-off of the Walt Disney Company, Web site. Available at: http://www.integrityarts.com/ideas.html. Accessed April 12, 2005.

14. Best Buy: Owner of eq-life. Available at www.eq-life.com. Accessed April 12, 2005.

15. Philips Web site. Available at: http://www.medical.philips.com/main/products/telemonitoring/products/telemonitoring/. Accessed April 15, 2005.

16. Arno PS, Levine C, Memmott MM. The economic value of informal caregiving. *Health Aff.* 1999;18:182-188.

17. A profile of caregiving in America. *The Pfizer Journal.* Fall 1997.

18. Schultz, R. et al. Psychiatric and physical morbidity effects of dementia caregiving: prevalence, correlates and causes. *Gerontologist.* 1995;35:771-91.

19. Grant I, Adler KA, Patterson TL, Dimsdale JE, Ziegler MG, Irwin MR. Health consequences of Alzheimer's caregiving transitions: effects of placement and bereavement. *Psychosom Med.* 2002;64:477-486.

20. First Annual Health Survey: Women Talk. National Women's Health Resource Center. May 2005.

21. Robinson JC. From managed care to consumer health insurance: the fall and rise of Aetna. *Health Aff* (Millwood). 2004;23:43-55.

22. Robinson JC. Reinvention of health insurance in the consumer era. *JAMA.* 2004;291:1880-1886.

TEACHING TOOLS

Policy Premises

1. The time has come to build a health care "carousel of progress."
2. Carousel designers should consider aging, health consumerism, and the internet.
3. We must recognize the caregiver revolution where most are third-generation women.
4. Many caregivers do not understand complex health care issues.
5. The health care value proposition is shifting from reactive intervention to proactive prevention.
6. There are 10 ideals for the ideal healthy home.
7. Voices are rising for health care reform.
8. Home-centered health addresses the needs of four- and five-generation families.
9. The home of the future will address the technological needs of these families.
10. Technology must reach its potential in order for home-centered health to be complete.
11. Universities, research and private institutions are developing new technological advancements to assist home-centered health care.
12. As we move toward a health care management team to provide care, the technological back up is necessary to facilitate it.
13. The power in health care is quietly shifting from hospital to office to home.
14. Most of today's family caregivers are third generation women managing aging parents and grandparents.
15. Women view health as multidimensional and integrated across life-spans.
16. Women highly value the health of their families and see themselves as health managers.
17. Women's needs as health managers are increasingly well-defined.
18. If we were to properly and formally support women as home health managers, quality, cost and participation would be postively impacted.

Review

1. Who plays the key role in a home-centered health scenario?
2. What impact does aging have on our health care system?
3. What is health consumerism, and how has it affected the patient-physician relationship?
4. How has caregiver knowledge changed recently?
5. What are the 10 concepts that should be integrated into home-centered health?
6. Who will be at the center of the ideal home-centered health scenario?
7. How will the American home change to adapt to home-centered health care?
8. What role will technology play, and which companies and institutions are already exploring the market?
9. Why are these groups interested in home health technology?
10. How will home-centered health care advance the health of all ages, not just the elderly?

Online Resources

  Access online resources with this book's CD.

Who are Family Caregivers?
http://www.thefamilycaregiver.org/who/caregivers.cfm

Healthy Web Surfing
http://www.nlm.nih.gov/medlineplus/healthywebsurfing.html

Family Matters
http://www.msnbc.msn.com/id/7528900/site/newsweek/

Mastering Effective Health Communication
http://www.healthypeople.gov/Document/HTML/Volume1/11Healt
hCom.htm

Aging Americans
http://www.aoa.gov/prof/Statistics/statistics.asp

Health Information Technology Review
http://www.e-health-insider.com/news/item.cfm?ID=1159

A Virtual Care Environment for Health Education
http://www.ilta.net/EdTech2004/papers/cannonhenrymunro.htm

Connecting for Health
http://www.connectingforhealth.org/news/pressrelease_011805.html

The Changing Home
http://architecture.mit.edu/house_n/intro.html

New Face of Elder Care
http://www.msnbc.msn.com/id/3076976/

Assisting the Aging Population
http://www.intel.com/pressroom/archive/releases/20040316corp.htm

Digital Home Technologies for Aging in Place
http://www.intel.com/research/exploratory/digital_home.htm

Understanding CAST
http://www.agingtech.org/mission.aspx

CAST Clearinghouse
http://www.agingtech.org/Browsemain.aspx

Home Assurance
http://geglobalresearch.com/01_coretech/homeAssurance.shtml

Tumbleweeds in the Bloodstream
http://science.nasa.gov/headlines/y2004/28oct_nanosensors.htm

Women and Health
http://www.healthywomen.org/content.cfm?L1=90&L2=9&RID=8
372

Health Politics Online

For Original Health Politics Programs and Slides:

The Emergence of Home-Centered Health – Part I:
Setting the Stage
http://www.healthpolitics.com/program_info.asp?p=Home_Health
Slide Briefing
http://www.healthpolitics.com/media/Home_Health/brief_Home_H
ealth.pdf

The Emergence of Home-Centered Health – Part II:
Turning Visions into Reality
http://www.healthpolitics.com/program_info.asp?p=home_health2
Slide Briefing
http://www.healthpolitics.com/media/home_health2/brief_home_he
alth2.pdf

The Emergence of Home-Centered Health — Part III:
Women and Family Caregiving
http://www.healthpolitics.com/program_info.asp?p=home_health3
Slide Briefing
http://www.healthpolitics.com/media/home_health3/brief_home_he
alth3.pdf

CHAPTER 1.5

Women's Health

UNDERSTANDING LIFESPAN MANAGEMENT

In the 21st century, we have come to realize that gender has a direct effect on health and well-being. We have a growing appreciation that women's health is not only affected by reproduction, but also by unique biological systems and complex social and economic roles.

What we see emerging is not only an expansion of knowledge and empowerment, but also an increasing effort to organize and prioritize needs in women's health. Key areas of focus now include the expansion of numbers of women in clinical trials, a concentration on accessible health care services available to women and their families, an expansion of informational empowerment, and an emphasis on lifespan management.

If there are challenges in prioritizing resources around women's health, those challenges are made all the more complex by major shifts presently occurring in the health care industry. First, we see a continued movement away from reactive treatment toward proactive prevention. Second, we are moving away from an organ-centric approach with a single focus on reproductive capabilities toward a broader, gender-based construct. And third, we are looking toward systems of insurance that are key to ensuring early access to lifelong continuums of care.

To effectively provide women with appropriate health care services, an awareness of lifespan is critical. Dr. Donna Dean of the National Institutes of Health recently said, "I do not know if the public truly understands that prevention needs to start very early in a woman's life. Osteoporosis is a good example. It is really a disease for which preventative steps need to start in childhood. If we started good health care practices at that age, we probably would not have as big a problem at the other end of the age spectrum."[1]

If a woman's lifespan is uniquely integrated, it is also uniquely segmented, with critical health needs and challenges at each stage. In the adolescent years, self-esteem is a critical health determinant. A study of 4,000 girls ages 14 to 18 conducted by *Seventeen* magazine revealed that 50 percent would consider cosmetic surgery, 50 percent were dissatisfied with their weight and shape, and 65 percent were tired, stressed and burned-out.[2] By age 15, girls were twice as likely as boys to experience a major depressive episode, a gender gap that is sustained through age 50.[3] Indeed, women attempt suicide two to three times as often as men.[4] And nearly 4 percent of young women suffered from a significant eating disorder.[5] In spite of those very real risks, teenage girls often have limited contact with physicians, falling between the cracks of pediatric and reproductive care.

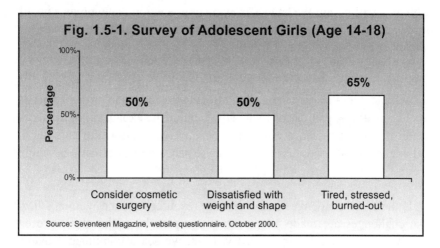

Fig. 1.5-1. Survey of Adolescent Girls (Age 14-18)

Source: Seventeen Magazine, website questionnaire. October 2000.

Leading health concerns among women 25 to 44 shift to childbearing and infertility. But other health concerns are often overlooked. In the 21st century, women are bearing children later in life and experiencing a higher incidence of infertility. In 1996, the percentage of childless women age 20 to 24 was 65 percent, age 25 to 29, 44 percent, and age 30 to 34, 26 percent.[6] A study, reported in 2002, found that 33 percent of professional women age 28 to 55 were childless, while only 14 percent wished to be child-free.[7] More than 6 million Americans suffer from infertility, half of them women.[8] The focus on reproduction in women age 25 to 44 tends to overshadow other health concerns, including important causes of death and disability such as cancer, accidents and violence, heart disease and HIV/AIDS.[6] The incidence of HIV among American women, for example, is on the rise and is now the fifth leading cause of death among Caucasian women, and the leading cause of death among African-American women.[9] The reproductive years provide greater contact with the health care system and, potentially, a unique opportunity to aggressively address these non-reproductive health care risks.

During the middle years, women encounter expanded responsibilities, menopause, and a number of serious health issues. Women spend more than one-third of their lives in the post-reproductive menopausal years. In the United States, the average age of menopausal onset is 51.[10] In addition to managing the physical and emotional symptoms of menopause, vigilance is required on a number of health fronts. One-third of 45- to 64-year-olds, and 55 percent of women over 65, experience arthritis. More than 50 percent will experience osteoporosis-related fractures during their lifetimes. Approximately 11 percent of 45- to 64-year-olds have heart disease, with one-third over 65 affected. And those over 50 are responsible for 77 percent of the new cases of breast cancer and 70 percent of the new cases of cervical cancer.[11,12,13,14,15] In all of these situations, prevention, early diagnosis, and effective treatment are life-enhancing and life-saving.

But women of this age group often find little time to care for themselves. Responsibilities for others — parents, grandparents, spouses, children and grandchildren — too often means that a middle-aged woman's own health comes last. There are more than 25 million family caregivers in the United States, with rates highest among women 45 to 64.[16] Women who are caregivers are more likely to have health problems, with 54 percent having one or more chronic conditions compared to 41 percent of non-caregivers, and 51 percent with high depressive symptoms compared to 38 percent of the control population.[17]

As the years advance, older women carry a disproportionate burden of chronic diseases, in part because they have longer lifespans than men.[18] Fully 22 percent of U.S. women will be over 65 by 2030.[19] In women 65 to 74, cancer is the leading cause of death, while heart disease dominates in those over 75.[6] As important, there is the ever-present risk of disability. Today, 23 million American women have osteoporosis.[20]

DISEASES AND RISK FACTORS

In women's health, knowledge alone does not equal power. Knowledge, combined with the willingness and ability to act on that knowledge, equals power. Dr. Andrea Pennington, the medical director for DiscoveryHealth.com, recently observed, "We are currently in a 'need-to-know' era in terms of health information. But tomorrow will bring the start of a 'need-to-act' era. Women need actionable instructions."

Relevant information is key. We know that a woman's health span is uniquely integrated across a lifetime, and uniquely segregated, with each phase of life containing its own distinct health concerns. That said, there are major risks and key diseases that represent a general threat across a woman's entire life spectrum.

The risk of cardiovascular disease is a major one that women "need to know" about and "act on." What are the risk factors for cardiovascular disease? First, smoking, which causes one-and-a-half times more deaths from heart disease than from lung cancer.[21] Smokers are two to six times more likely than non-smokers to suffer a heart attack.[21] Second, physical inactivity: 60 percent of women fail to meet moderate exercise requirements, and 25 percent do not exercise at all.[22] Third, nutrition: approximately one-third of American women are obese, and one-fourth have high cholesterol levels.[21,23] Fourth, high blood pressure: 52 percent of women over 45 have elevated blood pressure.[23] And finally, diabetes represents a more significant risk to women than men. Women with diabetes are nearly twice as likely as men to suffer from heart disease.[23]

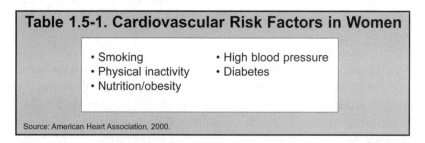

Table 1.5-1. Cardiovascular Risk Factors in Women

- Smoking
- Physical inactivity
- Nutrition/obesity
- High blood pressure
- Diabetes

Source: American Heart Association, 2000.

The additive effect of those risk factors creates a startling reality for women. In 1997, more than 500,000 women in the United States died of heart disease, compared to 450,000 men. Smoking and taking oral contraceptives after age 35 is an especially deadly combination. Currently, it is estimated that more than 20 percent of all U.S. women have cardiovascular disease. When women have heart attacks, they are more likely than men to die within a year — 42 percent compared to 24 percent. And African-American women's risk of a cardiovascular-related death exceeds that of white women by nearly 15 percent.[24]

A second major concern is cancer. While breast cancer remains the most common cancer among women, each year lung cancer is responsible for more women's deaths.[25,26] In fact, lung cancer deaths among men are dropping, even as rates among women rise.[25] In 1998, 22 percent of surveyed women smoked. Those numbers are increasing.[27] In 2000, 30 percent of high school senior girls smoked. Three million U.S. women have died from smoking-related causes since 1980, and it's estimated that more than 50 percent of those cancers were preventable.[27]

Depression is a third major threat to women across their entire lifecycle. The incidence of depression in women is twice that seen in men, affecting 12 percent versus 6 percent.[28] Teenage girls are especially vulnerable as they adjust to physical and hormonal changes, emerging sexuality and parental control issues. These all translate to higher rates of depression, anxiety, eating disorders and disruptive behaviors.[29] As women enter young adulthood, fluctuations in reproductive hormones affect levels of neurotransmitters and their circadian rhythms.[30] Adult women are also exposed to a wider array of adverse life events associated with depression, the most recent addition being adult caregiving responsibilities. Finally, women frequently outlive their husbands. About 800,000 women per year are widowed and left to sort through loneliness, feelings of abandonment and an array of complex management responsibilities and choices.[29]

A fourth major issue, often overlooked or swept under the rug, is violence and abuse. Studies show that 40 percent of all U.S. women have been subjected to violence.[17] Some 12 million women are victims of rape: 700,000 in a 12-month period, with 60 percent occurring before the age of 18, and 84 percent never being reported to the police.[31] Additionally, 31 percent of all women experience domestic violence. This is not simply confined to the poor. While one-half of all women with annual incomes less than $16,000 are affected by domestic violence, so too are one-third of those with incomes over $50,000.[17] Increasingly, the long-term connection between violence and poor health is being established. At least part of the story is tied to a higher incidence of secondary risk factors. Abused women are twice as likely to smoke as those not abused. They are also 40 percent more likely to drink and 34 percent more likely to be depressed.

The fifth major issue is HIV/AIDS and STDs among teenage girls and young women.[32] There are now three million cases of chlamydia annually, 45 million cases of genital herpes and 20 million cases of Human Papilloma Virus in women. While 9 percent were infected in 1989, by 1997, 15 percent were infected. In 2002, the number stood at 25 percent. Between 1989 and 1998, the incidence of HIV/AIDS among women ages 13 to 19 increased 18 times. Minority women carried most of that burden. While African-American and Hispanic-American women comprise 23 percent of America's female population, they represent 76 percent of all U.S. women infected with HIV/AIDS.[9,33]

There is, then, a "need-to-act" as well as a "need-to-know." What are the impediments to acting on our current knowledge of women's health?

OVERCOMING OBSTACLES

In the first two parts of this chapter we have examined the unique challenges encountered in women's health care. On the one hand, those challenges are tied to lifespans, which possess a high level of age-span segmentation. For example, the distinct challenges and risk factors in adolescence, compared to the very different health concerns of a woman in the middle years. On the other hand, a woman's health often involves a high level of integration. For example, the destructive seeds of elder osteoporosis are planted by poor nutrition habits set at an early age. We have also examined the major risk factors and disease entities that challenge women at different stages in their lives.

Now let's focus on the obstacles that must be overcome to advance women's health in the 21st century. Being healthy means different things to different women. The obstacles to health, therefore, are a function of the differing expectations of women. Nancy Fugate Woods, dean of the School of Nursing at the University of Washington, explored this issue in a study of 500 Seattle women. Those women, she noted, "said that being free of disease was just one part of good health. Many spoke about how being healthy meant being able to deal with the stresses and strains that were part of their daily lives, being able to perform optimally at whatever their roles were in society, whether that was going to work, taking care of their kids or being responsible for caregiving. And then there were some women who talked about health in a different way, as achieving a high level of wellness, really having a sense of feeling good."[34]

A primary and fundamental obstacle to the advancement of women's health is the fragmented nature of health care, itself. Approximately 37 percent of all adult women routinely see two different doctors for their health care. Communication between those caregivers is in no way ensured.[35] As Dr. Carol Weisman of the University of Michigan School of Public Health observes, "Women see multiple providers for primary care: OB-GYNs, family practitioners, general internists, advanced practice nurses and others." In many communities, different services are located in different places. Scheduling can be a problem too. The burden on women to access and coordinate their care is also likely to worsen as women age and develop multiple conditions.[1]

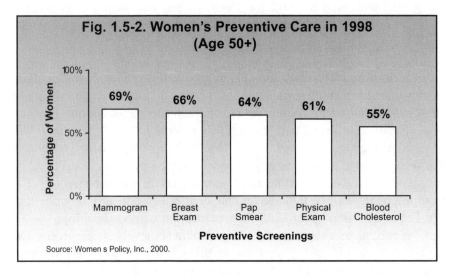

Fig. 1.5-2. Women's Preventive Care in 1998 (Age 50+)

Source: Women s Policy, Inc., 2000.

The business of being a healthy, 21st century woman takes a lot of work, and that work gets imposed on an already overworked and aging population. Dr. Evelyn Murphy, head of Women's Studies at Brandeis University, says, "Until we learn to match services with time constraints of the working woman, we cannot expect her to take the most simple precautionary measures, much less the more time-consuming ones, because it jeopardizes her job. Her job may already be in jeopardy if she is taking personal time off due to illness. Then she is nervous as well as ill. And of course, anxiety cannot be good for her health."[1]

A study commissioned by Women's Policy, Inc., and published in 2000, revealed that at best we were only two-thirds of the way to good, basic preventive health care for women. Only 61 percent of women over 50 had undergone a complete physical exam in the past year; 64 percent a pap smear; 66 percent a breast exam; 55 percent a blood cholesterol test and 69 percent a mammogram.

If the absence of time is a serious obstacle, the absence of money compounds the problem. Poverty is a significant determinant of poor health in women. Dr. Robert Rebar of the American Society for Reproductive Medicine states, "I honestly think that when it comes to providing health care for poor women, we did a better job 25 years ago than we do today."[1] Issues of poverty impact women of all ages. Poor women have higher levels of unintended and unattended pregnancies. They have higher levels of chronic diseases and disability. They have higher levels of depression and anxiety. More women are poorer than men, and time off for diagnosis and treatment is less often an option for poor women. And if time off is not an option when they are young, then the same is often true when they get old.[17]

Add to time and money the unique logistical demands of managing up and down the four- and five-generation American divide. Women now care for parents and grandparents as they tend to children and grandchildren. There are some 25 million informal family caregivers at work in the United States.[17] Of those, 70 percent are women 45 to 64. One-fifth of women caregivers change their work status to manage family responsibilities, 7 percent go part-time, 6.4 percent quit their jobs altogether and 11 percent take a leave of absence.[36] This is not the only sacrifice they make. One-quarter subsequently describe their own health as fair or poor. And their perception of poor health is "on the mark" according to a recent study of interleukin six levels in caregivers. This marker of stress and aging increased six times faster in caregivers of family members with dementia than in a non-caregiving matched cohort.[17]

The challenges are great. But leaders of the Women's Health Movement acknowledge progress, as well. One measure of this progress is the healthy output of congressional legislation. Here are a few representative examples. In the last few years, the NIH has been directed, through the Women's Health Reauthorization Act of 1998, to expand, intensify and coordinate cardiovascular research among women. A congressional commission has been created to examine the barriers to women entering health careers. The CDC has expanded its STD prevention budget to $148 million and conducted new research on the Human Papilloma Virus. The National Institute of Environmental Health Sciences has been directed to explore the links between the environment and breast cancer. And a national media campaign has been funded to educate young women on eating disorders.[37]

So women's health is very much a woman's issue. But success in defining and executing strategies to advance the health of America's women — the primary caregivers, health coordinators and wellness motivators of America's increasingly complex and aging family — will realize unparalleled benefits, not only to women, but to our society overall.

REFERENCES

1. Dean, DJ. Every Women's Health in the New Millennium. *The Pfizer Journal*. 5:1,2001, p.10.
2. S*eventeen Magazine*. Web site questionnaire, October 2000. www.seventeen.com.
3. Cyranowski JM, Frank E, Young E, Shear MK. Adolescent onset of the gender difference in lifetime rates of major depression: a theoretical model. *Arch Gen Psychiatry*. 2000; 57:21-27.
4. In Harm's Way: Suicide in America. *NIMH* publication No 01-4594. Available at: www.nimh.nih.gov/publicat/harmaway.cfm. Accessed 4 April 2001.
5. The Numbers Count. *NIMH* publication No 01-4584 Available at www.nimh.nih.gov. Accessed 27 April 2001.
6. Weisman CS. Women's health in perspective. In: *Women's Primary Care*. New York, NY: McGraw-Hill; 2000.
7. Hewitt, S. *Creating a Life: Professional Women and the Quest for Children*. New York, NY: Miramax; 2002.
8. American Society for Reproductive Medicine. www.asrm.org 2003.
9. Data Brief on Women and HIV/AIDS: The National Facts. Center for Women Policy Studies, Washington DC. Updated regularly.
10. Jacobs Institute of Women's Health. Guidelines for counseling women on the management of menopause, February 2000.
11. American Cancer Society. Breast cancer facts and figures 1996. Available at: www.cancer.org. Accessed 24 April 2001.
12. The National Women's Health Information Center. Older Women's Health Priorities. Available at: www.4woman.gov. Accessed 24 April 2001.
13. Older Women's League (OWL). Osteoporosis: a challenge for midlife and older women. Available at: www.owl-national.org. Accessed 24

April 2001.

14. Arthritis Foundation. Women and arthritis. Available at: ww.intelihealth.com. Accessed 27 April 2001.

15. Older Women's League. Women and heart disease: a neglected epidemic. Available at: www.owl-national.org. Accessed 24 April 2001.

16. Arno P, Levine C, Memmott M. The economic value of informal caregiving. *Health Aff.* 1999: 182-188.

17. The Commonwealth Fund 1998 Survey of Women's Health. Fact Sheet: Informal Caregiving. May 1999. Available at: www.cmwf.org.

18. Guralnik JM, Leveille SG, Hirsch R, et al. The impact of disability in older women. *JAMWA.* Summer 1997;52:113-120.

19. U.S. Census Bureau, population division. Available at: www.census.gov. Accessed 17 April 2001.

20. National Institutes of Health, Osteoporosis and Related Bone Diseases National Resource Center. Osteoporosis Overview. Available atwww.osteo.org/osteo.html. Accessed 10 June 2001.

21. NHBLI: Heart Disease & Women: Are You at Risk? NIH publication No 98-3654. August 1998.

22. Physical activity and health. A report of the Surgeon General. Centers for Disease Control. Available at: http://www.cdc.gov. Accessed March 30, 2001.

23. Mosca L, Manson E, Sutherland SE, et al. Cardiovascular disease in women: a statement for healthcare professionals from the American Heart Association. Circulation. 1997; 96: 2468-2482.

24. Women, Heart Disease and Stroke Statistics. American Heart Association, 2000. Available at: http://www.americanheart.org.

25. American Lung Association. Facts about lung cancer. Available at http://www.lungusa.org/diseases/lungcan.html. Accessed January 23, 2001.

26. American Cancer Society. Breast cancer: what is it? Available at http://www3.cancer.org. Accessed January 23, 2001.

27. Women and Smoking: A report of the Surgeon General-2001.Centers for Disease Control. Available at: http://www.cdc.gov. Accessed March 29, 2001.

28. Women Hold Up Half The Sky. NIMH publication No 99-4607. Available at: http://www.nimh.nih.gov. Accessed December 22, 2000.

29. Depression: What Every Woman Should Know. NIMH publication No 00-4779. August 2000. Available at: http://www.nimh.nih. Accessed December 2, 2000.

30. Parry BL, Haynes P. Mood disorders and the reproductive cycle. *The Journal of Gender-Specific Medicine.* 2000;3:53-58.

31. Kilpatrick DG, Edmunds CN, Seymour A. Rape in America: A Report to the Nation. National Victim Center: 1992.
32. Sexually transmitted diseases. Fact Sheet. National Institute of Allergy and Infectious Diseases. Available at: http://www.niaid.nih.gov. Accessed March 27, 2001.
33. Woman-Focused Response to HIV/AIDS. A Publication of the National AIDS Fund in collaboration with the Center for Women Policy Studies.
34. Woods N, Laffrey S, Duffy M, et al. Being healthy: women's images. Advances in Nursing *Science*. 1988; 1:36-46.
35. Collins KS, Schoen C, Joseph S, et al. Health concerns across a woman's lifespan. *The Commonwealth Fund* 1998 Survey of Women's Health, May 1999.
36. A Profile of Caregiving in America. *The Pfizer Journal*, Fall 1997.
37. Women's Policy, Inc. Women's Health Legislation in the 106th Congress. 1999-2000:85.

TEACHING TOOLS

Policy Premises

1. In the 21st century, we have come to realize that gender has a direct effect on health and well-being.
2. To provide appropriate health services for women an awareness of lifespan is essential.
3. Self-esteem is a critical health determinant in the adolescent years.
4. Childbearing and infertility are lead concerns in women 25 to 44 years, but other issues are a significant threat as well.
5. During the middle years, women encounter expanded responsibilities, menopause, and a number of serious health issues.
6. Older women carry a disproportionate burden of chronic disease in the United States.
7. In women's health, knowledge alone does not equal power. Knowledge combined with the willingness and ability to act on that knowledge equals power.
8. The risk of cardiovascular disease to woman is a major 'need to know' and 'need to act.'
9. While breast cancer remains the most common cancer in women, lung cancer is now responsible for more deaths in women.
10. Depression is a constant threat through a woman's entire life cycle.
11. Violence and abuse rates during a women's lifetime are high and have long-term health effects.
12. Minority teenage girls and young women are especially susceptible to STDs and increasingly HIV/AIDS.
13. Being healthy means different things to different women. The obstacles therefore are a function of the different expectations of women.
14. The fragmented nature of women's health care undermines the abilty to access coordinated preventive care.
15. Poverty is a significant determinant of poor health in women.
16. A wide range of senior care issues complicate personal health maintenance.
17. Recent congressional action suggests a more active approach to advancing women's health.

Review

1. How do major shifts occurring in health care affect women's health?
2. During the adolescent years, how is self-esteem critical in determining girls' health?
3. What are the leading health concerns among women between the ages of 25 and 44?
4. How does the caregiver role, frequently taken on by women, affect their health?
5. Why do older women carry a disproportionate share of chronic disease?
6. What are the five major risk factors for cardiovascular disease in women?
7. What type of cancer is responsible for the highest number of deaths in women each year?
8. Why are women more likely to suffer from depression than men?
9. What is the connection between domestic violence and poor health?
10. What percentage of young American women is infected with HIV/AIDS and STDs?
11. Why is women's health care often fragmented?
12. What percentage of women have undergone basic preventive health examinations?
13. How does poverty contribute to poor health among women?
14. Some 70 percent of all informal family caregivers are women. How does this role impact their health?
15. What recent congressional legislation advances improvement in women's health care?

Online Resources

Access online resources with this book's CD.

Women's Health
http://www.health.nih.gov/search.asp?category_id=28

Menopause Resource Guide
http://www.4woman.gov/owh/older.htm#Menopause%20Resource
%20Guide

Age and Female Infertility
http://www.theafa.org/aboutus/theaia.html

**Research Agenda for Psychosocial and Behavioral Factors in
Womens Health: Lifespan/Developmental Issues**
http://www.apa.org/pi/wpo/lifespan.html

Profile of Informal and Family Caregivers
http://www.careguide.com/modules.php?op=modload&name=CG_
Resources&file=article&sid=861

Women's Health Data Book
http://www.jiwh.org/Resources/Data%20Book%20Highlights%20
WoC.pdf

Depression: What Every Woman Should Know
http://www.nimh.nih.gov/publicat/depwomenknows.cfm

**Eating Disorders: Facts About Eating Disorders and the
Search for Solutions**
http://www.nimh.nih.gov/publicat/eatingdisorder.cfm

Women's Heart Health Education Initiative
http://hin.nhlbi.nih.gov/womencvd/whei/index.htm

**Information for Women on Food Safety, Nutrition and
Cosmetics**
http://vm.cfsan.fda.gov/~dms/wh-toc.html

United States HIV/AIDS Statistics
http://www.avert.org/womstata.htm

Divisions of HIV/AIDS Prevention
http://www.cdc.gov/hiv/stats.htm

National Center for Health Statistics
http://www.cdc.gov/nchs/fastats/womens_health.htm

**CDC National Prevention Information Network (NPIN)
Populations at Risk**
http://www.cdcnpin.org/scripts/population/women.asp

Women and Nutrition: A Menu of Special Needs
http://www.fda.gov/fdac/reprints/womnutri.html

**Facts About Lung Cancer Provided by the American Lung
Association**
http://www.lungusa.org/site/pp.asp?c=dvLUK9O0E&b=22542

HIV/AIDS Statistics — December 2002
http://www.niaid.nih.gov/factsheets/aidsstat.htm

**Women with Diabetes Face Greater Risk of Heart Disease —
October 2000**
http://www.nih.gov/news/WordonHealth/oct2000/story04.htm

Bill Summary & Status for the 105th Congress
http://thomas.loc.gov/cgi-bin/bdquery/z?d105:s.01722:

Caregiver Stress
http://www.4woman.gov/faq/caregiver.htm

American Society for Reproductive Medicine
http://www.asrm.org/index.html

**Family Caregiving in the U.S.— Findings from a National
Survey — June 1997**
http://www.caregiver.org/caregiver/jsp/home.jsp

**Access to Care and Use of Health Services by Low-Income
Women — Summer 2001**
http://www.ncbi.nlm.nih.gov/entrez/query.fcgi?cmd=Retrieve&db=
PubMed&list_uids=12378780&dopt=Abstract

Health Politics Online

For Original Health Politics Programs and Slides:

Women's Health: Part 1 – A Lifespan Issue
http://www.healthpolitics.com/program_info.asp?p=prog_11
Slide Briefing
http://www.healthpolitics.com/media/prog_11/brief_prog_11.pdf

Women's Health: Part 2 – Diseases and Risk Factors
http://www.healthpolitics.com/program_info.asp?p=prog_12
Slide Briefing
http://www.healthpolitics.com/media/prog_12/brief_prog_12.pdf

Women's Health: Part 3 – Overcoming Obstacles
http://www.healthpolitics.com/program_info.asp?p=prog_13
Slide Briefing
http://www.healthpolitics.com/media/prog_13/brief_prog_13.pdf

CHAPTER 1.6

Scientific Progress and Evidence-Based Medicine

WHAT IT MEANS FOR PATIENTS AND PHYSICIANS

Evidence-based medicine is a powerful tool that holds great promise if used properly. It has been defined as the conscientious, explicit, and judicious use of current best evidence in making decisions about the care of individual patients.[1] It has the potential to enhance the patient-physician relationship and improve patient care. Looking at a brief history of evidence-based medicine helps to clarify its potential.

The search for truth and physicians' desire to base their treatments and therapies on sound knowledge is as old as the medical profession itself. But medicine's first systematic randomized trials, which tested the use of streptomycin for tuberculosis, didn't occur until the 1940s.[2] Some 20 years later, in the wake of the thalidomide tragedy that caused birth defects in thousands of babies, the focus on "process" in medical research was greatly expanded. Beginning in 1962, new Food and Drug Administration regulations required "controlled trials" to demonstrate safety and effectiveness of new drugs as a condition of FDA approval.[3]

The focus remained on drugs, in relative exclusion of interventional treatment and diagnostics, until 1971 when Archie Cochrane, an epidemiologist, suggested that much of what modern medicine did lacked evidence and might indeed be harmful.[4] Further complicating the issue, critical research in 1974 documented that what we did know to be true about medicine was not systematically incorporated into textbooks or teaching materials in real time, creating a translational gap.[5] The 1980s and early 1990s focused on defining rules for systematic review of data and acquiring research funding to develop clinical practice guidelines.[6] The various guidelines from various sources typically took several years to develop, were often outdated by the time they were published, and often didn't represent real-world practice. Thus, adherence to guidelines was not optimal.[3]

It was within this context that David Sackett penned a classic article titled "Evidence Based Medicine: What it is and what it isn't" in 1996.[1] In the article, he clearly described that when used correctly, evidence-based medicine incorporates evidence, physician expertise, and patient values. In his words, "Good doctors use both individual clinical expertise and the best available external evidence, and neither alone is enough. Without clinical expertise, practice risks becoming tyrannized by evidence, for even excellent external evidence may be inapplicable to or inappropriate for an individual patient. Without current best evidence, practice risks becoming rapidly out of date, to the detriment of patients."

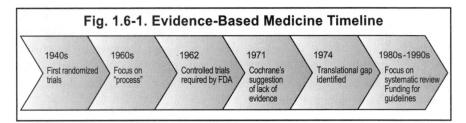

Fig. 1.6-1. Evidence-Based Medicine Timeline

1940s	1960s	1962	1971	1974	1980s-1990s
First randomized trials	Focus on "process"	Controlled trials required by FDA	Cochrane's suggestion of lack of evidence	Translational gap identified	Focus on systematic review Funding for guidelines

Sackett also says that evidence based medicine is not "cookbook" medicine. Because it requires a bottom-up approach that integrates the best external evidence with individual clinical expertise and patients' choice, it cannot result in "slavish cookbook" approaches to individual patient care.

Over the past decade, a critical examination of evidence-based medicine has begun to flesh out the complexity that Sackett highlighted. In caring for a patient, the physician attempts a precise identification of the problem, accesses information necessary to solve the problem, searches the literature, selects relevant studies, applies the rules of evidence to determine validity, applies this knowledge to the individual patient and clinical setting; and continually updates the knowledge, discarding what's old and out of date and adding what is new.[7]

Evidence evolves rapidly and has historically suffered in translation. The first gap is a delay from expert to practice, as evidenced by the multiple years it often takes to move knowledge from randomized trials to textbooks, review articles, or expert recommendations. The second gap, especially significant as the patient-physician relationship has evolved from paternalism to mutual partnerships, is the gap between physicians' continuous education and patients' educational empowerment. Clearly, with the benefit of new information technologies, we have identified the need to constantly evolve and update knowledge in a reliable and systematic manner and also to deliver knowledge to patients and their physicians simultaneously.

Adding to the complexity of evidence-based medicine, it is often inappropriately used as a cost-containment device.[8] Sackett defined the issue when he said, "Some fear that evidence-based medicine will be hijacked by purchasers and managers to cut the costs of health care. This would not only be a misuse of evidence-based medicine but suggests a fundamental misunderstanding of its financial consequences. Doctors practicing evidence-based medicine will identify and apply the most efficacious interventions to maximize the quality and quantity of life for individual patients. This may raise, rather than lower, the cost of care."[1]

Standards for evidence-based medicine must be consistent, transparent and applied to all parties. This means applying them equally to all health care interventions — diagnostic and therapeutic. It means standardizing evidence-based medicine use by all health care participants. It means having a process that is open not only to standard stakeholders but to the public as well. It means considering the clinical merits of recommendations that impact access, and independently considering cost. And it means up-to-date, ongoing evaluation by those with the greatest clinical expertise and real-world testing to advance doable applications.

Evidence-based medicine certainly benefits from clear definition and principled grounding. What are those principles? First, evidence-based medicine should support, not supplant, the decision-making function of the patient-physician relationship. Second, evidence-based medicine should enable the delivery of the best available patient care and consider the patient's individual condition and priorities. Third, financial impact studies should be decoupled and include the costs of the entire system of care and the entire treatment horizon. Fourth, evidence-based medicine must be reviewed regularly in light of evolving evidence, be shared with doctors and patients simultaneously, and evolve in a manner that preserves personalized medicine.

REFERENCES

1. Sackett DL, Rosenberg WMC, Gray JAM, Haynes RB, Richardson WS. Evidence based medicine: what it is and what it isn't. *BMJ*. 1996;312:71-72.
2. Colston J. Descending the Magic Mountain: how early clinical trials transformed the treatment of tuberculosis. National Institute for Medical Research. Available at: http://www.nimr.mrc.ac.uk/MillHillEssays/1998/clintrial.htm?setFont= LargeText. Accessed March 15, 2005.
3. U.S. Food and Drug Administration. The Evolution of U.S. Drug Law. Available at: http://www.fda.gov/fdac/special/newdrug/benlaw.html. Accessed March 15, 2005.
4. Cochrane AL. Random reflections on health services: Effectiveness and efficiency. 1971 (reprinted by RSM Press 1999).
5. Chalmers TC. The impact of controlled trials on the practice of medicine. *Mt Sinai J Med*. 1974;41:753-759.
6. Perfetto EM, Morris LS. Agency for Health Care Policy and Research clinical practice guidelines. *Ann Pharmacother*. 1996;30:1181.
7. Evidence-Based Medicine. A new approach to teaching the practice of medicine. Evidence-based Medicine Working Group. *JAMA*. 1992;268:2420-2425.
8. Soumerai SB. Benefits and risks of increasing restrictions on access to costly drugs in Medicaid. *Health Affairs*. 2004;23:141.

TEACHING TOOLS

Policy Premises

1. Evidence-based medicine is a powerful tool that holds great promise if used properly.
2. When used correctly, evidence-based medicine incorporates evidence, physician expertise and patient values.
3. Evidence evolves rapidly and has historically suffered in the translation.
4. Evidence-based medicine is not an appropriate cost-containment device.
5. Standards for evidence-based medicine must be consistent, transparent, and applied for all parties.
6. Evidence-based medicine benefits from clear definitions and being grounded in principle.

Review

1. What is evidence-based medicine?
2. Why was 1962 an important year for the concept of evidence-based medicine?
3. What are the three components of evidence-based medicine when it's used correctly?
4. How is evidence-based medicine inappropriately used?
5. How has information technology affected evidence-based medicine?

Online Resources

Access online resources with this book's CD.

EBM Basics
http://library.umassmed.edu/EBM/components.html

The Role of the Patient
http://www.muschealth.com/healthyaging/ebasedmed.htm

The Terms of Evidence-Based Medicine
http://www.cebm.net/glossary.asp

Evidence-Based Medicine Resource Center
http://www.ebmny.org/thecentr2.html

Making Evidence-Based Medicine Doable
http://www.aafp.org/fpm/20040200/51maki.pdf

Health Politics Online

For Original Health Politics Programs and Slides:

Evidence-Based Medicine: What It Means for Patients and Physicians
http://www.healthpolitics.com/archives.asp?previous=evi-dencemedicine
Slide Briefing
http://www.healthpolitics.com/media/evidencemedicine/brief_evi-dencemedicine.pdf

CHAPTER 1.7

Privacy

BALANCING THE BENEFITS AND THREATS

The majority of Americans take a pragmatic approach to the release of medical data. This is not to say that they take privacy lightly. It simply acknowledges that patients — and their doctors — realize that the daily evaluation, diagnosis and treatment of patient conditions requires the movement of a patient's medical information between individuals and organizations.

Dr. Amitai Etzioni, director of the Institute for Communication Policy Studies at George Washington University, said, "If you ask people the question, 'Do you want more privacy of personal information?' About 85 percent say 'Yes, of course.' If you put a price on it, then suddenly the amount of support drops sharply — though a segment of the public insists on keeping information private at any cost."[1] In one study on perspectives toward privacy, 25 percent rejected any benefits that require release of information. Twelve percent were unconcerned and did not care about giving away personal information or how it might be used. The majority, some 63 percent, when approached for personal information, balanced potential benefits and threats to releasing information.[2]

Currently, a wide range of individuals have access to patients' medical records. Medical information is frequently shared with consulting physicians, managed care organizations, health insurance companies, life insurance companies, employers, pharmacists, pharmacy benefit managers, blood laboratories, hospital accrediting organizations, medical information bureaus and state and federal agencies.[3]

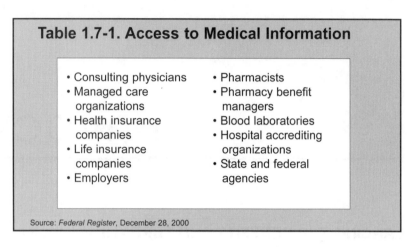

Table 1.7-1. Access to Medical Information

- Consulting physicians
- Managed care
  organizations
- Health insurance
  companies
- Life insurance
  companies
- Employers

- Pharmacists
- Pharmacy benefit
  managers
- Blood laboratories
- Hospital accrediting
  organizations
- State and federal
  agencies

Source: *Federal Register*, December 28, 2000

In the current era of electronic medical records, data moves and must be protected. How does one protect personal data? First, use non-identifiable data whenever possible. Second, use general consent forms, but not so general as to be meaningless or useless. Third, respect the original conditions of consent and safeguards, even if information is transferred to you and you're receiving it second hand. Fourth, have a well-thought-out, monitorable and enforceable security plan.[1]

Expanding approved access to medical data could yield significant patient benefits. Some of those benefits include convenience, efficiency, more coordinated care, remote monitoring of chronic health conditions and expanded participation in clinical research with advanced new discoveries and cures for patients in need.

If there is general agreement on the benefits of greater information exchange, what emotions hold us back? Peter Hutt, a Washington-based expert in privacy law, sites control issues and the need to balance personal freedom with societal need. In his words, "People want personal control over their data so that they can decide where it can and cannot be used, and how it can be used, to make sure that someone does not take control away from them — that is, does not take their privacy away from them."[4]

Regulatory and legislative bodies, in honoring citizens' wishes, must also consider societal needs. For example, in 1997 Minnesota required that patients give written authorization before their existing medical records could be released for an observational, non-interventional study intended to determine the risk of seizure with a newly marketed pain medication. The study was being conducted to provide ongoing information to the FDA regarding the risks and benefits of a drug already approved and available. But only 52 percent of the patients who were contacted responded, and of those, only 19 percent consented to allowing access to their records. In addition, the response rate was likely skewed to those with a related medical complication; people who were, therefore, motivated to respond. This, of course, impacted the accuracy of results. These and other issues caused the Minnesota legislature to amend its directive and allow implied authorization if patients did not respond to a written request within 60 days of two good faith attempts to obtain authorization.[5]

At the end of the day, there must be give and take. In negotiating this complex issue, technology can be a major asset.[6] A multifaceted approach to privacy offers the patient reliable, but not perfect protection. Patient privacy safeguards include user authentication or passwords; firewalls, or software barriers between the internal secure network and the unsecured public network; audits that track who looks at data, and when; coding technology that masks data before it is sent, leaving the identifiable data solely at the primary source site; and smart cards that store patient information and are under patient control.[6,7,8,9]

Is it possible to maintain progress in scientific research, in an age of consumer empowerment and expanded personal privacy rights?

THE HEALTH INSURANCE PORTABILITY AND ACCOUNTABILITY ACT (HIPAA)

Concerns about patient privacy and confidentiality are as old as the practice of medicine. Going back to the 6th century B.C., the oath of Hippocrates weighed in with these words, "Whatsoever things I see or hear concerning the life of men, in my attendance on the sick or even apart there from, which ought not be noised abroad, I will keep silence thereon, counting such things to be as sacred secrets."[10]

Most consumers agree, believing that confidentiality, especially when it comes to financial and health information, is of extreme importance. In one recent survey of 1,000 consumers, the Gallup Organization found that over 80 percent considered financial confidentiality very important, while nearly 80 percent considered health confidentiality very important. Concerns regarding employment and educational data were considerably less pronounced.[11]

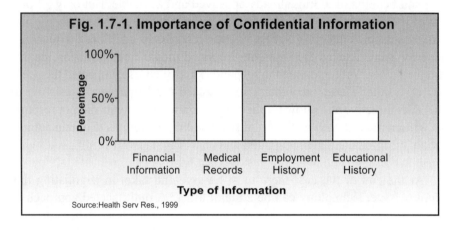

Fig. 1.7-1. Importance of Confidential Information

Source:Health Serv Res., 1999

Recognizing the sensitivity of both patients and physicians in our age of electronic transmission, Congress in 1996 passed the Health Insurance Portability and Accountability Act (HIPAA), which affects all health care providers, health plans and health education clearinghouses.[12] In amending the Internal Revenue Code, the bill was expected to increase efficiencies on the one hand and privacy on the other. And it was to do all of this at a savings. The savings, projected in mandated electronic billings, was $29.9 billion, while the cost of regulating new privacy provisions over a ten-year period was set at $17.6 billion. The projected net savings was estimated to be $12.3 billion.[13]

HIPAA, as designed, has a direct impact on doctors and patients. For patients, it is intended to lower the risk of losing health insurance, ease the ability of workers to switch health plans, allow the purchase of previously unavailable coverage by small groups, and limit companies from excluding coverage to patients with pre-existing conditions.[14]

For physicians, the impact is immediate. They must notify patients of their privacy policies and practices, obtain one-time consent from patients to share information with other clinicians, keep records of all who receive a patient's information, and use electronic files in standardized formats.[12,14,15,16,17] The failure to completely follow the letter of the law can immediately impact physician reimbursement for patient services.

While the new regulations will not completely ensure patient privacy, they have already raised consumer awareness. As Linda Golodner, president of the National Consumers League, has said, "The regulations put the health care system on notice to do something to prevent violations of confidentiality in the system. The regulations alert consumers that there may be problems with confidentiality of health information. That may prompt consumers to ask important questions about the confidentiality of health information."[18]

Table 1.7-2. Direct Impact of HIPAA

Patients	Physicians
• Lowers risk of losing health insurance • Eases the ability to switch plans without loss of insurance • Allows purchase of coverage when other coverage is unavailable • Limits exclusions for pre-existing conditions	• Must notify patients of privacy practices • Must obtain one-time consent from patient to share information with clinicians • Must keep records of all who receive patient information • Must use standardized electronic file formats

Source: HCFA. *HIPAA Insurance Reform: What is HIPAA?* ND.

Federal agencies like the FDA have a good track record on confidentiality. Still, implementation of HIPAA is expected to be difficult and costly.[19] Peter Hutt cites the FDA example. "Since 1962," he said, "the FDA has received, one way or another, data from every report of a clinical study that has been conducted in the U.S. to support the approval of a new drug, biological product, or medical device. It has also received much comparable data from abroad. This data often includes case report forms with patient information, which is, of course, at the heart of the study." In the early years, the data was patient specific and identifiable. To the credit of the FDA, there was never a breach of confidentiality. The FDA today is different, Mr. Hutt notes. "The FDA does not want patient-identifiable information. They want companies to blind data before sending it to the FDA."[19]

Concerns with the HIPAA remain however, if not about the ability of government to deliver, then about the burden of cost and implementation that often comes with unfunded or underfunded mandates. Much of the burden of the HIPAA falls squarely on the shoulders of physicians. As the AMA has said, "The HIPAA is complex and broad in scope" and has caused "major concerns about the cost and disruption of compliance."[20]

It will be incumbent upon policy makers to monitor the pressure points in the privacy debate as health consumer empowerment expands, and to adequately define the role of privacy in assuring the future success of clinical research and discovery.

REFERENCES

1. Balancing Medical Innovation and Patient Confidentiality. *The Pfizer Journal*. Vol 5:3. 2001. p.8.
2. Lester T. The Reinvention of Privacy. *Atlantic Monthly*. Mar 2001: 27-39.
3. DHHS. Standards for privacy of individually identifiable health information: final rules. Federal Register. Dec 28, 2000.
4. Balancing Medical Innovation and Patient Confidentiality. *The Pfizer Journal*. Vol 5:3. 2001. p.18.
5. McCarthy DB, Shatin D, Drinkard CR, et al. Medical records and privacy: empirical effects of legislation. *Health Serv Res*. 1999;34 (pt 2):417-25.
6. GAO. Medical Records Privacy: Access Needed for Health Research, but Oversight of Privacy Protections Is Limited. Washington, DC: *GAO*; Feb 1999. Publication GAO/HEHS-99-SS.
7. Barrows RC Jr, Clayton PD. Privacy, confidentiality, and electronic medical records. *J Am Med Inform Assoc*. 1996;3:139-48.
8. Etzioni A. Less privacy is good for us (and you). *Privacy J*. Apr 1999:3-5.
9. Berman JJ, Moore GW, Hutchins GM. U.S. Senate Bill 422: the genetic confidentiality and non-discrimination act of 1997. *Diagn Mol Pathol*. 1998;7:192-6.
10. Pear R. Bush accepts rules to guard privacy of medical records. *New York Times*. Apr 12, 2001.
11. McCarthy DB, Shatin D, Drinkard CR, et al. Medical records and privacy: empirical effects of legislation. *Health Serv Res*. 1999;34(pt 2):417-25.
12. Fitzmaurice JM, Rose JS. Cutting to the chase: what physician executives need to know about HIPAA. *Physician Exec*. 2000;26:42-9.
13. HHS Press Office. Protecting the privacy of patients' health information: summary of the final regulation. HHS Fact Sheet. Dec 20, 2000.
14. HCFA. HIPAA insurance reform: what is HIPAA? ND. Available at: www.fda.gov. Accessed December 4, 2000.
15. Despite leeway in sharing clinical data, definitions create operational

challenge. Report on Patient Privacy. 2001;1:1,5.

16. Maltz A. HIPAA: what is it and how do you comply? *Cyberounds*. 2000.

17. Etzioni A. New medical privacy rules need editing. *USA Today*. Feb 22, 2001:13A.

18. Balancing Medical Innovation and Patient Confidentiality. *The Pfizer Journal*. Vol 5:3. 2001. p.32.

19. Balancing Medical Innovation and Patient Confidentiality. *The Pfizer Journal*. Vol 5:3. 2001. p.26.

20. IDcide Inc. About IDcide. 2001.

TEACHING TOOLS

Policy Premises

1. The majority of Americans take a pragmatic approach to the release of medical data.
2. Currently a wide range of individuals have access to a patient's medical records.
3. In the current era of electronic medical records, data moves and must be protected.
4. Expanding approved access to medical data could potentially yield significant patient benefits.
5. Privacy is a personal control issue, and must balance personal freedom and societal need.
6. A multifaceted approach to privacy offers patients reliable but not perfect protection.
7. Caregivers' concerns about patient confidentiality are as old as the practice of medicine.
8. Most consumers believe that the confidentiality of financial and health information is important.
9. HIPAA was intended to increase the efficiency and effectiveness of the health care system while protecting confidentiality of health care information.
10. HIPAA has a direct impact on patients and their physicians.
11. The regulations will not completely ensure patient privacy but have raised consumer awareness.
12. Federal agencies like the FDA have a good track record on confidentiality, but HIPAA implementation will be difficult and costly.

Review

1. With whom is medical information frequently shared?
2. How can a patient protect his or her personal data?
3. How does expanded access to medical data improve patient benefits?
4. If access to medical data can provide benefits to patients, why don't some patients want to share their data?
5. What are some key patient privacy safeguards?

6. In a Gallup Organization poll of 1,000 consumers, what percentage considered financial confidentiality very important relative to those who considered health information very important?
7. What impact does HIPAA have on patients?
8. How has HIPAA raised consumer awareness?
9. What does HIPAA require of physicians?
10. Why is implementation of HIPAA expected to be difficult?

Online Resources

Access online resources with this book's CD.

Patient Confidentiality: Protecting Privacy and Preserving Innovation
http://www.advamed.org/publicdocs/innovation/patientconfidentiality.pdf

Impact of 1997 Minnesota Medical Record Law Amendment
http://www.cchconline.org/privacy/medreclaw.php3

Medical Records Privacy
http://www.cdt.org/privacy/medical/

Medical Privacy
http://www.epic.org/privacy/medical/

Patient Privacy and the Use of Medical Records in Research: Balancing the Principles of Confidentiality and the Need for Public Health Data - March 2003
http://www.meducator.org/archive/20030319/privacy.html

Health Politics Online

For Original Health Politics Programs and Slides:

The Privacy of Patient Data
http://www.healthpolitics.com/program_info.asp?p=prog_21
Slide Briefing
http://www.healthpolitics.com/media/prog_21/brief_prog_21.pdf

The Health Insurance Portability and Accountability Act (HIPAA)
http://www.healthpolitics.com/program_info.asp?p=prog_20
Slide Briefing
http://www.healthpolitics.com/media/prog_20/brief_prog_20.pdf

CHAPTER 1.8

Equity and Justice:
Class, Race and Health

THE CONNECTION BETWEEN CLASS, RACE AND HEALTH

A few years ago, the U.S. health care system received a shot across the bow from the World Health Organization. The WHO had been fast at work on a comparative study of national health systems. The study considered five standards — overall level of population health, health inequalities, overall health system responsiveness, distribution of responsiveness, and distribution of financial burden. Surprising to many U.S. leaders, our national system was ranked a dismal 37th, primarily because we scored comparatively low in distribution of resources and in distribution of financial burden.[1]

The report seemed to reveal the issue of feast or famine in U.S. health. The feast? According to a 2002 Institute of Medicine report, Americans today, compared to Americans in 1900, "are healthier, live longer, and enjoy lives that are less likely to be marked by injuries, ill health or premature death."[2] The famine? As stated by health policy experts Stephen Isaacs and Steven Schroeder in the *New England Journal of Medicine,* "Any celebration of these victories must be tempered by the realization that these gains are not shared fairly by all members of our society."[3]

The U.S. response has been to critically explore how best to expand health insurance and to critically examine racial disparities in our health system. Yet studying racial disparities in our health system isn't quite as straightforward as it may sound because, as Isaacs and Schroeder note, "Race and class are both independently associated with health status, although it is often difficult to disentangle the individual effects of the two factors."[3]

A few simple numbers illustrate this point. Whites have a median net worth in the United States that is 10 times greater than blacks.[4] While 11 percent of whites live below the poverty line, 27 percent of blacks struggle with poverty.[5] The life expectancy of blacks is seven years less than that of whites. And blacks suffer higher rates of cardiovascular disease, diabetes, hypertension, infant mortality, homicide, and a variety of cancers.[6] Are these differences due primarily to race or class?

It's clear that prejudice and discrimination, the hallmarks of racism, impact the health of minorities in America, but it is becoming increasingly obvious that low socioeconomic status, which is often a byproduct of racial discrimination, also has a significant impact on health. Looking at the number of deaths per 100,000 person-years in adult men with incomes under $10,000 per year, blacks have 21 percent more deaths than whites. This difference declines to 4 percent for those with incomes from $15,000 to $25,000. But when you turn the numbers sideways, comparing whites with incomes below $10,000 with whites with incomes of $15,000 to $25,000 per year, the lower income group has 2.4 times more deaths. A similar comparison among blacks shows 2.7 times more deaths among those with lower incomes.[3]

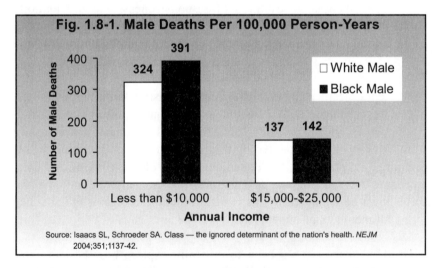

Fig. 1.8-1. Male Deaths Per 100,000 Person-Years

Source: Isaacs SL, Schroeder SA. Class — the ignored determinant of the nation's health. *NEJM* 2004;351;1137-42.

Besides income, other socioeconomic issues intersect with race to profoundly alter health.[7] People without a high school diploma are three times more likely to smoke than college graduates, and they're three times less likely to exercise.[8,9] And clerical civil servants in Britain have death rates from cardiovascular disease that exceed deaths rates of their administrators by 300 percent.[10]

Income, education, and employment are relatively blunt measures. But even these measures, and their relationship to a population's health, have not traditionally been captured in U.S. health policy research efforts. The United States does not systematically collect mortality and morbidity data stratified by social class.[3] Death certificates, for example, note race, but until recently did not capture employment, income, or education level.[3]

Experts debate which of these class factors primarily impacts health. Is it education, with its associated access to better jobs, embedded values, problem-solving skills and effect on self-esteem? Is it higher income, which allows for basic needs to be met, secures better neighborhoods and schools, and allows better access to services? Or is it employment, especially jobs that provide decent working conditions, security, health insurance, and moderate stress?

Likely, it's all of the above, playing off each other and not addressable solely through traditional health programming. But we know that some factors are associated with low socioeconomic status and poor health, such as poor nutrition, increased smoking, decreased exercise, increased stress and fear, unsafe neighborhoods with high crime levels, substandard housing, inaccessible and expensive services, environmental hazards, and poor schools.[3] So it is increasingly clear that significant investment in the short and medium term to address socioeconomic issues could favorably impact health and health care costs over the long term.

This favorable impact is likely because education, transportation, recreation, housing and tax policy all impact health policy. Studies have shown that expanding access to care, which certainly should be done, will only impact 10 percent to 15 percent of premature deaths.[11] Most of the remaining potential benefit is embedded in the expansion of healthy behaviors within individuals, families, and communities. The keys that unlock those doors are opportunity, security, and confidence in the future. Only by opening these doors will health care in the United States realize its full potential.

REFERENCES

1. World Health Organization Assesses the World's Health Systems [news release on World Health Organization Web site]. Available at: http://www.who.int/whr/2000/media_centre/press_release/en/print.htm l/html. Accessed November 30, 2004.
2. Committee on Assuring the Health of the Public in the 21st Century, *Institute of Medicine*. 2002. The Future of the Public's Health in the 21st Century. Available at: http://www.iom.edu/report.asp?id=4304. Accessed November 30, 2004.
3. Isaacs SL, Schroeder SA. Class - the ignored determinant of the nation's health. *NEJM* 2004;351;1137-42.
4. Williams DR. Race and health: trends and policy implications. In: Auerbach JA, Krimgold BD, eds. Income, socioeconomic status, and health: exploring the relationships. Washington, D.C.: National Policy Association, 2001:70. Cited in Isaacs SL, Schroeder SA.
5. U.S. Census Bureau. Poverty in the United States, 1997. Available at: http://www.census.gov/prod/3/98pubs/p60-201.pdf.Accessed November 30, 2004. Cited in Isaacs SL, Schroeder SA.
6. Thomas SB, Quinn SC. Eliminating health disparities. In: Braithwaite RL, Taylor SE, eds. Health issues in the black community. San Francisco: Jossey-Bass, 2001:543-63. Cited in Isaacs SL, Schroeder SA.
7. McDonough P, Duncan GJ, Williams DR, House J. Income dynamics and adult mortality in the United States, 1972 through 1989. *Am J Public Health* 1997;87:1476-83. Cited in Isaacs SL, Schroeder SA.
8. Health, United States. Hyattsville, Md.: National Center for Health Statistics, 2002:198. (DHHS publication no. (PHS) 2002-1232.) Cited in Isaacs SL, Schroeder SA.
9. Pratt M, Macera CA, Blanton C. Levels of physical activity and inactivity in children and adults in the United States: current evidence and research issues. *Med Sci Sports Exerc* 1999;31:Suppl:S527-S533. Cited in Isaacs SL, Schroeder SA.
10. Davey Smith G, Blane D, Bartley M. Explanations for socio-economic differentials in mortality: evidence from Britain and elsewhere. *Eur J Public Health* 1994;4:131-44. Cited in Isaacs SL, Schroeder SA.
11. McGinnis JM, Williams-Russo P, Knickman JR. The case for more active policy attention to health promotion. *Health Aff* (Millwood) 2002;21(2):78-93. Cited in Isaacs SL, Schroeder SA.

TEACHING TOOLS

Policy Premises

1. When judging varied nations' health, the WHO 2000 report ranked the U.S. 37th, primarily due to inequitable distribution of care.
2. The U.S. response has been to critically explore expansion of health insurance and racial disparities.
3. While racial prejudice is a social justice issue that impacts health, a wide range of socioeconomic issues intersect with race and profoundly alter health outcomes.
4. U.S. research focus on socioeconomic demographics in relation to health and premature death has been fundamentally lacking.
5. The socioeconomic factors impacting health are multiple and not addressable solely through health programming or policy.
6. Significant social investment in the short- and medium-term will favorably affect long-term health care costs.

Review

1. Where does the U.S. health care system rank among other national systems?
2. How did the United States respond to the results of the World Health Organization's study of national health systems?
3. Do college graduates have better health habits than those without a high school degree?
4. What are some of the socioeconomic factors that seem to impact health?
5. How can investment in these issues affect the long-term health of the U.S. population?

Online Resources

Access online resources with this book's CD.

Dare to Compare
http://www.census.gov/prod/2004pubs/p60-226.pdf

Health Disparities
http://www.cdc.gov/cancer/minorityawareness/index.htm

Race, Ethnicity, and Health: A Public Health Reader
http://www.josseybass.com/WileyCDA/WileyTitle/productCd-0787964514.html

A Snapshot of America's Families
http://www.urban.org/UploadedPDF/310969_snapshots3_no20.pdf

Children's Health
http://www.ajph.org/cgi/content/abstract/93/12/2105

Cholesterol Count
http://www.americanheart.org/presenter.jhtml?identifier=3026059

Bridging Cultures and Enhancing Care
http://www.hrsa.gov/financeMC/bridging-cultures/

Health Politics Online

For Original Health Politics Programs and Slides:

The Connection Between Class, Race and Health
http://www.healthpolitics.com/program_info.asp?p=class_race_health
Slide Briefing
http://www.healthpolitics.com/media/class_race_health/brief_class_race_health.pdf

CHAPTER 1.9

Cross-Sector
Partnerships

A BENEFIT TO THE GLOBAL SOCIETY

In 1999, Gro Brundtland, director general of the WHO, said, "Health is much more than survival…When resources are scarce — and they always are — we need methods to define what is most important."[1] She went on to emphasize that both the prioritization of need and the development of strategies to address our current health care crisis require cross-sector cooperation.

If this is true for HIV, malnutrition and maternal-fetal health around the world, it is no less true for the problems of the uninsured, for urban pockets of disease, or the outbreak of obesity, diabetes, or smoking-induced cardiovascular disease and lung cancer in women in the United States.

Today's challenges in health care — both globally and locally — require strong cross-sector partnerships to ensure successful outcomes. Health remains deeply siloed on both a macro and a micro level. The segregation is reinforced by different cultures, by language, by tradition, and by the power elite in each sector. On macro and micro levels in health, we have silos in developed and developing nations. We have silos in government, industry, academics and non-governmental organizations, hospitals, doctors, nurses, insurers and suppliers. Other silos include generalists, specialists, home-based caregivers, pharmacists and health educators. We also have silos with governance and financing, often strictly constrained within traditional and rigidly-defined boundaries.

Over the past two decades, we have seen emerge and collide two extraordinarily powerful external forces. The first is health consumerism, moving from emancipation, to empowerment, and on to active engagement. Coincident with this has been the explosion of the Internet, disregarding boundaries of geography, class, religion, race and politics, and carrying empowering health language and knowledge to a global population increasingly at risk for the health decisions of themselves and their families.

While these two forces have created demand for progress and new opportunities, they have also revealed glaring inequities in health care at home, the uninsured, safety in hospitals, or health disparities in minority populations. They have also created a globally connected population, reinforced by rapid air travel and overnight delivery, which is less tolerant of health disasters (like HIV or SARS) that were previously ignored, as they were perceived to occur in someone else's backyard.

Health consumers worldwide are quietly coalescing on an island of their own. They see around them the traditional health sectors, and acknowledge the validity and importance of historic checks and balances. But they believe as well that these can be preserved while, at the same time, cooperatively addressing a variety of significant health issues that reside on this "island of common stewardship."

The four major sectors in health care have well-defined historic purposes, roles and strategies for success. Governments have focused on governance and purpose, defined roles and responsibilities, invested in system redesign and re-engineering to advance efficiencies, and developed skills as bridgers and collaborators in an effort to share responsibility for the creation and execution of sound policy.

Academics have traditionally focused on a mission of service, education and research. Today, they confront diminishing resources and increasing demands for service and social action. In response, they have emphasized reengineering of patient-care processes to accomplish operational efficiencies, and constructive approaches to partnering, emphasizing trust and transparency, with a constant eye on institutional integrity.

Industry has focused on business performance, the delivery of customer service, the creation of wealth, the discovery of new markets, and the expansion and alignment of philanthropy as part of its social mission.

Non-governmental organizations, or NGOs, have focused on shaping attitudes and behaviors of government, industry and academics. This new mission has been layered upon traditional missions of service and activism. The enormous growth of NGOs over the past three decades is witness to a focus on and growing expertise in virtual communications, organization building and campaign execution, utilizing and synergizing Internet capability and high credibility within traditional media communities.

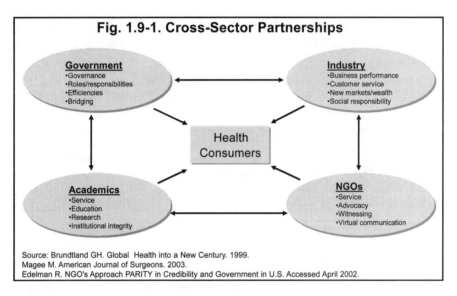

Fig. 1.9-1. Cross-Sector Partnerships

Source: Brundtland GH. Global Health into a New Century. 1999.
Magee M. American Journal of Surgeons. 2003.
Edelman R. NGO's Approach PARITY in Credibility and Government in U.S. Accessed April 2002.

Beyond the desire for collaboration, there must be environmental readiness to ensure success. Desire to truly collaborate is reflected in the various sectors' willingness to mutually plan, to align goals and objectives, to share risk, and to exhibit a good understanding of each other's strengths, weaknesses and capabilities. True readiness is evidenced by an appreciation that health care is a local phenomenon reflected in concrete and realistic planning, and in the design and management of the realities of time, place, people, institutions and target geography. Readiness also implies proactive involvement of all four sectors, right-sizing the effort or program to the challenges, possessing optimistic leaders, and having accurate baseline data on the front end.

If readiness and desire are present, success may hinge on a proper phase-in. Phased development helps overcome traditional obstacles, including absence of top leadership buy-in, disagreements on science, lack of strong prevention infrastructure, hidden political agendas, key sector exclusion, and failure to accurately identify key issues.

There are three phases to cross-sector collaborations. Phase I is creation. This generally begins with two individuals from two sectors with a common passion who seed a vision off-line. They subsequently enlist others and capture their enthusiasm and the vision grows.

Phase II is the launch phase, which builds consensus around science, scope, objective and timetable. The willingness to provide resources is confirmed, providing additional political stability. Relationships are established and training and communication efforts are launched. The vision finds context within the envelope of a fully fleshed out public health strategy.

Phase III is the sustainability phase, concentrating on clarity in governance, roles and responsibilities. Strong leadership is visible and instrumental in creating an ongoing community network of service and maintaining a reliable communication plan that sustains human and financial resources.

Fig. 1.9-2. Phased Development

I. Creation	II. Launch	III. Sustain
• Personal contact • Seed offline • Capture enthusiasm • Grow vision • Initial data	• Agree on science, scope, timetable • Resource project • Build relationship, training, communication • Comprehensive public health strategy	• Clear governance • Clear roles and responsibilities • Strong leadership • Community network • Reliable communication plan

Source: Magee M. *American Journal of Surgeons*. 2003.

Government, business, academics, and NGOs are increasingly overlapping in the areas of social purpose. The ability to organize their varied and often complementary skills and resources will significantly benefit our global and local societies.

REFERENCES

1. World Health Organization. The World Health Report 1999. Making a Difference. Geneva, Switzerland: WHO; 1999.

TEACHING TOOLS

Policy Premises

1. Today's challenges in health care — both globally and locally — require strong cross-sector partnerships to ensure successful outcomes.
2. Health care remains deeply siloed on both macro, micro and grassroots levels.
3. The emergence of health consumer empowerment and new information technologies are creating "islands of common stewardship" while preserving legitimate checks and balances.
4. The major sectors in health care have well-defined historic purposes, roles, and strategies for success.
5. Beyond the desire for collaboration, there must be environmental readiness to ensure success.
6. Phased development is as critical as proactively identifying the obstacles to success.

Review

1. What has been the impact of health consumerism and the Internet on health care?
2. What are some of the inequities that stand in the way of progress in health care?
3. What are the major sectors serving health consumers?
4. Is it possible to cooperate across sectors while preserving legitimate checks and balances?
5. What are the phases in developing successful cross-sector partnerships?

Online Resources

Access online resources with this book's CD.

Public-Private Partnerships in Public Health
http://www.hsph.harvard.edu/partnerships/

Red Cross President Highlights Public Health Partnerships
http://www.redcross.org/news/other/president/021119apha.html

WHO D-G Brundtland Emphasizes Importance of NGO Input Into Diet and Chronic Disease Strategy
http://www.who.int/mediacentre/news/statements/2003/statement7/en/

Health Politics Online

For Original Health Politics Programs and Slides:

Cross-Sector Partnerships in Healthcare
http://www.healthpolitics.com/program_info.asp?p=prog_07
Slide Briefing
http://www.healthpolitics.com/media/prog_07/brief_prog_07.pdf

CHAPTER 2

Risk
Management

*"Patients rarely do an analytic assessment of benefits and risks; they
follow their gut instincts about something. We have evolved to deal with
risks by trusting our senses, perceptions and feelings about whether a
situation looks good or bad or safe or dangerous. This very intuitive
process does not mix well with mathematical formulations of decision-
making that we have come to value as rational."*

— PAUL SLOVIC
Professor of Psychology
University of Oregon

CHAPTER 2.1

Major Risk Factors Affecting the Global Burden of Disease

CONTRIBUTORS TO THE PROBLEM

The cross-sector collaboration of the World Health Organization, the World Bank, and Harvard Medical School produced the landmark study, the Global Burden of Disease.[1] In the process, they created a mathematically acceptable measurement to understand the impact of disease and its connection to individual "health span" and "lifespan," and the impact on national productivity. The DALY, or Disability Adjusted Life Year, represents one year lost to poor health.

We have examined the study's design and basic findings and the environmental factors that have contributed to those findings. Before turning to considering concrete intervention, what are the major risk factors contributing to the global burden of disease?

Malnutrition alone accounts for nearly 16 percent of all DALYs and nearly 12 percent of deaths. Poor water and sanitation, another risk factor dominant in underdeveloped countries, is the second leading source of DALYs at nearly 7 percent and more than 5 percent of deaths. Unsafe sex and alcohol together account for 7 percent of all DALYs and approximately 4 percent of deaths.[1]

Tobacco is the most alarming trend when one looks at risks over the next two decades. By 2020, tobacco-related diseases are projected to kill more people than any single disease, including HIV.[2] What are some of the facts on global tobacco, increasingly marketed to developing countries? First, one in three people over the age of 15 worldwide currently uses tobacco.[3] Four million die each year from tobacco-related illness, and approximately 500 million people currently alive will die of tobacco-related illness, nearly half before the age of 69.[4, 5] China and India are the leading consumers of tobacco, and by 2020, 70 percent of tobacco deaths will be in the developing worlds.[3]

Table 2.1-1. Ten Major Risk Factors

	% Deaths	% DALYS
Malnutrition	11.7	15.9
Poor water/sanitation	5.3	6.8
Tobacco	6.0	2.6
Hypertension	5.8	1.4
Physical inactivity	3.9	1.0
Unsafe sex	2.2	3.5
Job injuries	2.2	2.7
Alcohol	1.5	3.5
Air pollution	1.1	0.5
Illicit drugs	0.2	0.6

Source: Murray CJL, Lopez AD. *Science* 1996;274:740-743.

The economic impact of tobacco on struggling economies is enormous when you consider loss in productivity and direct health care costs. Dr. Alan Lopez, lead researcher on the Global Burden of Disease study, has noted, "If current trends continue, every second person who begins smoking in adolescence and persists in smoking will die from a tobacco related illness. That is a 50 percent risk of dying." The threat is not exclusive by any means to developing nations. In the United States, tobacco use among kids is on the rise as well.[6]

If tobacco is the most alarming future trend, malnutrition is clearly the most persistent risk to global health. At least 500 million people worldwide are undernourished.[4] The impact of malnourishment on fetal and infant development creates a lifelong effect. For example, early malnutrition has been linked to cardiovascular disease in adulthood.[7]

But one need not look forward to uncover the risk. Gro Brundtland of the WHO has said, "Malnutrition is still haunting children in many corners of the world. Infections and malnutrition join in lethal alliance."[8] Malnutrition leads to poor health, blindness, stunted growth, mental retardation, low work productivity and more.[9] Literally, it touches everything, and at its core is poverty. In the developing world, about one in three or 1.3 billion people live on less than a dollar a day.[10]

Poor sanitation and unsafe sex together account for more than 10 percent of total DALYs. As Nils Daulaire, president of the Global Health Council, has said, "Several of the top diseases are still diseases of underdevelopment. Diarrhea and parasitic diseases are often attributed to poor water supply and sanitation as well as poor domestic and personal hygiene." The ability to address these issues requires stable cross-sector cooperation and resources. Infrastructure doesn't appear overnight, and there are plenty of examples to illustrate that political instability, warfare and nonsustainable external resources can rapidly reverse hard-fought gains.

The absence of stability and leadership clearly accelerates the risk of unsafe sex as well. Two percent of all deaths and 3.5 percent of all DALYs were attributable to unsafe sexual activity.[11] What is especially tragic is the fact that this burden is so disproportionately borne on the backs of women and children. In women of reproductive age, 12 percent of all deaths and 15 percent of all DALYs were the result of unsafe sex.[11] But the heaviest burden is likely felt by infants infected by a wide variety of disease, including HIV, during the birthing process.

Alcohol abuse, lack of exercise, environmental pollution and risk factors associated with the development of chronic diseases are not insignificant, and each deserves investment and long-term attention. One of the benefits of the Global Burden of Disease study is that it allows us to begin to prioritize and predict. How will the global burden of disease change over the next two decades?[8] The experts predict that death and disability from infection, diarrhea, famine, congenital anomalies and anemia will decline. But death and disability from mental illness, trauma, heart disease and stroke, lung cancer and emphysema from smoking, and HIV will rise.[11]

Table 2.1-2. Prospects on the Burden of Disease

Expected to Decrease	Expected to Increase
• Lower respiratory infections • Diarrheal disease • Perinatal conditions • Measles • Congenital anomalies • Malaria • Malnutrition • Anemia	• Depression • Heart disease • Cerebrovascular disease • Traffic accidents • Chronic obstructions/pulmonary disease • War, violence, suicide • HIV • Lung cancer

Source: Murray CJL, Lopez AD. *Science* 1996; 274:740-743.

If we know the risks and understand how they will likely grow or decline, we're in a much better position to use the data to inform investment in support of global health.

REFERENCES

1. Murray CJL, Lopez AD. Evidence-based health policy-lessons from the Global Burden of Disease Study. *Science*. 1996; 274:740-743.
2. Murray CJL, Lopez AD, eds. Summary: *The Global Burden of Disease*. Cambridge, Mass: Harvard University Press; 1996.
3. WHO declares global war against big tobacco. World Health News. [serial online]. Available at: http//www.worldhealthnews.Harvard.edu. Accessed November 16, 1999.
4. Brundtland GH. Global health into a new century; April 9, 1999. Available at: http://www.who.org/infdg/speeches/english/19990409_acc.html. Accessed June 1, 1999.
5. Peto R, Lopez AD, Boreham J, Thun M, Heath C Jr, Doll R. Mortality from smoking worldwide. *Br Med Bull*. 1996; 52:12-21.
6. Smoking is a big killer in Americas. New York, NY: Associated Press Report; September 28, 1999.
7. Reddy KS. Hypertension control in developing countries: generic issues. *J Human Hypertens*. 1996; 10(suppl 1):S33-S38.
8. Brundtland GH. Address to the XXII International Congress of Paediatrics; August 10, 1998. Available at: http://www.who.int/director-general/speeches/english/19980810_amsterdam.html. Accessed October 23, 1999.
9. World Health Organization. The World Health Report 1999. Making a Difference. Geneva, Switzerland: WHO; 1999.
10. World Health Organization. Infectious diseases are the biggest killer of the young. Available at http://www.who.int/infectious-disease-report/pages/ch1text.html#Anchor. Accessed December 16, 1999.
11. World Health Organization. First ever analysis of global disease burden of sexual activity and reproduction published [press release]. Available at: http://www.who.org/inf-pr-1998/en/pr98-86. html. Accessed January 10, 2000.

TEACHING TOOLS

Policy Premises

1. The causes of ill health are complex and often indirect.
2. Ten major risk factors account for more than one-third of the world's total disease burden.
3. Tobacco is the most alarming trend for the next two decades. By 2020 it will kill more people than any single disease including HIV.
4. Malnutrition is the risk factor responsible for the greatest loss of DALYs (15.9 percent).
5. Poor sanitation and unsafe sex together account for more than 10 percent of total DALYs.
6. New cross-sector health coalitions are emerging and, if successful, may alter future disease burden.

Review

1. What lifestyle habit is expected to create the most alarming risks over the next two decades?
2. What economic impact does tobacco have on struggling economies?
3. How many people worldwide are undernourished?
4. What is needed to address disease in underdeveloped countries?
5. How will the global burden of disease evolve over the next two decades?

Online Resources

Access online resources with this book's CD.

Burden of Disease Unit
http://www.hsph.harvard.edu/organizations/bdu/

New Vaccines Could Balance Global Burden of Disease —
Programs Often Depend as Much on Political Will as Scientific
Capacity
http://www.researchmatters.harvard.edu/story.php?article_id=206

Burden of Disease Project
http://www3.who.int/whosis/menu.cfm?path=evidence,burden&lan
guage=english

Health Politics Online

For Original Health Politics Programs and Slides:

Global Burden of Disease: Part 3 – Risk Factors
http://www.healthpolitics.com/program_info.asp?p=prog_03
Slide Briefing
http://www.healthpolitics.com/media/prog_03/brief_prog_03.pdf

CHAPTER 2.2

The Global Spread of Tobacco

INCREASED CONSUMPTION...INCREASED DEATH AND DISABILITY

Worldwide tobacco use is growing at an alarming rate. One-third of the world's population currently smokes tobacco. Today there are about 1.25 billion smokers around the globe, with numbers projected to rise by more than 30 percent to 1.64 billion in the next 20 years.[1] The burden of illness currently falls disproportionately on men. Forty percent of males over the age of 15 and 12 percent of females over age 15 smoke worldwide.[2]

Table 2.2-1. Worldwide Tobacco Consumption

	Worldwide Consumption	Male	Female
Developing World	65%	88%	12%
Developed World	35%	65%	35%

Source: ASH. Tobacco: global trends. Tobacco prevalence and consumption worldwide. 2001. Available at <http://www.ash.org.uk/html/international/html/globaltrends.html#_edn22>.

Following the Tobacco Master Settlement Agreement of 1998 in the United States, the attention of those promoting tobacco and those opposing its spread has turned distinctly global.[3] Clearly, the developing world has become the target of choice, not only for multinational tobacco giants, but also for state-owned tobacco monopolies.[4] The figures show us why. While tobacco use in the developed world is slowly declining by about one-half percent per year, tobacco use in the developing world is rising nearly 3½ percent per year.[2]

The developing world now consumes 65 percent of the world's cigarettes, males exceeding females 88 percent to 12 percent. By comparison, the developed world consumes only 35 percent of the world's cigarettes, with women consuming a more significant portion than in the developing world — 35 percent to men's 65 percent. If you are a tobacco executive, two targets for marketing, advertising, and growth are obvious — developing countries and women.[1,2]

As consumption has grown, so has death and disability. The harmful effects of smoking are no longer open to debate. More than 70,000 scientific articles have been published since 1950 documenting the harmful effects of tobacco. We now know that tobacco causes 90 percent of lung cancer deaths, 15 percent to 20 percent of all other cancer deaths, 75 percent of emphysema deaths, and 25 percent of all deaths from heart attack and stroke in men and women age 35 to 69.[5] Put this all together and the numbers are staggering: We lost an estimated 100 million lives to cigarettes in the 20th century. Multiply that by 10 and you have the deaths projected for the 21st century.[6]

The largest producer of cigarette tobacco in the world, surprisingly, is not the United States. In 1998, some 5.6 trillion cigarettes were produced worldwide. That's 2½ cigarettes per day for every human alive. China and its state-run tobacco monopoly produced more tobacco than the next six largest producers combined. Thirty-six percent of the world's tobacco originates in China, compared with 11 percent in the United States, 8 percent in India, six percent in Brazil, 3 percent in Turkey and Zimbabwe, and 2 percent in Indonesia.[2] China has grown a tobacco enterprise to meet its extraordinary demands. With 20 percent of the world's population, it is rapidly destroying the health of its future generations. Between 1970 and 1992, China's consumption of tobacco grew 260 percent.[1]

Table 2.2-2. Largest Producers of Cigarettes

	World Total
China	36%
United States	11%
India	8%
Brazil	6%
Turkey	3%
Zimbabwe	3%
Indonesia	2%

Source: ASH. Tobacco: global trends. Tobacco prevalence and consumption worldwide. 2001. Available at <http://www.ash.org.uk/html/international/html/globaltrends.html#_edn22>.

And poor health immediately followed. Deaths from tobacco in China now exceed 1 million per year, and will pass 2 million per year by 2025.[6] One in every three Chinese men below the age of 29 will die of a smoking-related illness.[7] Clearly, the costs in suffering, lost productivity, health care, and economic disruption will far exceed the profits of China's state-run tobacco cartel.

But even if enlightened health policy were to take hold in China, the multinationals would be more than happy to fill the void. Rothman tobacco executive Robert Fletcher, more than a decade ago, mused, "Thinking about Chinese smoking statistics is like trying to think about the limits of space."[8] Another leader at the Tobacco Industry Conference in 1990 was more direct when he said, "We should not be depressed simply because the total free world markets appear to be declining. Within the total market, there are areas of strong growth, particularly in Asia and Africa."[8] And indeed, a look at global market share data some seven years later reveals that the familiar names were listening closely. At the top of the list were Philip Morris, with 18 percent market share; British American Tobacco, with 14 percent; R.J. Reynolds, with 6 percent; Japan Tobacco, with 6 percent; and Rothman, with 4 percent.[9]

Aided by the addictive properties of its product, the tobacco industry has made tremendous inroads in the developing world. But the experience of the developed world proves this trend can be turned around. Here is what is required at home, and as part of a highly coordinated global campaign. Number one, begin global mass media education. Two, ban all tobacco advertising and promotion. Three: put dramatic graphic warnings — as used effectively in Canada — on cigarette packaging. Fourth, increase taxation on cigarettes. Fifth, restrict the use of cigarettes in the workplace. And sixth, diversify crops and provide grants to allow countries to shift away from dependence on this highly lethal, drug-producing plant.

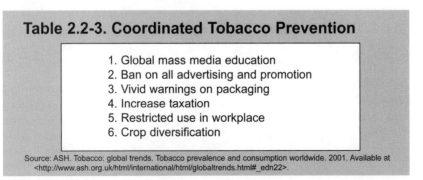

Table 2.2-3. Coordinated Tobacco Prevention

1. Global mass media education
2. Ban on all advertising and promotion
3. Vivid warnings on packaging
4. Increase taxation
5. Restricted use in workplace
6. Crop diversification

Source: ASH. Tobacco: global trends. Tobacco prevalence and consumption worldwide. 2001. Available at <http://www.ash.org.uk/html/international/html/globaltrends.html#_edn22>.

REFERENCES

1. ASH. Tobacco: global trends. Tobacco prevalence and consumption worldwide. 2001. Available at http://www.ash.org.uk/html/international-al/html/globaltrends.html#_edn22. Accessed on 3/10/04.
2. World Health Organization Tobacco or Health Programme.Tobacco or Health: A global status report.1997. Cited in ASH.
3. American Cancer Society. Spending tobacco settlement money. Available at: http://www.cancer.org/docroot/NWS/content/NWS_1_1x_Spending_T obacco_Settlement_Money.asp. Accessed on 3/10/04. Cited in ASH.
4. Frankel G. Vast china market key to smoking disputes. Washington Post. November 20, 1996. Cited in ASH.
5. The World Health Organization. The World Health Report 1999: Making a Difference. Geneva, Switzerland;1999. Cited in ASH.
6. Peto R. and Lopez A. The future worldwide health effects of current smoking patterns. In: Global Health in the 21st Century. In Press.
7. Bo-Qi Liu, Peto R. et al. Emerging tobacco hazards in China: 1. retrospective proportional mortality study of one million deaths. *BMJ.* 1998;317:1411-22. Cited in ASH.
8. ASH. Tobacco Explained. Available at http://www.ash.org.uk/html/conduct/html/tobexpld1.html. Accessed 3/10/04. Cited in ASH.
9. The World Bank. Curbing the Epidemic. Governments and the Economics of Tobacco Control. 1999. Cited in ASH.

TEACHING TOOLS

Policy Premises

1. Tobacco use worldwide is growing at alarming rates.
2. The developing world is the target of choice.
3. As consumption grows, so does death and disability. Harmful effects are no longer open for debate.
4. The largest producer of cigarettes is surprisingly not the United States.
5. U.S. and U.K. tobacco producers are aggressively competing for growth in the developing world.
6. Uniform global approaches are required to combat tobacco.

Review

1. What are the new growth markets for the tobacco industry?
2. How many lives were lost to tobacco-related illness in the 20th century?
3. Which countries are the major producers of tobacco?
4. Why is the consumption of tobacco so high in China?
5. What measures could slow down or reverse the rise in tobacco consumption in the developing world?

Online Resources

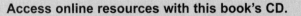 **Access online resources with this book's CD.**

A Vicious Circle
http://www.who.int/tobacco/communications/events/wntd/2004/tobaccofacts_families/en/

Global Progress
http://www.who.int/features/2003/08/en/

World Health Organization: Tobacco Free Initiative
http://www.who.int/tobacco/en/

The World Bank: The Economics of Tobacco Use & Tobacco Control in the Developing World
http://europa.eu.int/comm/health/ph/programmes/tobacco/world_bank_en.pdf

Tobacco: Global Trends
http://www.ash.org.uk/html/international/html/globaltrends.html

Tobacco Control Country Profiles 2003
http://www.who.int/tobacco/global_data/country_profiles/en/

New Study Shows State Tobacco Control Programs Cut Cigarette Sales
Http://www.cdc.gov/od/oc/media/pressrel/r030918.htm

Health Politics Online

For Original Health Politics Programs and Slides:

Tobacco's Deadly Global Grip
http://www.healthpolitics.com/program_info.asp?p=prog_45
Slide Briefing
http://www.healthpolitics.com/media/prog_45/brief_prog_45.pdf

U.S. Tobacco Settlement

A MISSED OPPORTUNITY

The Tobacco Master Settlement Agreement of 1998 was viewed as a landmark public health victory. Signed on November 23, 1998, it directed $246 billion in tobacco assets to 46 participating states over the following 25 years. Mississippi, Texas, Florida and Minnesota were excluded due to prior settlements. In return for the money, the states halted all lawsuits for health damages against the tobacco industry. The intent was to cover the states' past Medicaid costs related to tobacco injuries. The understanding was that between 20 percent and 25 percent of the settlement dollars to each state would be spent on tobacco prevention programming targeted at children. In addition, the tobacco industry agreed to restrict certain types of marketing directed at children.[1,2]

The plan sounded good, but now, reality has set in. Collectively, the 46 participating states pledged $1.6 billion for tobacco prevention programming in 2003. But only one-third of that, or $541 million, was actually spent. Fulfilling the pledge would have meant dedicating just 8 percent of the revenues the states obtained through tobacco taxes and the settlement. They only managed 2.6 percent. Surveys have found that most of these states' citizens believed that 25 percent or more of the settlement dollars should have been spent on tobacco prevention.[1]

The states' record in fulfilling their commitment to childhood tobacco prevention has been abysmal. As Matthew Myers of the Campaign for Tobacco Free Kids has said, "The twin promises of the 1998 tobacco settlement were to significantly increase how much the states spend on programs that protect children from tobacco and to reduce kids' exposure to tobacco marketing. Neither promise has been kept."[1]

In fact, only four states have spent at the recommended level — Maine, Delaware, Mississippi and Arkansas. And they have reaped benefits beyond good will. For example, in Maine, smoking in high schools has dropped 48 percent since 1997 and in middle schools has declined 59 percent. The story in Mississippi is the same. High school smoking has decreased 29 percent since 1999 and middle school use is down 48 percent. The long-term economic and social benefits to these states will be many times greater than their original investment. All the more surprising is that in 2002, 12 states invested less than 1 percent of their tobacco revenues on childhood smoking prevention.[1]

Most states have failed to keep their promise in spite of record revenues from the settlement and taxes on tobacco. In 2003, 32 states increased tobacco taxes over 2001 levels, yielding $19.5 billion in combined revenues.[2] These dollars were largely directed elsewhere — due, in part, to a nationwide budget crisis. Severe cuts in preventive programming occurred in Florida, Massachusetts and Oregon; moderate cuts compromised progress in Indiana, Maryland, Minnesota, Nebraska and New Jersey.[1]

In the meantime, the tobacco industry has moved to fill this gap, expanding its overall marketing investment in the United States and worldwide. The settlement required tobacco companies to restrict marketing through billboards and transit ads, cartoon characters, branded merchandise and event sponsorship. But these activities at the time represented less than 20 percent of tobacco's marketing budget. Since the settlement, more dollars have been thrown into marketing, with expansion of store displays, price discounts, free gifts with purchase, and increased advertising in non-U.S. markets.[1]

What is the resulting 2003 U.S. scorecard? Four hundred thousand people died of tobacco-related illnesses. The direct health care cost of tobacco in 2003 was $75 billion, primarily borne by employers and state and federal governments. More importantly, 4,000 kids continue to become new smokers each day, and 2,000 remain permanently hooked. Looking down the road, each day 670 of those 2,000 have committed themselves to a premature death.[1]

The solution is obvious. Leaders must step up and lead. Fulfilling the 1998 commitment is good social, economic and health policy. So say the experts. From John Seffrin, chief executive officer of the American Cancer Society: "What we have here is a real missed opportunity to reduce and prevent suffering from tobacco related illness."[1] From M. Cass Wheeler, chief executive officer of the American Heart Association: "Tobacco prevention programs work — reducing smoking and deadly illnesses that result, like cardiovascular disease." From John Kirkwood, chief executive officer of the American Lung Association: "Funding prevention programs makes both good health sense and good fiscal policy."[1]

From me: "We could do better; much, much better!"

REFERENCES

1. http://tobaccofreekids.org/Script/DisplayPressRelease.php3?Display=708.
2. http://www.cancer.org/docroot/NWS/
   content/NWS_1_1x_Spending_Tobacco_Settlement_Money.asp.

TEACHING TOOLS

Policy Premises

1. The Tobacco Master Settlement Agreement of 1998 was viewed as a landmark public health victory.
2. Now the reality has settled in.
3. The states' record in fulfilling their committment to childhood tobacco prevention is abysmal.
4. Most states have failed to keep their promise in spite of record revenues from the settlement and cigarette taxes.
5. The tobacco industry, moving in the cracks, has expanded its marketing dollars in the United States and worldwide.
6. Fulfilling the 1998 committment is good social, economic and health policy.

Review

1. What were the main provisions of the 1998 Tobacco Master Settlement Agreement?
2. How much money did states pledge to advance the cause of tobacco prevention?
3. How much did states actually spend on tobacco prevention?
4. What are some ways tobacco companies continued marketing to kids after the settlement?
5. Which states have appropriately funded tobacco-prevention programs, and what have the results been?

Online Resources

 Access online resources with this book's CD.

Still Addicting Kids
http://tobaccofreekids.org/reports/addicting/

Cutting Prevention
http://www.cdc.gov/tobacco/research_data/youth/mm5314a1_Press Release.htm

Chronology of Significant Developments Related to Smoking and Health
http://www.cdc.gov/tobacco/overview/chron96.htm

New Study Shows State Tobacco Control Programs Cut Cigarette Sales
http://www.cdc.gov/od/oc/media/pressrel/r030918.htm

State Tobacco Settlement
http://tobaccofreekids.org/reports/settlements/

National Association of Attorneys General: Tobacco Project
http://www.naag.org/issues/issue-tobacco.php

Tobacco Use Behavior Research Survey
http://ssdc.ucsd.edu/tobacco/

World Health Organization Country Report: The United States of America
http://www.who.int/tobacco/media/en/USA.pdf

What You(th) Should Know about Tobacco
http://www.cdc.gov/tobacco/educational_materials/KIDTIPS4sm2.pdf

Health Politics Online

For Original Health Politics Programs and Slides:

The U.S. Tobacco Settlement of 1998: A Missed Opportunity
http://www.healthpolitics.com/program_info.asp?p=prog_46
Slide Briefing:
http://www.healthpolitics.com/media/prog_46/brief_prog_46.pdf

The Real Story Behind Obesity

IT'S TIME TO TAKE A FRESH LOOK

Obesity in America has set off all the traditional alarms — it's an urgent epidemic with catastrophic implications.[1,2] But to date, the discussion about obesity lacks context. Apparently, the war on obesity is to be waged on old battlegrounds, and the solutions being offered are more adaptive than prescriptive.

In 2003, there were more than 103,000 gastric bypass surgeries for morbid obesity in the United States. The complication rate was 7 percent.[3] If I were morbidly obese, with my quantity and quality of life slipping away, I've no doubt I would grasp on to the last straw of gastric bypass, too. But what an admission of failure for our health care system, where intervention continues to trump prevention, diseases are siloed as if unlinked by physiologic and pathophysiologic processes, and disease burden segregates by gender and race.

If you don't believe gastric bypass surgery at least in part signals the acceptance of the inevitability of obesity, let's consider other measures. Take, for instance, the Puget Sound ferry seats, which were recently widened from 18 inches to 20 inches. Or the Colorado ambulances that are now equipped with a hydraulic winch capable of lifting a 1,000-pound human. Or Indiana's new super-sized casket — it's 38 inches rather than 24 inches wide.[3]

How should we be thinking about obesity? First, the science of obesity is complex and in its infancy. The hormone leptin, which is produced by fat cells and provides the chemical message to the brain that helps control excessive caloric intake, was first discovered at Rockefeller University just 10 years ago in 1994.[4] With that discovery, researchers and social scientists took a fresh look at obesity. Was it simply a reflection of greed and weak will, or something more? Dr. Michael Schwartz of the University of Washington defined scientists' new way of thinking when he said, "We like to think that eating is a voluntary act. But the amount you eat is controlled in part by how much fat you have."[5]

The fat cell is a veritable endocrine factory. In addition to leptin, it makes adiponectin, which enhances insulin's effect and reduces inflammation; resistin, which dampens insulin's effect and encourages inflammation; angiotensinogen, which leads to vascular constriction; IL-6 and TNF-Alfa, which both contribute to chronic inflammation; cortisol, which comes from the adrenal glands but converts to active form in the fat cell; and stored triglycerides, which are broken down to fatty acids and, when released in large amounts, can clog liver, heart, and muscle cells.[5]

The logical question: why is there so much activity in the fat cell? Part of the answer is that fat cells, like the brain, stomach, liver, pancreas, and thyroid, are continually absorbing or releasing substances in response to the body's energy needs.[5] But these systems evolved millions of years ago, so it seems that fat cells are better adapted to preserving calories than shedding them. That appears to have been their historic mission.

The fat cell's work begins early in life, and that helps explain why obesity is an increasingly common early childhood condition. Over the past three decades, the percentage of U.S. children between 6 and 11 years old with obesity has risen from 4 percent to 13 percent, and the rate in 12 to 19 year olds has increased from 5 percent to 14 percent.[6] Children who are obese at age 6 have a 50 percent chance of being obese for life, and those who are obese at age 13 have a 75 percent likelihood of lifelong obesity.[7] Blacks and Mexican Americans, age 6 to 19, are 50 percent more likely to be obese than their white counterparts.[8]

Obesity loves inequity. Those with a body mass index of greater than 25 are defined as overweight; those over 30 are obese; those over 40 are morbidly obese. Blacks and Mexican Americans are generally more at risk than whites, and women are more at risk than men. The numbers of obese black women and obese Mexican American women, as well as black morbidly obese women, are especially high.[9] Socioeconomics appears to have a tie-in, as does level of education. In fact, incidence of obesity and diabetes steadily climbs

Table 2.4-1. Demographics of Overweight and Obese Americans

	Gender	BMI > 25: Overweight	BMI > 30: Obese	BMI > 40: Morbidly Obese
Black	Male	60%	29%	4%
	Female	78%	50%	15%
Mexican American	Male	74%	29%	2%
	Female	72%	40%	6%
White	Male	68%	28%	3%
	Female	58%	31%	5%

	No High School	High School	Some College	College
Obese	27%	23%	21%	16%
Diabetic	13%	8%	8%	13%

Source: American Obesity Association. Obesity in Minority Populations. Available at: http://www.obesity.org/subs/fastfacts/Obesity_Minority_Pop.shtml. Accessed October 26, 2004.
2001 Obesity and Diabetes Prevalence Among U.S. Adults by Selected Characteristics. CDC. Nutrition and Physical Activity. Obesity Trends. Available at: http://www.cdc.gov/nccdphp/dnpa/obesity/trend/obesity_diabetes_characteristics.htm. Accessed October 13, 2004.

as number of years of schooling drops.[10]

Being obese doesn't mean you're a bad person, but it virtually guarantees bad health. Obese individuals have a higher-than-normal rate of hypertension, type 2 diabetes, high lipids, cardiovascular disease, gallbladder disease, osteoarthritis, strokes, respiratory disease and some types of cancers.[1] As the fat cell executes its evolutionary mission, in a land of plenty it does so with little knowledge of or feedback on the havoc it is creating. As Dr. Bruce Spiegelman of Harvard Medical School has stated, "For most of evolution, getting enough to eat was a driving force for survival. How many individuals were lost to morbid obesity?"[5]

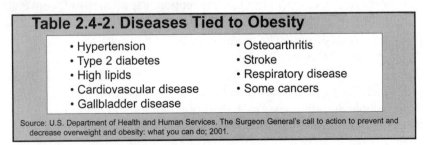

Table 2.4-2. Diseases Tied to Obesity

- Hypertension
- Type 2 diabetes
- High lipids
- Cardiovascular disease
- Gallbladder disease
- Osteoarthritis
- Stroke
- Respiratory disease
- Some cancers

Source: U.S. Department of Health and Human Services. The Surgeon General's call to action to prevent and decrease overweight and obesity: what you can do; 2001.

But times have changed. Today, there are as many over-nourished people as undernourished around the world.[3] For obesity to be properly addressed, we need to target the individual less, and target the molecule, the cell, and the population more. On the chemical level, Dr. Gökhan Hotamisligil of the Harvard School of Public Health, thinks strategically: "In the human body, as in the world, if you control fuel resources, you influence a lot of other things as well." According to researchers, fat is not a by-product of individual greed and guilt but rather an active organ in its own right, worthy of a significant scientific effort to uncover its complex chemical and biological mysteries that will allow its evolutionary mission to adjust to 21st century realities.[5]

On a population level, increased prosperity has meant increased calories. Compared to 1971, U.S. women now consume an additional 335 calories per day, and men consume an added 168 calories per day.[3] Advances in technology mean less exertion, and more indoor entertainment options have brought more sedentary behavior. Finally, the marketing of poor food in large quantities has added fuel to the fire.[1]

What's the real story behind obesity? Before we go full speed ahead, investing in the problem rather than the solution, we should consider the following. How can scientists help the lipid cell adjust to population-wide over-nourishment? How can we promote decreased quantity and increased quality in the American diet? How do we get Americans outdoors again? Why are children, women, and minorities targets for obesity? And are investments in gastric bypass surgery, wider ferry seats, ambulance winches, and bigger caskets really the way to go?

REFERENCES

1. U.S. Department of Health and Human Services. The Surgeon General's call to action to prevent and decrease overweight and obesity: what you can do; 2001.
2. Centers for Disease Control and Prevention. Prevalence of Overweight and Obesity Among Adults: United States, 1999-2002. Available at: http://www.cdc.gov/nchs/products/pubs/pubd/hestats/obese/obse99.htm. Accessed October 13, 2004.
3. Newman C. Why Are We So Fat? *National Geographic*. August 2004.
4. Rockefeller Researchers Clone Gene for Obesity. December 1, 1994. Available at: http://www.rockefeller.edu/pubinfo/ob.nr.html. Accessed October 13, 2004.

5. Underwood A, Adler J, Hand K, Ulick J. What You Don't Know About Fat. *Newsweek*. 2004;144:40-47.

6. National Center for Health Statistics. National Health and Nutrition Examination Survey (NHANES). Hyattsville, MD: U.S. Department of Health and Human Services. 1999.

7. Moran R. Evaluation and treatment of childhood obesity. *Am Fam Physician*. 1999;59:758, 761-762.

8. Hedley AA, Ogden CL, Johnson CL, Carroll MD, Curtin LR, Flegal KF. Prevalence of overweight and obesity among US children, adolescents, and adults, 1999-2002. *JAMA*. 2004;291:2847-2850.

9. American Obesity Association. Obesity in Minority Populations. Available at: http://www.obesity.org/subs/fastfacts/Obesity_Minority_Pop.shtml. Accessed October 26, 2004.

10. 2001 Obesity and Diabetes Prevalence Among U.S. Adults by Selected Characteristics. CDC. Nutrition and Physical Activity. Obesity Trends. Available at: http://www.cdc.gov/nccdphp/dnpa/obesity/trend/obesity_diabetes_characteristics.htm. Accessed October 13, 2004.

TEACHING TOOLS

Policy Premises

1. All of the alarms have been set off on obesity. But to date the solutions are more adaptive than prescriptive.
2. The science of obesity is complex and in its infancy.
3. Obesity is an early childhood condition.
4. Obesity loves inequity.
5. Obesity virtually guarantees bad health.
6. Obesity must be addressed more on the molecular, cellular and population levels and less on the individual level.

Review

1. What is leptin and what does it do?
2. What kind of activity occurs in the fat cell?
3. What percentage of American children are obese?
4. Obese individuals have a higher rate of which diseases?
5. Has prosperity affected the prevalence of obesity in America?

Online Resources

Access online resources with this book's CD.

Time for a Change
http://familydoctor.org/788.xml

Childhood Obesity
http://www.obesity.org/subs/childhood/

Overweight and Obesity
http://www.cdc.gov/nccdphp/dnpa/obesity/faq.htm

Marketing Food to Children
http://whqlibdoc.who.int/publications/2004/9241591579.pdf

Food and Nutrition Information Center
http://www.nal.usda.gov/fnic/

Getting Fit Whenever, Wherever
http://americanheart.org/presenter.jhtml?identifier=2155

American Dietetic Association
http://www.eatright.org/Public/index.cfm

Gastric Bypass A-Z
http://my.webmd.com/hw/weight_control/hw252819.asp

Health Politics Online

For Original Health Politics Programs and Slides:

The Real Story Behind Obesity
http://www.healthpolitics.com/program_info.asp?p=prog_71
Slide Briefing
http://www.healthpolitics.com/media/prog_71/brief_prog_71.pdf

Exercise and Childhood Obesity

CHARTING A CORRECTIVE COURSE

The airwaves have been filled with two public health pronouncements that are increasingly linked by cause and effect. The first is that physical activity has a profound positive physiological effect on the body. The second is that childhood obesity is growing in epidemic proportions.

That childhood obesity is on the rise is undeniable. The rates have been advancing steadily for the past 35 years, with obesity growing from 4 percent to 13 percent in 6- to 11-year-olds and from 5 percent to 14 percent in 12- to 19-year-olds. In just two decades, the number of obese children has doubled.[1]

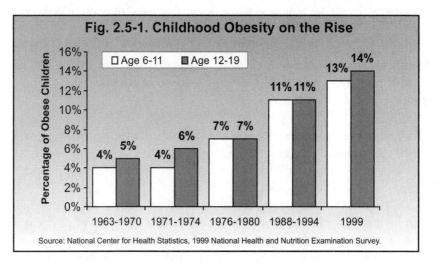

Fig. 2.5-1. Childhood Obesity on the Rise

Source: National Center for Health Statistics, 1999 National Health and Nutrition Examination Survey.

A sedentary lifestyle is a known major contributor to obesity and poor health. Almost half of all young people between ages 12 and 21 get no vigorous exercise at all on a daily basis.[2] Sedentary children are more likely to be obese, and obese children have higher blood pressure, higher cholesterol levels and a greater incidence of type 2 diabetes.[3]

Obese children are very likely to become obese adults, troubled for life by a wide variety of chronic diseases. Young women and minorities are at special risk. The probability of becoming an obese adult if obese at age 6 is 50 percent. The chances rise to 70 percent or 80 percent if the child is still obese at age 13.[3] In young women, inactivity and obesity go hand in hand. Twenty-five percent of American women do not exercise at all, and 60 percent do not exercise at recommended moderate levels during the day.[4] In their earliest years, boys and girls exercise at similar rates. But by adolescence, rates in girls are already entering a steep decline. By high school, only two-thirds of girls are involved in moderate exercise, compared with 80 percent of boys; 15 percent of girls do little or no exercise, compared with 8 percent of boys.[5]

According to Dr. Jay Cookley, professor of the Sociology of Sport at the University of Colorado, "This is due, in part, to the media-saturated culture in which women grow up. Exercise is not a high priority in the lives of most teenage girls, and many of those who do exercise tie it to a desire to be physically attractive rather than to its health benefits."[6] Dr. James Sallis, professor of psychology at San Diego State University, adds, "With young women, we've got to help them connect health-related physical activities to their identities, to their relationships, and to the things that are important in their lives."[7]

If women are at special risk for inactivity and obesity, so are African Americans and Hispanic Americans. Compared to Caucasians, sedentary lifestyle rates are 7 percent higher among Hispanic Americans and 6 percent higher among African Americans.[8]

Uninformed public school policy and unsafe, barrier-laden environments contribute significantly to childhood obesity.[9] Just when we ought to be expanding opportunities for kids to be active, many of our school districts are cutting back on physical education. In at least 37 states, elementary school physical education is managed by homeroom teachers. Nationwide, a majority of high school students are required to take only one year of physical education in spite of the fact that the national guideline is two years.[9] Too often, tightening the budget means benching the student. Where there is activity, it is most often fashioned into competitive sports, leaving a general absence of non-competitive exercise options with health, rather than glory, as the reward. Add to this a generally unenlightened and non-nutritious, fast food-laden school cafeteria, and it's little wonder that scales are rising and activity falling.

On the public policy side, we see similar limitations in leadership and funding. Crime-ridden neighborhoods, the absence of sidewalks, and danger-ous and unmanaged parks conspire to keep urban children indoors for safety's sake. Poverty, limited childcare assistance, and transportation challenges fur-ther complicate the picture and prevent at-risk kids from getting to safe loca-tions for exercise and socialization.[10,11,12]

The problem of kids' inactivity and obesity, then, is well enough under-stood to begin a corrective course. But to do so requires that families and com-munities take an active role in challenging this unhealthy culture. Here are ten tips to get us all started:

1. Limit fast foods and soft drinks. Parents control a kid's nutrition. They buy the food.
2. Limit TV, movies and video games to a maximum of two hours at the same time each day.
3. Give children household jobs and chores that require physical exer-tion, including household cleaning and yard work.
4. Walk to destinations whenever safe and possible.
5. Advocate at your school for an active physical education program, and for a nutritionally sound cafeteria, including no vending machines.
6. Encourage your kids to participate in school sports and activities, and, if feasible, make them a nutritional lunch to carry.
7. Encourage active, outside time when your children return from school, and before they start their homework. If you are not at home, try to enroll them in an activity or after-school club.
8. Investigate city recreational opportunities. If there's a neglected park that's redeemable, form a civic association to reclaim and manage it.
9. Choose fitness-oriented gifts for your children like jump ropes, skates and bikes.
10. Plan family outings and vacations in the fresh air. This problem is fixable!

REFERENCES

1. National Center for Health Statistics. 1999 National Health and Nutrition Examination Survey (NHANES). Hyattsville, MD: U.S. Dept of Health and Human Services. 1999.
2. The Medical Center of Central Georgia. Cardio-vascular Disorders. Available at: www.mccg.org/childrenshealth/cardiac/index.asp. Accessed April 11, 2001.
3. Moran R. Evaluation and treatment of childhood obesity. *Am Fam Physician.* 1999;59:861-8, 871-3.
4. U.S. Dept of Health and Human Services. Physical Activity and Health: A Report of the Surgeon General. Atlanta, GA: U.S. Dept of Health and Human Services, CDC, National Center for Chronic Disease Prevention and Health Promotion; 1996.
5. Schoen C, Davis K, Collins KS, et al. *The Commonwealth Fund Survey of the Health of Adolescent Girls.* November 1997.
6. Coakley, J. Exercise and Health. *The Pfizer Journal.* Vol 6:1, 2002. p.13.
7. Sallis, J. Exercise and Health. *The Pfizer Journal.* Vol 6:1, 2002. p. 13.
8. CDC. MMWR Special Focus: Behavioral Risk Factor Surveillance - United States, 1991. Atlanta, GA: U.S. Dept of Health and Human Services. August 27, 1993.
9. National Association for Sport and Physical Education. Shape of the Nation Report. Princeton, NJ: Opinion Research Corporation International of Princeton, NJ; 2001.
10. Parr RB. Exercise or overweight kids. *The Physician and Sportmedicine.* 1998; 26:109.
11. Curtis MJ. Students help bridge the gap between poverty and good health. Brown University. Available at: www.brown.edu/Administration/George_Street_Journal/vol25/25GSJ0 f.html. Accessed November 28, 2001.
12. Icon Broadcasting Network. Kids are a lifetime investment. Available at: www.innercitygames.org/mission.html. Accessed November 28, 2001.

TEACHING TOOLS

Policy Premises

1. Childhood obesity has reached epidemic proportions in America and is on the rise.
2. A sedentary lifestyle is a major contributor to obesity and poor health.
3. Obese chidren are very likely to become obese adults with a variety of chronic diseases. Young women and minorites are at increased risk.
4. Exercise contributes to effective weight control, lowers the risk of diabetes, protects the heart and improves mental health.
5. Uninformed public school policy and unsafe barrier-laden environments contribute significantly to childhood obesity.
6. Families and communities have a role to play in addressing the culture of inactivity and childhood obesity.

Review

1. What is a major contributor to obesity and poor health in children?
2. What is the probability of becoming an obese adult if one is already obese at age 6?
3. Why is exercise not a high priority for many teenage girls?
4. How do public school policies toward exercise affect teenagers?
5. Name five ways that families and communities can help correct childhood obesity and inactivity.

Online Resources

Access online resources with this book's CD.

Physical Activity Fundamental to Preventing Disease - June 2002
http://aspe.hhs.gov/health/reports/physicalactivity/index.shtml

U.S. Obesity at an All-time High
http://healthlink.mcw.edu/article/1031002183.html

Physical Educators Buoyant over Parents' Support in American Obesity Association Survey
http://www.aahperd.org/naspe/pdf_files/whatsnew-obesity.pdf

Obesity, Individual Responsibility, and Public Policy — July 2003
http://www.aei.org/publications/pubID.18073,filter.economic/pub_detail.asp

Chartbook on Trends in the Health of Americans — 2002
http://www.cdc.gov/nchs/data/hus/hus02cht.pdf

Prevalence of Overweight Among Children and Adolescents: United States, 1999-2000
http://www.cdc.gov/nchs/products/pubs/pubd/hestats/overwght99.htm

Statistics Related to Overweight and Obesity
http://www.niddk.nih.gov/errors/Redirect.asp?URL=http://win.niddk.nih.gov/statistics/index.htm

Overweight and Obesity: The Surgeon General's Call to Action to Prevent and Decrease Overweight and Obesity
http://www.surgeongeneral.gov/topics/obesity/

Health Politics Online

For Original Health Politics Programs and Slides:

Exercise and Childhood Obesity
http://www.healthpolitics.com/program_info.asp?p=prog_18
Slide Briefing
http://www.healthpolitics.com/media/prog_18/brief_prog_18.pdf

CHAPTER 2.6

Eating Disorders Among College Women

CONFRONTING THE PROBLEM HEAD-ON

Every spring across the United States, many female high school seniors finalize their plans for college as their parents consider the financing and how best to deal with an empty nest. But many students and their parents aren't prepared for one issue they'll face: Eating disorders are extremely common among college women in America.

The problem has grown in recent years and is now a focus of National Eating Disorders Awareness Week, which is sponsored by the National Eating Disorders Association each year to help health care providers, teachers, social workers, and students promote healthy body image and prevent eating disorders. The yearly observance makes an important point: In order to address eating disorders, we have to confront them head on. Eating disorders are real illnesses affecting millions of Americans.

According to Dr. Doug Bunnell, president of the National Eating Disorders Association, "The stigma associated with eating disorders has long kept individuals suffering in silence, inhibited funding for crucial research, and created barriers to treatment."

Surveys indicate that nine out of every 10 college women attempt to control their weight with dieting.[1] Thirty-five percent of those who begin as "normal dieters" become "pathologic dieters," and, of these, about one-quarter will develop partial or full-blown clinical eating disorders.[2] One study of 682 non-anorexic college women, with a body mass index (BMI) greater than 18.5, found that only one-third demonstrated normal nutritional behavior. Sixty-one percent had intermediary nutritional disorders and 3 percent had bulimia nervosa, a secretive style of binge eating followed by purging or vomiting.[3]

Major eating abnormalities have their origins in childhood in America. Forty-two percent of girls age 6 to 9 "want to be thinner."[4] Eighty-one percent of 10-year-old girls are "afraid of being fat." In the pre-teen years, approximately 50 percent exercise to lose weight; 50 percent diet to lose weight; and 5 percent take diet pills or laxatives to lose weight.[5,6,7] Many even smoke to suppress their appetite, and tobacco advertising targets this population.[6,8]

Young girls generally aren't alone in their obsession with weight, since 85 percent of American families are "sometimes" or "often" on a diet.[1] The fact is, nearly 15 percent of young women head into college already burdened by substantially disordered eating attitudes and behaviors.[3]

The most serious eating disorders rarely appear independent of other psychiatric conditions. Anorexia nervosa, characterized by self-starvation and excessive weight loss below a BMI of 18.5, has a lifetime prevalence of .5 percent in women, while bulimia nervosa has a lifetime prevalence in women of 1 percent to 3 percent. Both conditions are 10 times more common in women than in men.[10] In a study of women with one of these two conditions, 42 percent had a history of one or more childhood anxiety disorders. The rate of obsessive compulsive disorder was particularly high at 23 percent (compared with 3 percent in the general population).[3]

About 30 percent of women with anorexia nervosa or bulimia nervosa abuse alcohol or drugs, and 86 percent battle depression. In a study of 246 women with one of these eating disorders, 30 percent attempted suicide, and 4.5 percent died.[10]

College campuses are unique breeding grounds for eating disorders in women. The contributors are multiple. The environment is stressful and filled with change. Loneliness, depression and sleep disorders are common. Substance abuse is deeply embedded in the culture, and peer pressure for women to be thin is enormous.[1] On the other hand, access to excellent nutrition and a continuum of personalized nutrition counseling for students is relatively uncommon. Those seeking the right foods, in the right portions, at the right times, face a frustrating challenge. On most college campuses, fitting in good nutrition is inconvenient, especially for a sizable portion of the population with poor habits already deeply entrenched.

We still don't know a great deal about eating disorders, but there is general consensus that the causes are multifactorial. Dr. Walter H. Kaye, a psychiatrist who studies eating disorders, said, "We think genes load the gun by creating behavioral susceptibility such as perfectionism or the drive for thinness. Environment then pulls the trigger."[10] And, sadly, women are between the crosshairs. For example, women's magazines have 10 times more ads promoting weight loss than men's magazines; and the weight of Miss America has steadily declined by a full 12 percent over the past 75 years, with one recent contestant having a BMI of 16.[9,11,12,13]

A continuum of strategies is needed to create healthier nutritional behaviors for college women. Parents, students, and colleges all have a role to play. Parents should begin early by examining their own prejudices and biases regarding food, nutrition, weight, and body image. What behaviors are you modeling for your children? Parents need to manage and advance good nutrition as part of a healthy inheritance. Eating should be encouraged in response to hunger. Self-worth and self-esteem should be constantly reinforced, as should open communication and critical thinking about human values. Finally, exploring nutrition during college campus visits and raising the topic of nutrition early and often places the issue on everyone's radar screen.[14]

For students, particularly females, recognize you are vulnerable, and, through discussion with family and peers, come up with a realistic nutrition plan. Choose a college that will support your needs. Do not abuse substances. Do not smoke. Focus on balance, self-worth, and reaching your full potential.[14]

Colleges: Understand you have a responsibility to your students. Recognize publicly the seriousness of eating disorders. Consider formally monitoring BMI each semester through student health services. Offer full nutritional counseling with registered dieticians who will personalize nutrition plans when necessary — if BMI is outside the 20-30 corridor. Integrate mental health support where appropriate. Create a preventive, programmatic focus and consider making nutrition leadership a center of excellence for your institution.[14]

In the words of Dr. Bunnell, "It's time to unmask the problem and spread awareness about the realities of eating disorders."

REFERENCES

1. National Eating Disorders Association. Information about NEDAW 2005. Available at: http://www.nationaleatingdisorders.org/p.asp?WebPage_ID=337. Accessed February 22, 2005.
2. Bunnell D. Personal Communication, 2005.
3. Shisslak CM, Crago M, Estes LS. The spectrum of eating disturbances. *International Journal of Eating Disorders*. 1995;18:209-219.
4. Mintz LB, Betz, NE. Prevalence and correlates of eating disordered behaviors among undergraduate women. *Journal of Counseling Psychology*. 1988;35:463-471.
5. Collins ME. Body figure perceptions and preferences among pre-adolescent children. *International Journal of Eating Disorders*. 1991;10:199-208.
6. Mellin L, McNutt S, Hu Y, Schreiber GB, Crawford P, Obarzanek E. A longitudinal study of the dietary practices of black and white girls 9 and 10 years old at enrollment: The NHLBI growth and health study. *Journal of Adolescent Health*. 1997;20:27-37.
7. Serdula MK, Collins E, Williamson DF, Anda RF, Pamuk E, Byers TE. Weight control practices of US adolescents and adults. *Annals of Internal Medicine*. 1993;119:667-671.
8. Picard CL. The level of competition as a factor for the development of eating disorders in female collegiate athletes. *Journal of Youth & Adolescence*. 1999;28:583-594.
9. Gustafson-Larson AM, Terry RD. Weight-related behaviors and concerns of fourth-grade children. *Journal of American Dietetic Association*. 1992;92:818-822.
10. Lamberg L. Advances in eating disorders offer food for thought. *JAMA*. 2003;290:1437-1442.
11. Study Reveals Childhood Vulnerabilities that May Lead to Eating Disorders. Press Release, December 1, 2004. National Eating Disorders Association. Available at: www.nationaleatingdisorders.org/p.asp?WebPage_ID=774. Accessed February 22, 2005.
12. Andersen AE, DiDomenico L. Diet vs. shape content of popular male and female magazines: a dose-response relationship to the incidence of eating disorders? *International Journal of Eating Disorders*.1992;11:283-287.

13. Rubinstein S, Caballero B. Is Miss America an undernourished role model? *JAMA*. 2000;283:1569.
14. Perfect Illusions: Eating Disorders and the Family. Available at: www.pbs.org/perfectillusions/eatingdisorders/print_preventing_strategies.html. Accessed February 22, 2005.

TEACHING TOOLS

Policy Premises

1. Eating disorders are extremely common among college women.
2. These eating abnormalities have their origins in childhood.
3. Eating disorders rarely appear independent of other psychiatric conditions.
4. College campuses are breeding grounds for eating disorders.
5. The causes of eating disorders are poorly understood but appear multifactorial.
6. A continuum of strategies is needed to create healthier nutritional behavior for college women.

Review

1. What is the purpose of National Eating Disorders Awareness Week?
2. How many college women attempt to control their weight with dieting?
3. How many normal dieters become pathologic dieters, and then develop an eating disorder?
4. Why are college campuses rife with eating disorders?
5. Is depression common among women with eating disorders?

Online Resources

Access online resources with this book's CD.

Healthy Eating On Campus
http://www.healthpolitics.com/eating_disorders.asp

Eating Disorders Awareness Week
http://www.nationaleatingdisorders.org/p.asp?WebPage_ID=767

Facts and Solutions
http://www.nimh.nih.gov/publicat/eatingdisorders.cfm

At Risk
http://www.4woman.gov/BodyImage/bodywise/bp/AtRisk.pdf

Beyond Anorexia Nervosa and Bulimia Nervosa
http://www.anred.com/defslesser.html

Health Politics Online

For Original Health Politics Programs and Slides:

Eating Disorders Among College Women
http://www.healthpolitics.com/program_info.asp?p=eating_disor-
ders
Slide Briefing
http://www.healthpolitics.com/media/eating_disorders/brief_eat-
ing_disorders.pdf

CHAPTER 2.7

Unhealthy Alcohol Use

UNDETECTED AND UNADDRESSED

Unhealthy alcohol use is a significant public health problem in the United States and around the world. Annually in the United States, there are 85,000 alcohol-related deaths, as well as substantial disability from the medical, psychological and trauma-related effects of alcohol use.[1,2,3] Despite this, drinking alcohol is somewhat common in our culture, and unhealthy use often gets ignored or goes undetected.

The spectrum of alcohol behaviors in our country extends from abstinence to dependency. Approximately 30 percent of Americans are abstinent, 30 percent are low-risk alcohol users, 30 percent are risky with their alcohol use, and 10 percent are abusive or dependent.[1] Risky use is defined as more than seven drinks per week, or three per occasion, in women, and more than 14 drinks per week, or four per occasion, in men, with no alcohol-related consequences — at least not yet.[1] According to a study in the *New England Journal of Medicine*, those suffering from alcohol abuse have experienced recurrences of the following situations in the last 12 months: failure to fulfill major role obligations, alcohol use in hazardous situations, alcohol-related legal problems, or social or interpersonal problems resultant from alcohol. Those with alcohol dependency suffer "clinically significant impairment or distress in the presence of three or more of the following: tolerance; withdrawal; a great deal of time spent obtaining alcohol, using alcohol, or recovering from its effects; reducing or giving up important activities because of alcohol; drinking more or longer than intended; a persistent desire or unsuccessful efforts to cut down or control use; continued use despite having a physical or psychological problem caused or exacerbated by alcohol."[1]

While moderate use of alcohol may have mild health benefits — namely, some protection from ischemic heart disease and stroke — the effects of moderate use impact people differently based on their age, sex, genetics, and other factors. The benefit of a reduced risk of heart disease and stroke is often counterbalanced by the wide range of harmful effects, including liver disease, pancreatitis, motor vehicle accidents, gun-related trauma, hypertension, hemorrhagic stroke, and cancer of the esophagus, larynx and mouth. For men under age 34 and women under age 45, those who do not drink alcohol at all have the lowest death rates. For men 35 or older, those who have five or fewer drinks a week have the lowest death rates. For women over 45, those who take two or fewer drinks per week live the longest.[1]

How does one know if their alcohol use is unhealthy? Two tests in particular are useful for self-evaluation and clinical screening — they're known as CAGE and AUDIT.[4] CAGE asks four questions: Have you ever felt you should cut down on your drinking? Have people annoyed you by criticizing your drinking? Have you ever felt bad or guilty about your drinking? Have you ever had a drink first thing in the morning to steady your nerves or get rid of a hangover? One or two affirmative answers indicates a high likelihood of unhealthy alcohol use.

The AUDIT test includes 10 questions with multiple choice answers scaled 0 to 4. For example, the first question — "How often do you have a drink containing alcohol?" — provides the following answers and scores: never (0), monthly or less (1), 2 to 4 times a month (2), 2 to 3 times a week (3), 4 or more times a week (4). Some of the other questions are: How many drinks of alcohol do you have on a typical day when you are drinking? How often do you have six or more drinks on one occasion? How often during the past year have you found you were not able to stop drinking once you had started? How often during the past year have you failed to do what was normally expected from you because of drinking? Has a relative, friend, doctor or other health worker been concerned about your drinking or suggested you cut down? After answering all 10 questions, a score of 8 or more is associated with a high likelihood of unhealthy alcohol use.[1]

As for treatment, three types have demonstrated similar success rates — cognitive behavior therapy, 12-step programs, and motivational-enhancement therapy. Cognitive behavior therapy emphasizes the learning of skills to cope with situations that precipitate heavy drinking.[1] Twelve-step programs emphasize that alcoholism is a disease, and they encourage active involvement in Alcoholics Anonymous (AA). And motivational-enhancement therapy involves motivational interviewing that's outlined in written guides. How successful are these plans? A recent study found that at one year, participants reported that 85 percent of their days were abstinent, versus 20 percent to 30 percent of their days when the study began. At three years, some two-thirds of participants were still abstinent.[1]

Prevention of long-term disability from unhealthy alcohol use in a patient or loved one requires intervention, tailored treatment plans, and supportive follow-up. To get involved and address a suspected problem, here are nine steps to follow:

1. Gather information. Ask — "What do you think about your drinking?"
2. Express concern.
3. Provide specific feedback, such as, "Alcohol use is very common, but fewer than 1 in 10 people your age drink the amount you're drinking."
4. Express empathy — "Quitting is difficult, but you are a strong person."
5. Offer help — "Would you like more information on how to cut down?"
6. Know local referral options — "There are many resources. Here are two contacts that can help."
7. Reinforce self-worth — "Please think about your drinking because there are many people who care deeply about you."
8. Assist with a plan — "Let me help you make an appointment with an expert."
9. Follow-up — "Let's schedule time to get together on a regular basis to monitor your success."[5,6]

The most unhealthy thing about unhealthy alcohol use is that we allow it to remain largely undetected and unaddressed.

REFERENCES

1. Saitz R. Unhealthy Alcohol Use. *NEJM*. 2005;352:596-607.
2. Mokdad AH, Marks JS, Stroup DF, Gerberding JL. Actual causes of death in the United States, 2000. *JAMA*. 2004;291:1238-1245. Cited in Saitz R.

3. Harwood HJ. Updating estimates of the economic costs of alcohol abuse in the United States: estimates, update methods, and data. Bethesda, Md.: National Institute on Alcohol Abuse and Alcoholism, 2000. Cited in Saitz R.

4. Fiellin DA, Reid MC, O'Connor PG. Screening for alcohol problems in primary care: a systematic review. *Arch Intern Med.* 2000;160:1977-1989. Cited in Saitz R.

5. Helping patients with alcohol problems: a health practitioner's guide. Rockville, Md.: National Institute on Alcohol Abuse and Alcoholism, January 2003. (NIH publication no. 03-3769.) Cited in Saitz R.

6. Screening and behavioral counseling interventions in primary care to reduce alcohol misuse: recommendation statement. *Ann Intern Med.* 2004;140:554-556. Cited in Saitz R.

TEACHING TOOLS

Policy Premises

1. Unhealthy alcohol use is a common problem that is infrequently addressed in our current health care system.
2. There is a wide spectrum of behavior, ranging from abstinence to dependency.
3. While alcohol use has mild health benefits, risks are significant.
4. Screening tests for unhealthy alcohol use are useful for self-evaluation and clinical screening.
5. Various treatments have demonstrated similar success rates.
6. Prevention of long-term disability from unhealthy alcohol use requires intervention and tailored treatment plans.

Review

1. How many alcohol-related deaths occur each year in the United States?
2. What percentage of Americans abstain from drinking alcohol?
3. What is considered risky alcohol use?
4. How can a person find out if his or her alcohol use is unhealthy?
5. How successful is treatment for alcohol abuse?

Online Resources

Access online resources with this book's CD.

April: Alcohol Awareness Month
http://www.mentalhealth.org/highlights/april2005/alcoholawareness/default.asp

Alcohol and Public Health
http://www.cdc.gov/alcohol/faqs.htm

The Numbers
http://www.cdc.gov/alcohol/factsheets/general_information.htm

What About Moderate Drinking?
http://www.niaaa.nih.gov/publications/ModerateDrinking-03.htm

Screening for Alcohol Abuse
http://healthlink.mcw.edu/article/1031002170.html

American Council on Alcoholism
http://www.aca-usa.org/index.htm

Health Politics Online

For Original Health Politics Programs and Slides:

Addressing Unhealthy Alcohol Use
http://www.healthpolitics.com/program_info.asp?p=Alcohol
Slide Briefing
http://www.healthpolitics.com/media/Alcohol/brief_Alcohol.pdf

Healthy Waters

A PUBLIC TRUST

"In the vastness of the planet's oceans and the pureness of its rivers lies the very basis of life itself" states a United Nations healthy waters study.[1] One might wonder, since 70 percent of the earth is covered by water, why should we worry about running out of it? Here are the facts: 97 percent of the earth's water is salt water. Only 3 percent is pure and most of that is trapped in glaciers, icebergs and snow. Only 1 percent of the earth's water is both fresh and available either on the surface or in underground aquifers.[2]

As Dr. Kerstin Leitner of the World Health Organization has noted, "We're not running out of water; we're running out of fresh water."[3] Why is this the case? Let's start from the beginning. Human beings are critically dependent on water for life. Seventy percent of the human body is water. An average human consumes 2.3 liters of water a day — .5 liters goes to sweat, .3 liters is released through respiration, and 1.5 liters is excreted as waste. If we lose 1 percent of water, we become thirsty. If we lose 5 percent, a mild fever develops. Lose 10 percent, we're immobilized. And if we lose 12 percent, we die.[2]

As critical as water is to life itself, one-sixth of the planet's human population, some 1.1 billion people, lack reliable access to clean water.[4,5] The source points of all water are complex, interdependent and fragile. The oceans' seawater is 80 times as dense as air and provides many species with complete support, including nutrition and reproductive needs. The oceans support the growth of 50 billion tons of living creatures per year. They deliver 90 million metric tons of fish to humans each year. They also annually absorb 8 billion tons of carbon dioxide, acting as a safeguard against global warming. The sea provides a secure environment for biologic cells, it's a chemical buffer, a good solvent, and a barrier against severe external temperature gradients.[6]

Feeding the oceans are streams, river basins, lakes and wetlands, which join together to form hundreds of distinct watersheds. These networks cover 45 percent of the earth's land and nourish locations that support 60 percent of our global population. The coexistence of these watersheds and human populations has created growing challenges. Two hundred sixty-one of these watersheds cross two or more countries' jurisdictional boundaries. The Nile crosses nine countries; the Danube 13; and the Mississippi passes through 31 states.[1,6,7] Poor management and policy upstream invariably means trouble downstream. Raw sewage, pollutants from unregulated industry, poor land management, and agricultural runoff all contribute, at times irreversibly, to the growing water crisis.[4]

Between mountaintop and sea, water suffers at every turn. To begin with, 40 percent of the world's population, some 2.5 billion people, lack access to proper sanitation. In Bangladesh, 60 percent have no access to bathrooms.[2] Human waste, joined by agricultural and industrial waste, easily finds its way into surface and underground water.

With pollution comes disease, accessed through unhealthy behaviors. For example, in Varanasi, India, a sacred site on the Ganges River, 60,000 people bathe in the polluted waters each day.[2] Infected water and lack of public health education both contribute to 4 billion cases of diarrhea a year worldwide, which results in 2.2 million deaths, mostly among young children. In fact, these deaths represent approximately 15 percent of all deaths of children under five in developing countries.[5]

While demand for fresh water is increasing, our limited supply is further diminished by waste and ignorance. The World Health Organization standards state that 75 liters of water per day are necessary to protect against household disease, and 50 liters are necessary for basic sanitation.[4] But individual consumption around the world varies widely. A member of the Masai tribe in Africa survives on approximately 4 liters per day, while a typical resident of Los Angeles uses 500 liters per day.[2]

But individuals are small consumers compared to agriculture. Farmers use 70 percent of all fresh water. Using standard irrigation, 50 percent never

gets to the roots of plants. With newer drip technologies, 90 percent is well utilized. Increasingly, we will have to think of food in water terms. For example,
a typical ton of wheat is really 1,000 tons of water with sun and soil thrown
in.

Industry is the next largest water consumer. Yet, only 10 percent of the
water that industries use actually ends up in products. Ninety percent is discarded, often permanently fouled and on its way downstream.[2]

On the demand side, the world's population of more than 6 billion is due
to double by 2050. And the imbalance of supply and demand for water is especially acute in certain regions. For example, the Middle East has only .9 percent of the earth's fresh water but 5 percent of the world's population.[2] By
2020, more than 50 nations will have severe water shortages, and by 2025,
more than a dozen nations will face a severe need for water from a hostile
neighbor.[2]

Ensuring healthy waters requires wise policy and grassroots activation of
health care and governmental leaders. The Aral Sea debacle is a useful cautionary tale. In the 1950s, Khrushchev diverted two Russian rivers to supply
profitable cotton fields in the region. Using open-ditch irrigation, 80 percent
of the water was lost to evaporation and seepage. Over the next few decades,
the Aral Sea shrunk to half its size, salinity rose, and fish died. Sixty thousand
citizens living off the sea were impacted immediately. With the passage of
time, dust from the sea's contaminated seabed, picked up by winds, spread
across the globe, was ingested by penguins in the Antarctic, and deposited on
Himalayan peaks where the salt caused early melting of snow. One ill-advised
policy choice created a lasting negative impact around the world.[2,8]

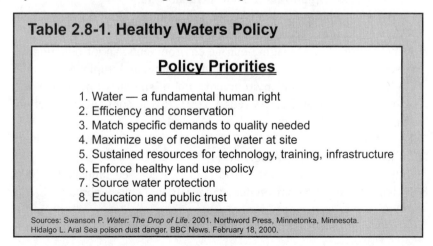

Table 2.8-1. Healthy Waters Policy

Policy Priorities

1. Water — a fundamental human right
2. Efficiency and conservation
3. Match specific demands to quality needed
4. Maximize use of reclaimed water at site
5. Sustained resources for technology, training, infrastructure
6. Enforce healthy land use policy
7. Source water protection
8. Education and public trust

Sources: Swanson P. *Water: The Drop of Life*. 2001. Northword Press, Minnetonka, Minnesota.
Hidalgo L. Aral Sea poison dust danger. BBC News. February 18, 2000.

With such a complex and expansive challenge, where does one begin? First, we recognize water as a fundamental human right. Second, focus on efficiency and conservation of what all agree is a limited resource. Third, match specific demands to the quality of water needed rather than supplying all the same quality water from a single centralized outlet. Fourth, maximize the use of reclaimed water as close to site usage as possible. Fifth, commit private and public resources in a sustained manner for technology, training, and infrastructure growth. Sixth, enforce healthy land use policy, carefully segregating water sources from sanitation systems. Seventh, focus special attention on agriculture and industry. Finally, let's emphasize water education and water as the ultimate human resource.[7] Water is a health and public trust.

REFERENCES

1. Protecting International Waters: Sustaining Livelihoods. United Nations Development Programme. Available at: http://www.undp.org/gef/undp-gef_publications/publications/intlwaters_brochure2004.pdf. Accessed January 11, 2005.
2. Swanson P. Water: The Drop of Life. 2001. Northword Press, Minnetonka, Minnesota.
3. Leitner K. Personal communication, October 15, 2004.
4. Water for Health: WHO's Guidelines for Drinking-Water Quality. Geneva, World Health Organization, 2004. Available at: http://www.who.int/water_sanitation_health/dwq/waterforhealth3/en/. Accessed January 11, 2005.
5. Global Water Supply and Sanitation Assessment 2000 Report. Geneva, World Health Organization, 2000. Available at: http://www.who.int/docstore/water_sanitation_health/Globassessment/GlobalTOC.htm. Accessed January 11, 2005.
6. Kenchington RA. Managing marine environments: an introduction to issues of sustainability, conservation, planning and implementation. In: Conserving marine environments: out of site out of mind. Pat Hutchings and Dan Lunney (eds.). 2003. Royal Zoological Society of New South Wales. Mosman, NSW Australia.
7. From Source Water to Drinking Water. Workshop Summary. Institute of Medicine, 2004. Available at: http://www.iom.edu/report.asp?id=23325. Accessed January 11, 2005.
8. Hidalgo L. Aral Sea poison dust danger. BBC News. February 18, 2000.

TEACHING TOOLS

Policy Premises

1. The earth is a water world with the future of mankind rising and falling in the balance.
2. Human beings are critically dependent on water for life.
3. Water bodies are complex, interdependent, and fragile.
4. Various waste products easily find their way into our supply.
5. While demand is expanding, limited supply is further diminished by waste and ignorance.
6. Ensuring healthy waters requires wise policy and grassroots activism.

Review

1. How much of the earth's water is both fresh and available?
2. How many people don't have access to clean water?
3. What happens when our bodies lose water?
4. What percentage of the available fresh water is used for agriculture?
5. What can be done to improve the global water situation?

Online Resources

Access online resources with this book's CD.

After the Tsunami
http://www.fao.org/ag/tsunami/assessment/assess-water-a.html

Healthy Water, Healthy People
http://www.healthywater.org/

World Ocean Forum
http://www.worldoceanforum.org/

United Nations Environment Programme to Protect Water
http://www.unep.org/dpdl/water/

Bottled Water
http://www.nrdc.org/water/drinking/nbw.asp

Global WASH Campaign
http://www.wsscc.org/dataweb.cfm?edit_id=57&CFID=663036&C
FTOKEN=1684229

The Nile Basin Initiative
http://www.worldbank.org/afr/nilebasin/

Health Politics Online

For Original Health Politics Programs and Slides:

Healthy Waters: A Public Trust
http://www.healthpolitics.com/program_info.asp?p=healthy_water
Slide Briefing
http://www.healthpolitics.com/media/healthy_water/brief_healthy_
water.pdf

CHAPTER 2.9

Lead Poisoning

EXPOSING HEALTH CARE SYSTEM WEAKNESSES

In the United States, we have been fast to build overlapping, redundant, reactive, and non-integrated health systems, but slow to advance the cause of health in a reliable and verifiably equitable way. Lead poisoning is an excellent case that illustrates this point.[1]

In 1908, an Australian scientist first recognized an epidemic of lead poisoning in children. It took European nations just one year to make a connection with lead-based paints and ban their use. Australians verified the connection in medical journals in 1912. But in the United States, it would take nearly 70 more to ban lead in paints, due mostly to the effective lobbying action of the Lead Industries Association.[1] As the group's president boasted in 1984, "Our victories have been in the deferral of implementation of certain regulations."[2]

Once the weight of the facts and the actions of other nations drove regulatory bodies to action, those actions were still timed and incremental. Take, for example, the definition of lead poisoning in the United States. In 1970, a blood lead level of greater than 60 micrograms per deciliter made the diagnosis. One year later, the level was lowered to 40. It would take 7 more years to drop it to 25. Not until 1991 did we reach the current level of 10 micrograms per deciliter as the definition of lead poisoning.[1,3]

Large portions of the U.S. population benefited from new regulations that banned lead paint and progressively decreased the amount of lead in our gasoline. In 1970, 88 percent of all U.S. children under age 6 had blood lead levels above 10 micrograms per deciliter. By 1991, that number was down to only 5 percent.[4,5] Even so, significant numbers of children are still affected. A study from 1999 to 2001 found that 430,000 kids, or 2.2 percent of the under age 6 population had lead poisoning.[6] The numbers were higher among poor kids with rates topping 6 percent in one Medicaid study. Also, lack of proper follow-up post-diagnosis is extremely common. A study published in 2005 found that out of about 3,600 Medicaid-enrolled children in Michigan with lead poisoning, 46 percent did not receive appropriate follow-up testing.[7]

Looking across the nation, high variability in risk remains evident. Urban environments, especially in the Northeast and Midwest, are highly vulnerable areas. Poor children in old rental properties and rich children in rehabilitated old properties often turn up positive.[1] Up until 1997, population-wide testing was the rule. But as incidence rates fell nationwide, the Centers for Disease Control recommended a more targeted approach with testing recommended only in high-risk populations in the hope that more focused and concentrated funding would carry the incidence of lead poisoning below 2 percent. However, the 2005 study illustrates that even when we make the diagnosis, we are largely ineffective in basic follow-up because of the weak linkages between health clinics who make the diagnoses and public health professionals who are charged with treating confirmed cases and advocating for regulatory processes that address issues such as lead poisoning, asthma, safety, and now bioterrorism on a population basis.[7]

It is not that we are disinterested, but rather disintegrated and conflicted. The story of lead poisoning illustrates that failed leadership in health can carry extraordinarily long-term costs. Lead poisoning in children has a well-established association with reading delays, school failure, delinquency and criminal behavior, independent of other associated risk factors.[1] And as the effected kids turn into adults, the picture worsens. We now know that lead-poisoned children become chronically ill adults with high rates of cardiovascular disease, renal disease, cognitive decline, spontaneous abortion, tooth decay, and cataracts. As pediatric and environmental health expert Dr. Bruce Lanphear recently stated, "Lead toxicity may underlie some of the prevalent health disparities found in socially disadvantaged children."[1]

My point is not to simply run on about lead poisoning, which in its own right needs careful attention — certainly if you're the parent of a preschooler in an urban environment, you need to have your child tested, and if the test is positive, make sure appropriate follow-up occurs. Your involvement protects your child and helps clinicians retool systems and processes that are too often error-prone.

But beyond the parochial interests of this particular population, we need to shine a light on the inherent system weaknesses of U.S. health care that lead poisoning so well illustrates. What are the lessons learned? First, we are too slow to the draw in facing difficult policy choices on health, especially when organized economic interests are at stake. Whether its lead, tobacco, or seat-belts, it takes too long to do what everyone knows in their heart is the right thing to do. Second, we are too risk-averse in organizing the care. Because we fear over-centralization of power and purchasing and adversely impacting innovation, choice and progress, which are real concerns, we too often choose disintegration and broken systems that we know will fail. We need to find a way to preserve entrepreneurship while expanding universality and high qual-ity equity and justice. Third, we too often stick our head in the sand, ignoring the long-term costs of failed early health management.

Investing across multiple generations of life, rather than on a single episode, is long overdue.

REFERENCES

1. Lanphear BP. Childhood lead poisoning prevention: too little, too late. *JAMA*. 2005;293:2274-2276.
2. Reich P. The Hour of Lead: A Brief History of Lead Poisoning in the United States. Washington, DC: Environmental Defense Fund; 1992. Cited in Lanphear BP.
3. Centers for Disease Control. Preventing Lead Poisoning in Young Children: A Statement by the Centers for Disease Control. Atlanta, Ga. US Dept of Health and Human Services; 1991. Cited in Lanphear BP.
4. Annest JL, Pirkle JL, Makuc D, Neese JW, Bayse DD, Kovar MG. Chronological trend in blood lead levels between 1976 and 1980. *NEJM*. 1979;300:689-695. Cited in Lanphear BP.
5. Pirkle JL, Kaufmann RB, Brody DJ, Hickman T, Gunder EW, Paschal DC. Exposure of the U.S. population to lead, 1991-1994. Environ Health Perspect. 1998;106:145-150. Cited in Lanphear BP.
6. Meyer PA, Pivetz T, Dignam TA, Homa DM, Schoonover J, Brody D. Surveillance for elevated blood lead levels among children - United

States, 1997-2000. *MMWR*. 2003;52:1-21.

7. Kemper AR, Cohn LS, Fant DE, Dombkowski DJ, Hudson SR. Follow-up testing among children with elevated screening blood lead levels. *JAMA*. 2005;293:2232-2237.

TEACHING TOOLS

Policy Premises

1. The story of lead poisoning prevention in the United States is sad and instructive.
2. Once forced to confront the facts, regulatory bodies took an incremental approach.
3. Large portions of the population benefited by national regulation.
4. Significant portions of our vulnerable populations remain at risk.
5. The impact is lifelong and may contribute to health disparities.
6. Lessons learned from lead should inform health care transformation in the United States.

Review

1. What year did the United States ban lead use in paints?
2. Which populations are at the highest risk for lead poisoning?
3. How does lead poisoning affect children and adults?
4. What should you do if your child tests positive for lead poisoning?
5. What does the story of lead poisoning teach us about our system weaknesses?

Online Resources

Access online resources with this book's CD.

Barriers to Care
http://www.med.umich.edu/opm/newspage/2005/lead.htm

Lead and Your Health
http://www.niehs.nih.gov/oc/factsheets/lyh/lyh.htm

Predicting and Reducing Lead Poisoning in Urban Youth
http://ehp.niehs.nih.gov/press/030305.html

Lead Poisoning FAQ
http://www.epa.gov/region02/faq/lead_p.htm

The Lead Test
http://www.labtestsonline.org/understanding/analytes/lead/test.html

Is Lead a Problem in Your Home?
http://www.aiha.org/GovernmentAffairs-PR/html/OOlead.htm

Goal: Safer Drinking Water
http://yosemite.epa.gov/opa/admpress.nsf/b1ab9f485b098972852562e
7004dc686/a62e69cba4424f9e8525702100629612!OpenDocument

Health Politics Online

For Original Health Politics Programs and Slides:

Lead Poisoning
http://www.healthpolitics.com/program_info.asp?p=Lead_poisoning
Slide Briefing
http://www.healthpolitics.com/media/lead_poisoning/brief_lead_po
isoning.pdf

Ozone Effects

A STORY OF GOOD AND BAD

Ozone is a very small part of our atmosphere, but its presence has significant effects — good and bad — on our health. To understand this concept, one first needs to understand ozone itself. Ozone was first discovered in a laboratory experiment in the mid-1800s. The word ozone comes from the Greek word ozein, meaning "to smell." Ozone is a pungent blue gas, detectable in small amounts. It is composed of three oxygen atoms linked together and is signified chemically as O_3.[1]

Ozone is highly reactive with many chemicals. Its reactivity is part of what makes ozone both good and bad. This explanation must begin with a word or two about the earth's atmosphere, separated broadly into the troposphere and the stratosphere. The troposphere is the portion of our atmosphere closest to earth. It extends from our surface upward approximately 10 kilometers (km). Mount Everest, the highest mountain on earth, at 8.8 km high, nearly reaches to its limit. Almost all of earth's weather occurs in the troposphere. Temperatures decline with altitude since warm air cools as it rises, dropping back to earth.[1,2]

The stratosphere is earth's upper atmosphere. It extends from 10 km above our surface to 50 km. The stratosphere's temperature rises with increased altitude. This is largely due to ozone's ability to absorb the sun's ultraviolet radiation. This effect leads to a horizontal separation of atmosphere with warm above and cool below, and far less vertical mixing of components than in the troposphere.[1,2]

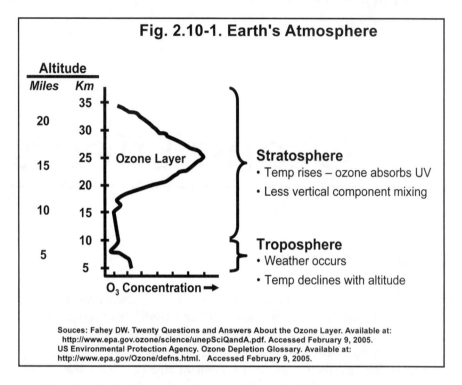

Fig. 2.10-1. Earth's Atmosphere

Ninety percent of ozone exists in the "ozone layer" in the stratosphere. This ozone is naturally formed in chemical reactions involving ultraviolet sunlight and oxygen molecules, which make up 21 percent of the atmosphere. That said, ozone is relatively uncommon in the atmosphere, with only 12,000 molecules per billion air molecules in the stratosphere, and only 20 to 100 molecules per billion air molecules in the troposphere.[1] While most of the ozone that is present in the upper atmosphere is naturally occurring, most ozone in the lower atmosphere is the result of human pollution. Ozone above shields humans from the harmful effects of ultraviolet radiation and stabilizes global weather. Ozone below irritates the heart and lungs and traps heat, which contributes to global warming.[1,3]

In the mid-1970s, it was discovered that some human-produced chemicals can destroy ozone. Chlorine-containing compounds like chlorofluorocarbons (CFCs), which are very stable in the troposphere, are readily broken down by ultraviolet radiation in the stratosphere. Such compounds were commonly used in refrigeration, air conditioning, foam blowing, and industrial cleaning. The released chlorine atoms break the ozone molecule apart, decreasing human protection from cancer-causing ultraviolet radiation and disrupting normal weather patterns.[1,2] And bromine-containing compounds,

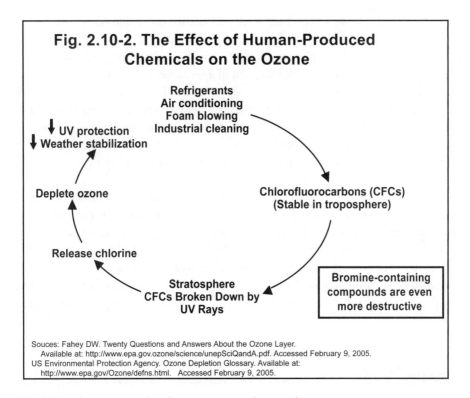

Fig. 2.10-2. The Effect of Human-Produced Chemicals on the Ozone

Refrigerants
Air conditioning
Foam blowing
Industrial cleaning

↓ UV protection
↓ Weather stabilization

Deplete ozone

Chlorofluorocarbons (CFCs)
(Stable in troposphere)

Release chlorine

Stratosphere
CFCs Broken Down by
UV Rays

Bromine-containing
compounds are even
more destructive

Souces: Fahey DW. Twenty Questions and Answers About the Ozone Layer.
   Available at: http://www.epa.gov.ozone/science/unepSciQandA.pdf. Accessed February 9, 2005.
US Environmental Protection Agency. Ozone Depletion Glossary. Available at:
   http://www.epa.gov/Ozone/defns.html. Accessed February 9, 2005.

like halon, have proved to be even more destructive.

In the lower atmosphere, the problem is different. Here, fossil fuel combustion leads to the release of hydrocarbons and nitric oxides. When these are exposed to sunlight, ozone is produced. Exposure to ozone at high levels is known to be associated with increased rates of hospitalization, increased emergency department visits, exacerbation of chronic respiratory disease, decreased lung function, and increased death rates. Little good comes of this ozone, identical chemically to its naturally occurring stratosphere cousin, because it exists in very small quantities and has difficulty rising to that level. On the surface, it is naturally degraded by other chemicals, soil, and plants.[1]

High ozone levels in the troposphere, independent of other variables such as temperature or particulate matter, are now known to increase premature death.[3] The current ozone limit set by the U.S. government is a daily maximum eight-hour standard of 80 parts per billion (ppb).[4] A study of 95 U.S. cities from 1987 to 2000 showed an average daily ozone concentration of 26 ppb. Tracking death rates several days before and after ozone spikes uncovered that daily mortality increased by .52 percent for every 10 ppb increase in surface ozone. The risk increased to .7 percent for those age 65 to 75.[3]

New York City is clearly number one for ozone-instigated premature deaths.[2] Looking at the 95 cities studied in aggregate, there were 3,767 premature deaths per year due to ozone levels. The top five cities were New York City, Newark, Philadelphia, Cincinnati, and Dallas. The increased risk of premature death for every 10 ppb increase in ozone in these five cities was 1.7 percent, 1.3 percent, 1.3 percent, 1.2 percent, and 1.1 percent, respectively. In New York City alone, this translates into 319 premature deaths each year.[3]

What do we now know about ozone and its effects on health? Ozone in the upper atmosphere is good. Ozone in the lower atmosphere is bad. And both are under human control. Enlightened policy and regulation can decrease the invasion of the stratosphere by unstable bromine- and chlorine-containing compounds that are destroying its protective layer. Sound government policy can also control the release of primarily auto-emitted hydrocarbons and nitric oxides that create a deadly ozone brew for humans when exposed to surface sunlight.

REFERENCES

1. Fahey DW. Twenty Questions and Answers About the Ozone Layer. Available at: http://www.epa.gov/ozone/science/unepSciQandA.pdf. Accessed February 9, 2005.
2. US Environmental Protection Agency. Ozone Depletion Glossary. Available at: http://www.epa.gov/Ozone/defns.html. Accessed February 9, 2005.
3. Bell ML, McDermott A, Zeger SL, Samet JM, Dominici F. Ozone and short-term mortality in 95 US urban communities, 1987-2000. *JAMA*. 2004;292:2372-2378.
4. US Environmental Protection Agency. National Ambient Air Quality Standards for ozone, final rule. Federal Register. 1997;62:38855-38896. Cited in Bell ML, McDermott A, Zeger SL, Samet JM, Dominici F.

TEACHING TOOLS

Policy Premises

1. Ozone was first discovered in laboratory experiments in the mid-1800s.
2. Ozone is a very small part of our atmosphere, with most residing in the upper portion.
3. In the mid-1970s, it was discovered that some human-produced chemicals could destroy ozone.
4. The amount of ozone in the lower atmosphere is primarily a function of pollutants.
5. High ozone levels in the troposphere independent of other variables such as temperature or particulate matter increase the risk of premature death.
6. New York City is number one in ozone-instigated premature death among 95 U.S. cities.

Review

1. When and where was ozone discovered?
2. What is the ozone layer, and how was it formed?
3. What are the health effects of ozone in the lower atmosphere?
4. Which city suffers from the highest increased risk of premature death due to ozone levels?
5. How can we lower the harmful levels of bad ozone in our atmosphere?

Online Resources

Access online resources with this book's CD.

Ozone and You
http://www.epa.gov/docs/ozone/resource/indiv.html

Understanding Global Warming
http://www.ncdc.noaa.gov/oa/climate/globalwarming.html

Ozone Alerts
http://www.niehs.nih.gov/oc/factsheets/ozone/ozonevalu.htm

The Deadly Brew
http://www.lungusa.org/site/pp.asp?c=dvLUK9O0E&b=22542

Arctic Ozone May Drop to New Low
http://news.bbc.co.uk/2/hi/science/nature/4217329.stm

Ozone Problems
http://users.rcn.com/jkimball.ma.ultranet/BiologyPages/O/Ozone.html

Climate Change
http://www.newscientist.com/channel/earth/climate-change

Health Politics Online

For Original Health Politics Programs and Slides:

Ozone's Effects on Health: A Story of Good and Bad
http://www.healthpolitics.com/program_info.asp?p=ozone
Slide Briefing
http://www.healthpolitics.com/media/ozone/brief_ozone.pdf

CHAPTER 2.11

Consumer Risk Management

PERCEPTION VERSUS REALITY

Though the health consumer movement is barely 20 years old in the United States, it is already entering its third phase. The first phase was emancipation — the realization and recognition that individuals have responsibility for their own health decisions and health management. The second phase, health empowerment, witnessed a move away from paternalistic patient-physician relationships toward mutual partnership models consummated by patient empowerment through education. Phase three is now underway as, together, patients and caregivers reorganize care delivery, moving toward prevention, outpatient care, and team support in both clinical and educational arenas.[1]

This third phase of the health consumer movement has placed the burden of benefit/risk decisions squarely on the patient's shoulders, and U.S. patients appear up to the challenge. Fully 94 percent agree that they must be more involved in health decisions, 92 percent agree that they must be in control of their own health, 89 percent agree that they need to take more responsibility, and 82 percent believe that, faced with a health challenge, they should be presented several treatment options with varying degrees of risk.[2]

Perceptions of risk are often overestimated or underestimated by the public. A National Academy of Science study conducted in 1995 found that accidents, pregnancy, tornados, botulism, cancer, fire, snake bite and homicide were the most frequently overestimated risks, and small pox vaccination, diabetes, stomach cancer, lightning, stroke, tuberculosis, asthma and emphysema were the most underestimated risks.[3]

Table 2.11-1. Public Perceptions of Risk	
Most Overestimated	**Most Underestimated**
• Accidents	• Small pox vaccination
• Pregnancy	• Diabetes
• Tornados	• Stomach cancer
• Botulism	• Lightning
• Cancer	• Stroke
• Fire	• Tuberculosis
• Snake bite	• Asthma
• Homicide	• Emphysema

Source: Nat. Center for Health Statistics 2001. Nat. Acad. Sciences 1995.

The point is, we consumers often get it wrong. The numbers are increasingly clear, if not widely available to the average citizen. For example, the chances of death from heart disease are 1 in 385; from cancer, 1 in 519; from stroke, 1 in 1,752; from an accident, 1 in 2,929; from suicide, 1 in 9,170; from Alzheimer's, 1 in 12, 458; from homicide, 1 in 14,857; from fire, 1 in 83,333; and from a bike accident, 1 in 369,881.[4]

But in the field of health consumer risk management, knowing the numbers is not enough, because science and self blend in risk assessments. Professor Paul Slovic, one of the nation's leading experts on risk, explains it this way, "Patients rarely do an analytic assessment of benefits and risks; they follow their gut instincts about something. We have evolved to deal with risks by trusting our senses, perceptions and feelings about whether a situation looks good or bad, or safe or dangerous. This very intuitive process does not mix well with mathematical formulations of decision-making that we have come to value as rational."[5]

Dr. Slovic's research points out that our everyday risk assessments, including those in health, are affective responses. If an activity is liked, people under-judge its risks and over-judge its benefits. If an activity is disliked, risks are over-weighted and benefits under-weighted.[6]

How information is framed can also effect decisions and outcomes. For example, studies show that a "1-in-10" possibility of a poor outcome is seen as much more frightening than a stated "10 percent" risk of a poor outcome.[5] And while air travel, on a per-mile basis, is 50 times safer than automobile travel, it is only five times safer on a per-hour-of-exposure basis.[7]

Finally, there is the classic experiment with lung cancer patients asked to select radiation or surgery as therapy. When told that 10 percent die from the surgery, more than 40 percent chose radiation. Yet fewer than 20 percent chose radiation when told that 90 percent survive surgery.[8]

Those assisting patients in health decision-making must take care not to bias the patient by how questions or issues are framed. They must be equally aware of problems with health numeracy. Health numeracy is the ability to understand the mathematics and statistics of health. Consider the fact that only one in five high school graduates can convert 0.1 percent to 1 in 1000, let alone comprehend "P value," a common measure of statistical probability that results are tied to cause and effect, not just to chance.[9] A "P value" of less than 0.01 means that there is a less than a 1 percent probability that the result occurred by chance. A "P value" of less than 0.05 means that there is a less than 5 percent probability that the result occurred by chance.[10] Consumer risk management requires improvements in health numeracy, and the creation of statistics for non-statisticians.

One thing is absolutely clear: Risk communications should be carefully designed in concert with patients. What do the experts say are the keys to success? First, drain emotion from words. Attempt to present choices in a neutral format. Second, whenever possible, simplify. Use pictures, images, and simple math. Third, be mindful of your own prejudices. This is the patient's decision. Give them the opportunity to make the decisions fairly. Fourth, define risk in absolute terms, the actual number of cases or outcomes expected in the target population. Fifth, remember that, while there is a risk to action, there is also a risk to inaction.

REFERENCES

1. Magee M and D'Antonio M. *The Best Medicine*. 1999.
2. Magee M. Health Consumer Risk Management: Patients Perceptions of Pharmaceuticals and Health Risks (A Harris Poll). 2000. Available at: www.positiveprofiles.com. 2003.
3. Baruch Fischhoff. Managing Risk Perceptions. Issues in Science and Technology. Fall, 1995: 2 (1) (c) National Academy of Sciences.
4. National Center for Health Statistics. 2001. Available at: http://www.cdc.gov/nchs/about/major/dvs/mortdata.htm.
5. Solive P. Assessing and Communicating Risks and Benefits. *The Pfizer Journal*. Vol 4:5, 2001. p. 12.

6. Finucane ML, Alhakami A, Slovic P, Johnson SM. The affect heuristic in judgments of risks and benefits. *J Behav Dec Making*. 2000; 13:1-17.

7. No author listed. Living by the numbers: how to gauge your risks. UC Berkeley Wellness Letter. June 2000:4-5.

8. McNeil BJ, Pauker SG, Sox HC Jr, Tversky A. On the elicitation of preferences for alternative therapies. *N Engl J Med*. 1982; 306:1259-1262.

9. Schwartz LM, Woloshin S, Black WC, Welch HG. The role of numeracy in understanding the benefit of screening mammography. Ann Intern Med. [serial online.] 1997;127:966-972. Available at: http://www.acponline.org/journals/annals/01dec97/numeracy.htm. Accessed Nov 28, 2000.

10. Greenhalgh, T. How to read a paper: statistics for the nonstatistician. *BMJ*. 1997;315:422-425.

TEACHING TOOLS

Policy Premises

1. The health consumer empowerment movement has placed the burden of benefits-risk decisions on the patient's shoulders.
2. Perceptions of risk are often overestimated or underestimated by the public.
3. Science and self blend in risk assessments.
4. How information is framed can affect decisions and outcomes.
5. Health numeracy — the ability to understand mathematics and statistics about health — is a requirement for informed decision making.
6. Risk communications should be carefully designed in concert with patients.

Review

1. How does the consumer health movement place the burden of benefit-risk decisions on patients?
2. According to a National Academy of Science study conducted in 1995, what are some of today's most underestimated health risks?
3. According to research reported in the NEJM, which is perceived as more frightening to patients: a 1 in 10 possibility of a poor outcome or a 10 percent risk of a poor outcome?
4. What is health numeracy?
5. What are the keys to success in communicating health risks to patients?

Online Resources

Access online resources with this book's CD.

Numeracy and the Medical Student's Ability to Interpret Data
http://www.acponline.org/journals/ecp/janfeb02/sheridan.htm

A Consumer's Guide to Taking Charge of Health Information
http://www.health-insight.harvard.edu/guide.html

Evidence-based Medicine: Useful Tools for Decision Making
http://www.ncbi.nlm.nih.gov/entrez/query.fcgi?cmd=Retrieve&db=
PubMed&list_uids=11280698&dopt=Abstract

The Meaning of 6.8: Numeracy and Normality in Health Information Talks
http://www.ncbi.nlm.nih.gov/entrez/query.fcgi?cmd=Retrieve&db=
PubMed&list_uids=97058908&dopt=Abstract

Be an Active Member of Your Health Care Team
http://www.pueblo.gsa.gov/cic_text/health/active-
member/active_member.htm

The World Health Report 2002
http://www.who.int/whr/en/

Health Politics Online

For Original Health Politics Programs and Slides:

Consumer Risk Management
http://www.healthpolitics.com/program_info.asp?p=prog_14
Slide Briefing
http://www.healthpolitics.com/media/prog_14/brief_prog_14.pdf

CHAPTER 3

Infectious Diseases

"Unfortunately, much of the ground work for the burden of disease in 2020 has already been laid in infants born in poverty or at low-birth weights, who are then malnourished or unprotected from infection as children. We need to end this continuum."

— A.C. ACHUTTI
Chair
World Heart Federation

"Several of the top diseases are still diseases of underdevelopment. Diarrhea and parasitic diseases are often attributed to poor water supply and sanitation as well as poor domestic and personal hygiene."

— NILS DAULAIRE
President & CEO
Global Health Council

CHAPTER 3.1

Fighting Infectious Diseases Worldwide

150 YEARS OF LEARNING

Since the Middle Ages, societies have struggled to develop effective and well-coordinated responses to infectious diseases. Outbreaks of bubonic plague first led to nation-state responses in Europe, including the tracking of migration of food and goods, the establishment of quarantine authority, and the closure of ports to isolate cities from entry of disease. But these earliest efforts were frequently compromised by a lack of cooperation across borders over concerns that responding effectively to disease would have severe consequences on trade and economics. Not only was disease regularly imported, it was also actively exported, fueled by colonial and evangelical zeal. The demise of native peoples of the Americas, victimized by infectious disease carried by the Spanish conquistadors, is a particularly well-documented example.[1,2,3]

By 1851, the first international health platforms began to appear. They were stimulated by a cholera epidemic that had devastated Asia in the first half of the 19th century. The first International Sanitary Conference was convened in Paris and included 11 European nations. Friction lines rapidly appeared as issues of sovereignty and economics played out in contrast to clear imperatives for transparency and protective measures. Still, the foundation had been laid for future networking of governments and scientists on behalf of public health.[4]

Advances in scientific understanding and commitment to regional coordination took hold in the late 19th and early 20th centuries. United States' involvement came to the forefront in 1881 when the International Sanitary

Conference was convened in Washington, D.C., partly in response to an outbreak of Yellow Fever in the Mississippi River Valley. By 1890, participants
had agreed to a common scientific lexicon, had accepted the germ theory, and
agreed to sanitary and quarantine controls. In 1892 and 1897, the first
International Sanitation Conventions were signed. In 1902 the Pan American
Sanitary Bureau, committed to a regional approach to infectious diseases
(especially yellow fever) was created, subsequently becoming PAHO or the
Pan American Health Organization. A similar regional body was created in
Europe in 1907, followed by the post-World War I League of Nations Health
Committee in 1920.[1]

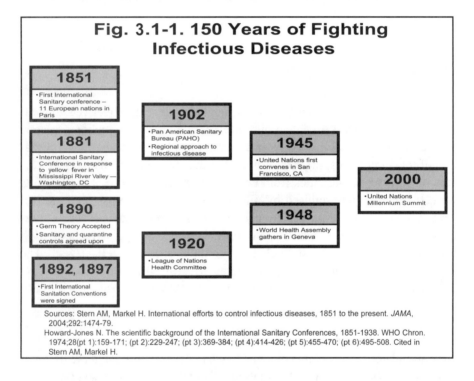

Fig. 3.1-1. 150 Years of Fighting Infectious Diseases

1851
• First International Sanitary conference – 11 European nations in Paris

1881
• International Sanitary Conference in response to yellow fever in Mississippi River Valley – Washington, DC

1890
• Germ Theory Accepted
• Sanitary and quarantine controls agreed upon

1892, 1897
• First International Sanitation Conventions were signed

1902
• Pan American Sanitary Bureau (PAHO)
• Regional approach to infectious disease

1920
• League of Nations Health Committee

1945
• United Nations first convenes in San Francisco, CA

1948
• World Health Assembly gathers in Geneva

2000
• United Nations Millennium Summit

Sources: Stern AM, Markel H. International efforts to control infectious diseases, 1851 to the present. *JAMA*,
2004;292:1474-79.
Howard-Jones N. The scientific background of the International Sanitary Conferences, 1851-1938. WHO Chron.
1974;28(pt 1):159-171; (pt 2):229-247; (pt 3):369-384; (pt 4):414-426; (pt 5):455-470; (pt 6):495-508. Cited in
Stern AM, Markel H.

With World War II looming, the last International Sanitary Conference
convened in 1938. By then, the forum's accomplishments included the sharing of scientific discoveries (notably bacteriology), a canon of quarantine
regulations, a commitment to the medical inspection of travelers and goods,
a disease classification and surveillance system, and standardization of laboratory testing.[1]

The atrocities of World War II helped stimulate an expansion of international cooperation and helped redefine health in broad, humanistic terms. In

1945, the United Nations was first convened in San Francisco. Its constitution was signed the following year in New York, and its World Health Assembly gathered for the first time in Geneva in 1948. Out of the United Nations emerged a new vision of health that included a coordinated multinational approach to disease treatment and prevention; a commitment to holistic well being, including physical, mental and social dimensions; advocacy for health as a human right; and a strong endorsement of health as fundamental to peace and security. For all of this, the United Nations' power has remained in moral persuasion rather than in international law.[5,6]

So what are the lessons we have learned over the past 150 years? Some, of course, are obvious. Geographic borders do not naturally contain disease any more than they contain people and products in an age of transatlantic flight, the Internet, and overnight delivery. To combat infectious diseases, humans must outsmart and outwork microorganisms. This means cooperative surveillance, testing, and early response systems. And it means continuous research and development of therapies and vaccines against new and old threats alike. Finally, it means investment in health infrastructure, nutrition, clean water, safety, and economic development to help nations and individuals rise up from poverty and reach their full potential.

The U.N. Millennium Summit of 2000 outlined the challenges in three observations. First, our current disease burden not only threatens vulnerable populations but also our global economics and global security. Second, absent a more effective response, millions more will die. And third, investment of .1 percent of developed nations' GNP, effectively applied, could make a real difference.[7]

More than 150 years of work has taught us that international cooperation, appropriate incentives to fight infectious diseases, cross-sector partnering, transparency, and accountability are all critical, and as we saw with the SARS threat, they are indispensable to our global public health.

REFERENCES

1. Stern AM, Markel H. International efforts to control infectious diseases, 1851 to the present. *JAMA*, 2004;292:1474-79.
2. World Health Organization. Six diseases cause 90 percent of infection disease deaths. Available at: www.who.int/infectious-disease-report/pages/ch2text.html. Accessed December 1, 2004. Cited in

Stern AM, Markel H.

3. Crosby AW. The Columbian Exchange: Biological and Cultural Consequences of 1492. Westport, Conn: Greenwood Publishing Co; 1972. Cited in Stern AM, Markel H.

4. Howard-Jones N. The scientific background of the International Sanitary Conferences, 1851-1938. *WHO Chron.* 1974;28(pt 1):159-171; (pt 2):229-247; (pt 3):369-384; (pt 4):414-426; (pt 5):455-470; (pt 6):495-508. Cited in Stern AM, Markel H.

5. Howard-Jones N. The World Health Organization in historical perspective. *Perspect Biol Med.* 1981;24:467-482. Cited in Stern AM, Markel H.

6. Charles J. Origins, history, and achievements of the World Health Organization. *BMJ.* 1968;4:293-296. Cited in Stern AM, Markel H.

7. Sachs JD. Investing in health for economic development. Project Syndicate Web site. Available at: http://www.project-syndicate.org. Accessed December 1, 2004. Cited in Stern AM, Markel H.

TEACHING TOOLS

Policy Premises

1. Infectious diseases — new and old — continue to affect citizens worldwide.
2. Since the Middle Ages, societies have struggled to develop effective and well-coordinated responses to infectious diseases.
3. Formal international platforms first appeared in 1851.
4. Advances in scientific understanding and regional coordination took hold in the late 19th and early 20th centuries.
5. The atrocities of WWII helped stimulate an expansion of international cooperation and redefined health in broad humanistic terms.
6. Lessons learned over the past 150 years need to be applied to modern challenges.

Review

1. When was the first international health organization established?
2. What did this forum accomplish before the beginning of World War II?
3. Did the United Nations play a role in changing the world's view on health?
4. What are some of the challenges of our current global burden of disease?

Online Resources

Access online resources with this book's CD.

Risk Control
http://www.who.int/csr/ihr/en/

Diseases: Old and New
http://www.niaid.nih.gov/publications/microbes.htm#k

All About Infectious Diseases
http://www.cdc.gov/ncidod/diseases/

On a Mission
http://www.nfid.org/

Disease Outbreak News
http://www.who.int/csr/don/en/

The Continual Challenge of Emerging Infectious Diseases
http://www2.niaid.nih.gov/newsroom/releases/infectious_diseases_04.htm

Global Travel: Advance Planning Can Prevent Illness
http://www.mayoclinic.com/invoke.cfm?id=HQ00760

Health Politics Online

For Original Health Politics Programs and Slides:

Fighting Infectious Diseases Worldwide: 150 Years of Learning
http://www.healthpolitics.com/program_info.asp?p=fighting_infectious_diseases
Slide Briefing
http://www.healthpolitics.com/media/fighting_infectious_diseases/brief_fighting_infectious_diseases.pdf

CHAPTER 3.2

AIDS —
24 Years Later

STILL GROWING

Twenty-four years after the disease made its first appearance, the HIV/AIDS pandemic continues to explode. Over the past 24 years, more than 20 million people have died from AIDS worldwide.[1] A snapshot of recent numbers tells the story. An estimated 38 million people currently have HIV, and 4.8 million of them became infected for the first time in 2003. About 2.9 million people died of AIDS last year, and more than 2 million women with HIV gave birth, passing the infection along to 630,000 infants.[2]

HIV/AIDS has certainly established a worldwide foothold, but sub-Saharan Africa, where the disease first exploded, remains the most massively affected region because it includes eight of the nine countries that have the most HIV-infected people. These countries, with more than 13 million infected people combined, are South Africa, Nigeria, Zimbabwe, Tanzania, the Congo, Ethiopia, Kenya, and Mozambique. Other countries with a significant HIV/AIDS-infected population include the United States with 950,000 cases, the Russian Federation with 860,000, China with 840,000, Brazil with 680,000, and Thailand with 570,000.[3]

Table. 3.2-1. Top HIV/AIDS-Infected Countries

Sub-Saharan Africa		
1. South Africa	5. The Congo	9. United States
2. Nigeria	6. Ethiopia	10. Russian Federation
3. Zimbabwe	7. Kenya	11. China
4. Tanzania	8. Mozambique	12. Brazil
		13. Thailand

Source: Steinbrook, R. The AIDS epidemic in 2004. *NEJM*. 2004, 351:115-117.

The modes of transmission of HIV/AIDS are well understood. The most predominant, according to the World Health Organization, is unprotected intercourse — both heterosexual and homosexual.[1] Injection drug use, other unsafe injections, blood transfusions and direct blood contact also transmit the virus. Finally, transmission from mother to child during pregnancy, at birth, or through breast-feeding is a serious risk, especially in developing countries.[3]

HIV/AIDS continues to disproportionately affect those most at risk in the developing world. Limitations in health infrastructure and limited access to effective therapies have both contributed to the continued growth and spread of the disease. Compare, for example, the 6,000 AIDS deaths last year in Western Europe, where retroviral treatment for HIV/AIDS is readily available, with sub-Saharan Africa's 2.2 million deaths. Less than 7 percent of people in developing countries in need of anti-retroviral drugs receive them, and treatment of infected pregnant women remains uncommon.[1]

Children are uniquely vulnerable. In sub-Saharan Africa in 2003, the 2.2 million deaths from AIDS resulted in 12.1 million orphaned children. HIV-infected women in this region gave birth to 550,000 infected infants, whose fate, if things remain the same, is sealed. About 1.9 million African children under age 15 have HIV — that's 90 percent of the world's total. Of these African children, 440,000 died last year.[2,3]

Despite the challenges, we have made some progress over the last 24 years. There is greater funding, a global focus, increased political will, and a cross-sector effort to make resources and anti-retrovirals more widely available. Yet problems remain. We continue to struggle with denial. We lack a vaccine. We are challenged by poor health infrastructure and unenlightened health policy. We lose focus easily, fighting each other rather than fighting the disease.

We know the answer is prevention in the form of education, behavioral modification, and awareness campaigns such as World AIDS Day. We know as well that anti-retrovirals work and can be delivered with greater efficiency and effectiveness than we once thought. And lastly, we know how to protect infants and children from the disease.

Knowing all these things, the question remains — can we act upon them? The WHO's goal is "3 by 5 " — to provide antiretroviral treatment to 3 million people in developing countries by the end of 2005. That would mean that instead of 7 percent receiving these life-saving therapies today, 50 percent would be receiving them at the end of 2005.[2] If we could accomplish that, the 25th year of the HIV/AIDS pandemic would look considerably brighter than the 24th.

REFERENCES

1. 2004 Report on the global AIDS epidemic. Geneva: Joint United Nations Program on HIV/AIDS, July 2004.
2. The world health report 2004: changing history. Geneva: World Health Organization, May 2004. Available at www.who.int/whr/2004/en/. Accessed November 17, 2004.
3. Steinbrook R. The AIDS epidemic in 2004. *NEJM*. 2004;351:115-117.

TEACHING TOOLS

Policy Premises

1. Twenty-four years after making its appearance, the AIDS pandemic continues to explode.
2. HIV/AIDS first gained a foothold in sub-Saharan Africa, but is now a worldwide reality.
3. The modes of transmission are now well understood and have varied somewhat from culture to culture.
4. The greatest impact of HIV/AIDS remains in the developing world.
5. Children are uniquely vulnerable to HIV/AIDS.

Review

1. How many people have died of AIDS worldwide?
2. Which region of the earth has the most infected people?
3. What percentage of HIV/AIDS-infected people in developing countries currently receive antiretroviral treatment?
4. What type of progress has been made toward controlling HIV/AIDS?
5. If the World Health Organization's "3 by 5" initiative is successful, what will occur?

Online Resources

Access online resources with this book's CD.

The "3 By 5" Initiative
http://www.who.int/3by5/en/

HIV/AIDS in Africa
http://www.worldbank.org/afr/aids/

Working Together
http://www.unaids.org/en/default.asp

HIV & AIDS: For Your Information
http://www.aids.org/

Advancing HIV Prevention: New Strategies for a Changing Epidemic
http://www.cdc.gov/hiv/partners/ahp.htm

World AIDS Day
http://www.worldaidsday.org/

HIV and Pregnancy
http://familydoctor.org/093.xml

Health Politics Online

For Original Health Politics Programs and Slides:

AIDS: Still Growing, 24 Years Later
http://www.healthpolitics.com/program_info.asp?p=aids
Slide Briefing
http://www.healthpolitics.com/media/aids/brief_aids.pdf

CHAPTER 3.3

HIV Testing

TOO LITTLE, TOO LATE?

A large percentage of U.S. citizens with HIV are unaware of their condition. In fact, out of about 950,000 individuals who are HIV positive, 280,000 — or 30 percent — don't know it.[1,2] According to recent statistics, out of those who have been diagnosed with HIV, 1 in 5 already have symptoms of AIDS at the time of diagnosis, reflecting well-advanced damage to their immune systems. About 41 percent of HIV-positive patients develop AIDS symptoms within one year of diagnosis. This simply shows that we routinely make the diagnosis of HIV too late in its clinical course. As a result, the disease takes hold, and the damage is done. Ideally, we would like to make a diagnosis when the specialized protective immune cells in the body, called CD4 cells, are relatively high — at 350 or greater cells per cubic millimeter. However, currently, some 41 percent of patients have a CD4 level below 200 at the time of their diagnosis.[1]

Being unaware of silent HIV places both the patient and the general population at increased risk. For the patient, every day the infection goes undetected is another day for the virus to compromise immune cells that protect the body. Treatment with highly active anti-retroviral therapy, or HAART, which is a well-coordinated regime of medicines, provides chronic protection and maintains quality of life. The sooner the treatment, the better. Making a diagnosis when one's CD4 count is 350 rather than 175 offers a survival advantage of 1.5 years.[1]

Protecting the patient also protects the general population. Patients who know their diagnosis are less likely to engage in risky behavior. Knowledge impacts number of partners, types of behavior, and use of condoms. When people are aware they're HIV-positive, they are 20 percent less likely to pass it on to someone else. Even if one were to engage in risky sexual behavior, HAART treatment lowers infectivity and decreases the likelihood of transmission by 12 percent.[1]

The high rate of silent HIV in the U.S. population reflects a relatively conservative approach to testing. As noted in a recent *New England Journal of Medicine* article: "The Centers for Disease Control recommends health care providers consider the type of setting, prevalence of HIV, and behavioral and clinical HIV risk of individual patients when they are deciding between targeted screening and routinely recommended screening. The CDC guideline suggests that a prevalence of 1 percent can be used as a general threshold for recommending routine screening, but it also notes that routine screening may be recommended at lower prevalences depending on available resources and circumstances."[1] Translation: if you live or work in an area where HIV positivity is present in 1 in 100 citizens, you are more likely to be offered HIV testing. But, the question is, why is our approach on the conservative side? Is it a cost issue?

Two recent studies have clearly documented that it would actually be health beneficial and cost-effective to finance expanded testing when one considers the money that would be saved by caring for HIV-positive patients who are diagnosed early and avoiding the cost of caring for others who might be infected by untreated HIV carriers.[1,3]

In the first study, conducted by Duke, Stanford, and the University of Toronto, patients diagnosed early began treatment at CD4 counts of 350 cells per cubic millimeter versus the more common situation of lower CD4 counts. Upon financial analysis, the earlier treatment at higher counts reached conventional levels of cost-effectiveness even when the additional benefits of reduced transmission to sexual partners was not considered.[1]

The second study, conducted by Yale, Harvard, and Boston University, used computer simulation to analyze the benefits of testing populations with a 3 percent, 1 percent and .1 percent prevalence rate of undiagnosed HIV.[3] In the high-risk population, diagnosis with testing was set at a CD4 level of 210. In terms of cost-effectiveness, the study found that populations barely meeting the CDC's thresholds compared favorably with many commonly used screening interventions for chronic conditions, including breast cancer, colorectal cancer, diabetes and hypertension.[3,4]

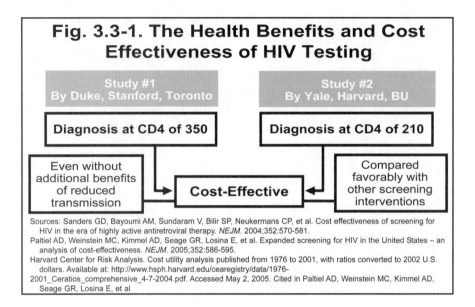

Fig. 3.3-1. The Health Benefits and Cost Effectiveness of HIV Testing

Sources: Sanders GD, Bayoumi AM, Sundaram V, Bilir SP, Neukermans CP, et al. Cost effectiveness of screening for HIV in the era of highly active antiretroviral therapy. *NEJM*. 2004;352:570-581.
Paltiel AD, Weinstein MC, Kimmel AD, Seage GR, Losina E, et al. Expanded screening for HIV in the United States – an analysis of cost-effectiveness. *NEJM*. 2005;352:586-595.
Harvard Center for Risk Analysis. Cost utility analysis published from 1976 to 2001, with ratios converted to 2002 U.S. dollars. Available at: http://www.hsph.harvard.edu/cearegistry/data/1976-
2001_Ceratios_comprehensive_4-7-2004.pdf. Accessed May 2, 2005. Cited in Paltiel AD, Weinstein MC, Kimmel AD, Seage GR, Losina E, et al

The bottom line is that timely HIV detection is critical, and voluntary testing should be greatly expanded because current approaches to testing are falling short. Study results reinforce this opinion. According to the first study: "In all but the lowest risk populations, routine voluntary screening for HIV once every three to five years is justified on both clinical and cost-effectiveness grounds."[3] According to the second study: "The cost-effectiveness of routine HIV screening in health care settings, even in relatively low prevalence populations, is similar to that of commonly accepted interventions, and such programs should be expanded."[1]

Considering that it would save money and lives, HIV testing should increasingly be the rule rather than the exception.

REFERENCES

1. Sanders GD, Bayoumi AM, Sundaram V, Bilir SP, Neukermans CP, et al. Cost effectiveness of screening for HIV in the era of highly active antiretroviral therapy. *NEJM*. 2004;352:570-581.
2. Advancing HIV prevention: new strategies for a changing epidemic – United States, 2003. *MMWR Morb Mortal Wkly Rep*. 2003;52:329-332. Cited in Sanders GD, Bayoumi AM, Sundaram V, Bilir SP, Neukermans CP, et al.
3. Paltiel AD, Weinstein MC, Kimmel AD, Seage GR, Losina E, et al.

Expanded screening for HIV in the United States – an analysis of cost-effectiveness. *NEJM.* 2005;352:586-595.

4. Harvard Center for Risk Analysis. Cost utility analysis published from 1976 to 2001, with ratios converted to 2002 U.S. dollars. Available at: http://www.hsph.harvard.edu/cearegistry/data/1976-2001_CEratios_comprehensive_4-7-2004.pdf. Accessed May 2, 2005. Cited in Paltiel AD, Weinstein MC, Kimmel AD, Seage GR, Losina E, et al.

TEACHING TOOLS

Policy Premises

1. A large percentage of U.S. citizens with HIV are unaware of their condition.
2. Being unaware of silent HIV places the patient and the population at increased risk.
3. The high silent HIV population in the United States is the result of a relatively conservative testing recommendation.
4. Expansion of voluntary HIV testing has now been shown to be cost-effective.
5. HIV meets all the criteria of the U.S. preventive services task force for targeted screening.
6. Timely HIV detection is critical and voluntary testing should be greatly expanded.

Review

1. How many people with HIV are unaware of their infection?
2. What happens when an HIV diagnosis is made too late?
3. What is our current approach to HIV testing?
4. How does one's knowledge of his/her HIV status usually affect his/her behavior?
5. How does expanded HIV testing compare to commonly used screening interventions for chronic conditions such as colorectal cancer, hypertension and diabetes?

Online Resources

Access online resources with this book's CD.

Rapid HIV Testing
http://www.cdc.gov/hiv/rapid_testing/

HIV Therapy: What is HAART?
http://suntimes.healthology.com/webcast_transcript.asp?b=suntimes&f=hiv&c=hiv_haart&spg=FIF

Getting Tested
http://www.hivtest.org/subindex.cfm?FuseAction=FAQ

Who's at Risk?
http://my.webmd.com/hw/health_guide_atoz/aa124835.asp?navbar=hw4961

Routine HIV Testing Urged for Nearly All Americans
http://msnbc.msn.com/id/6941258/

Saving Lives
http://mediresource.sympatico.ca/channel_health_news_detail.asp?channel_id=16&menu_item_id=4&news_id=5949

Know Your Status
http://www.omhrc.gov/omh/aids/2k4/4702_2C1.htm

Health Politics Online

For Original Health Politics Programs and Slides:

HIV Testing: Too Little, Too Late?
http://www.healthpolitics.com/program_info.asp?p=hiv_testing
Slide Briefing
http://www.healthpolitics.com/media/hiv_testing/brief_hiv_testing.pdf

CHAPTER 3.4

Blood Safety

WILL IT EVER BE RISK FREE?

Blood is safer than ever, especially in the United States and other developed countries, and many lives are saved each year through blood transfusions.

However, as noted by blood expert Dr. Harvey Klein, like many good things, blood does come with risks. And while it seems that developed countries have come to demand absolute freedom from transfusion-transmitted infection, we've simultaneously conceded that zero-risk transfusion is unlikely to ever be achieved.[1]

Many years ago, the American Red Cross positioned blood as "the gift of life." According to 2001 data, the most recent available, 15 million units of this gift were donated in the United States and 14 million units were transfused to nearly 5 million patients. The volume of blood transfused is increasing at the rate of 6 percent per year.[2] Yet, today, the Red Cross and other blood-related organizations are engaged in an ongoing battle for public confidence. A multi-layer safety net has been created to include donor education, selection and deferral criteria, increasingly sophisticated testing of donated blood, post-donation product quarantine, and donor tracing when blood is rejected.[1]

In addition, much of the research effort surrounding blood is now safety focused and includes characterizing new pathogens, data collection to measure infection rates in donor and recipient populations, exploring the immuno-silent period of early viral and parasitic infection, assessing the risk and benefit of increasingly restrictive donor eligibility, and developing efficient and sensitive automated blood testing.[3]

From the public's point of view, none of this is an overreaction. All we need to do is look back 20 years, and we'll discover that up to 1 in every 100 units of blood tragically transmitted HIV or the hepatitis C virus (HCV) to blood recipients in the United States.[4] Now fast forward to 2005, and most will agree that time spent focusing on blood safety was time well spent. Standard serologic testing to detect antibodies to HIV or HCV in donated blood was a dramatic safety improvement. This lowered the risk of transmission of HIV and HCV to 1 in 1.5 million and 1 in 276,000, respectively.[4,5]

In 1998, nucleic-acid amplification testing, or NAT, was introduced in the United States. It was used to screen volunteer blood donors for HCV and HIV RNA, which was a major breakthrough.[3,6] Why? Because for all infections, there is a delay period between introduction of the microorganism into the body and the body mounting a challenge with immune defense cells. During this "window period" the infection that is present is undetectable with sero-logic tests. Thus, infected donors may slip through the cracks of an imperfect detector system. The NAT test pushes the clock back on the vulnerability time. For example, the "window period" for HIV-1 decreased from 22 days with serology testing to 11 days with NAT, and HCV moved from 70 days of expo-sure to just 10 days.[3] The net impact is that, today, HIV and HCV slip through the cracks only once in every 2 million blood units with NAT mini-pool test-ing, which tests a pool of 25 to 30 units rather than each unit.[4,5]

While progress in blood safety in the developed world is real, the devel-oping world continues to face special challenges. Approximately 70 percent of all nations worldwide do not have policies in place to ensure a safe blood sup-ply. This deficiency reflects a myriad of problems, including lack of financial resources, inadequate numbers of trained health care personnel, underdevel-oped health infrastructure, and competing national priorities. About 13 million blood donations worldwide are not tested for HIV or HCV, and most of these occur in areas with high-risk populations for these diseases. Add to this the pressing need for blood in these areas, and the tragic cycle is near complete. Consider, for example, that 25 percent of all maternal deaths related to preg-nancy in the developing world are associated with blood loss.[1]

Of course, the developing world's problems are not contained within geographic borders. Global travel and migration means, for all practical pur-poses, a globally connected blood supply. This ensures an unlimited supply of new threats. What are the current concerns? One is malaria, which shows up at a rate of .25 cases per million units donated. A second is Trypanosoma cruzi, the parasitic agent that causes Chagas disease, which is relatively common in Hispanic donors. Six cases of transfusion-transmitted Chagas disease have been reported in North America over the last 20 years. Third, variant Creutzfeldt-Jakob disease, the human version of mad cow, has affected more than 100 Europeans, but, as yet, has never been proven to be transmitted in blood. Fourth, the hepatitis B virus (HBV), which is more difficult to detect than HCV, is transmitted to 1 in every 220,000 U.S. blood recipients. And finally, there is the potential threat of bio-terrorism and emerging new organisms.[3,4]

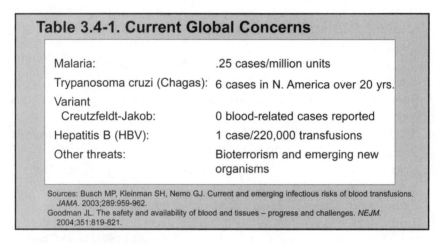

Table 3.4-1. Current Global Concerns

Malaria:	.25 cases/million units
Trypanosoma cruzi (Chagas):	6 cases in N. America over 20 yrs.
Variant Creutzfeldt-Jakob:	0 blood-related cases reported
Hepatitis B (HBV):	1 case/220,000 transfusions
Other threats:	Bioterrorism and emerging new organisms

Sources: Busch MP, Kleinman SH, Nemo GJ. Current and emerging infectious risks of blood transfusions. *JAMA*. 2003;289:959-962.
Goodman JL. The safety and availability of blood and tissues – progress and challenges. *NEJM*. 2004;351:819-821.

Five current points of focus for risk prevention include studying and better understanding the "window period" when infection is silent; predicting new and emerging blood-borne infections; developing a detection strategy for antibody negative carriers; eliminating screening errors; and developing cost-efficient and effective plans for areas where no screening is currently done.[3]

With such significant challenges, cost certainly comes into play. As we continue to decrease blood risk, the cost of the improvements increases. For example, the serology tests that were the mainstay in the United States up until 1998 were cost neutral. The introduction of NAT "mini-pool" testing saved additional lives, but at a cost of approximately $1 million dollars per infection prevented. The critical question, then, is how much will we spend for additional improvements, and what other pressing health care issues may be left unaddressed in the process?[3]

The next steps for "the gift of life" would likely include new tests to detect HBV and the implementation of NAT testing on every unit donated. Pursuing methods to inactivate pathogens in blood and sterilizing units already donated without impairing blood function would make good sense. And, since retroviruses, protozoa, and other exotic agents will certainly continue to appear long term, creating engineered blood substitutes drawn from the laboratory rather than from civic-minded volunteers would break new ground.[1]

REFERENCES

1. Klein HG. Will blood transfusions ever be safe enough? *JAMA*. 2000;284:238-240.
2. National Blood Data Resource Center. FAQs. Available at: www.nbdrc.org/faqs.htm. Accessed February 15, 2005.
3. Busch MP, Kleinman SH, Nemo GJ. Current and emerging infectious risks of blood transfusions. *JAMA*. 2003;289:959-962.
4. Goodman JL. The safety and availability of blood and tissues - progress and challenges. *NEJM*. 2004;351:819-821.
5. Jackson BR, Busch MP, Stramer SL, AuBuchon JP. The cost-effectiveness of NAT for HIV, HCV, and HBV in whole-blood donations. *Transfusion*. 2003;43:721-729. Cited in Goodman JL.
6. Busch MP, Dodd RY. Nucleic acid amplification testing and blood safety: what is the paradigm? *Transfusion*. 2000:40:1157-1160. Cited in Busch MP, Kleinman SH, Nemo GJ.

TEACHING TOOLS

Policy Premises

1. Blood is safer than ever, but still not safe enough for a risk-averse public.
2. The American Red Cross "Gift of Life" program, engaged in a long-term battle for public confidence, now carries multiple layers of security.
3. New discoveries have vastly improved safety.
4. The developing world faces special challenges when it comes to blood safety.
5. Globalization markedly complicated the blood safety picture.
6. As risks decrease, the cost per unit of safety success will increase exponentially, forcing new paradigms.

Review

1. How much blood is donated and transfused each year in the United States?
2. How have blood research efforts changed over the last few decades?
3. What is nucleic-acid amplification testing?
4. What percentage of the world's nations do not have policies in place to ensure a safe blood supply?
5. What are the current threats to our blood supply?

Online Resources

Access online resources with this book's CD.

All About Blood
http://www.givelife2.org/aboutblood/default.asp?thisHB=02/15/20
05%2014:11:48

Understanding NAT
http://www.nih.gov/news/pr/aug2004/nhlbi-18.htm

The Search for a Blood Substitute
http://www.americasblood.org/download/bulletin_v7_n1.pdf

Women and Blood Donation
http://www.healthywomen.org/content.cfm?L1=2&CID=103&Blist
=5&PubType=6

Blood Safety
http://www.fda.gov/cber/faq/bldfaq.htm

Blood: From A to Z
http://www.aabb.org/All_About_Blood/FAQs/aabb_faqs.htm

Transfusing Red Blood Cells, Platelets, and Fresh Frozen Plasma
http://www.nhlbi.nih.gov/health/prof/blood/transfusion/transfin.htm

Health Politics Online

For Original Health Politics Programs and Slides:

Examining Blood Safety
http://www.healthpolitics.com/program_info.asp?p=blood_safety
Slide Briefing
http://www.healthpolitics.com/media/blood_safety/brief_blood_saf
ety.pdf

Syphilis

HISTORIC, ANCIENT, AND ON THE REBOUND

As the world has struggled with and focused on HIV-AIDS over the past 24 years, a well-known microorganism is quietly gaining steam and mounting a resurgence. The bug is Treponema pallidum, and the disease is syphilis.[1]

In the 21st century, HIV and syphilis are increasingly appearing in tandem. Transmitted by sexual contact and advanced through risky behavior, syphilis causes a breakdown of the skin and mucosal membranes that makes infection with the HIV virus more likely.

Syphilis advances through several phases. In the early phase, it is marked by ulcerative lesions that occur at the site of inoculation then heal and disappear with or without treatment. Several months later, secondary lesions become widespread on skin and mucosal membranes, once again resolving without treatment. The disease then enters a latent period when all seems well, only to appear much later, having progressed throughout the body, infecting the nervous system, the heart and blood vessels, and seeding inflammatory masses in other organs. Throughout the entire process, including the latent periods, mothers remain infective and are able to pass the disease to newborn infants.[1]

The World Health Organization says that approximately 12 million new cases of syphilis appear each year. One-third of these are in sub-Saharan Africa, one-third are in South and Southeast Asia, and one-fourth are in Latin America and the Caribbean. About 90 percent of the cases occur in developing nations.[2]

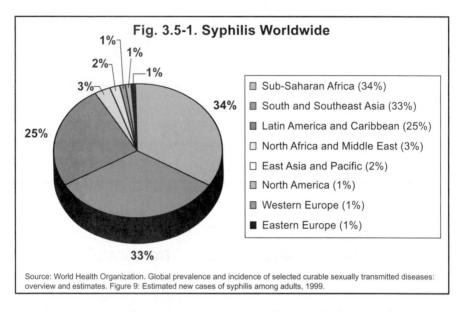

Fig. 3.5-1. Syphilis Worldwide

- ☐ Sub-Saharan Africa (34%)
- ■ South and Southeast Asia (33%)
- ■ Latin America and Caribbean (25%)
- ☐ North Africa and Middle East (3%)
- ☐ East Asia and Pacific (2%)
- ☐ North America (1%)
- ☐ Western Europe (1%)
- ■ Eastern Europe (1%)

Source: World Health Organization. Global prevalence and incidence of selected curable sexually transmitted diseases: overview and estimates. Figure 9: Estimated new cases of syphilis among adults, 1999.

Treponema pallidum is both stealthy and sturdy, having persisted for centuries, surviving by spreading with sexual contact and eluding broad, population-wide prevention and treatment strategies. It is a one-on-one, grassroots disease, with the capacity to go silent under the radar screen while still maintaining, from mother to child, its transmission capability. According to experts, many infants in developing nations still die of congenital syphilis, despite the fact that current serologic tests cost less than 50 cents, and one dose of long-acting benzathine penicillin costs 23 cents.[1]

For decades, syphilis has been effectively treated with a single intra-muscular, somewhat painful injection of penicillin. Over the years, resistance to this drug has not developed. The medicine maintains bacteria-killing levels for weeks, which is important since Treponema pallidum grows and reproduces slowly. The only problem with the therapy is its somewhat painful nature, and the fact that trained personnel are required to perform the injections. The discovery that the oral medication azithromycin is effective against the disease has been met with great enthusiasm. However, recent studies raise a caution since some mutated forms of the microorganisms can be resistant to this new therapy.[3]

A second issue is detection. Detecting the microorganisms under a microscope requires special equipment and training. Clinicians have utilized serologic blood testing since the 1930s to detect the presence of Treponema pallidum in the body. The test is simple, sensitive and inexpensive, but it is primarily a clinic-based test. The wait for the result prevents treatment during the initial visit, and there are false positives. The third issue revolves around health infrastructure in developing nations, where most of the new cases occur. Effective treatments require that clinicians go to the people rather than wait for the people to seek help.[1]

A decentralized, point-of-care effort, augmented by strong awareness and prevention is what's needed. To make this possible, experts are working on the development of rapid, on-site testing and effective, low resistance oral therapy. This will, in turn, fully support a decentralized public health outreach that simultaneously educates, raises awareness, diagnoses, and treats patients attacked by this remarkably persistent invader.

REFERENCES

1. Hook EW III, Peeling RW. Syphilis control - a continuing challenge. *NEJM*. 2004;351:122-124.
2. World Health Organization. Global prevalence and incidence of selected curable sexually transmitted diseases: overview and estimates. Figure 9: Estimated new cases of syphilis among adults, 1999. Available at: www.who.int/docstore/hiv/GRST1/pdf/figure09.pdf. Accessed Sept. 29, 2004. Cited in Hook EW III, Peeling RW.
3. Lukehart SA, Godornes C, Molini BJ, et al. Macrolide resistance in Treponema pallidum in the United States and Ireland. *NEJM*. 2004;351:154-158.

TEACHING TOOLS

Policy Premises

1. While the name syphilis is well-known throughout history, complete control remains elusive.
2. Syphilis is a stealthy survivor.
3. Treponema pallidum, the microorganism causing the disease, is built to spread and increases the risk of contracting HIV.
4. Syphilis is resurging in developing nations where it is of special risk to infants.
5. Available approaches to treatment have their limitations.
6. A decentralized "point-of-care" approach, as well as prevention and awareness are required.

Review

1. Why are HIV and syphilis increasingly appearing in tandem?
2. What occurs during the early phases of syphilis?
3. During which stage can untreated mothers infect newborn children with syphilis?
4. How is syphilis usually treated?
5. Why is syphilis more prevalent in developing countries?

Online Resources

Access online resources with this book's CD.

The Facts About Syphilis
http://www.cdc.gov/std/Syphilis/STDFact-Syphilis.htm

Testing for Syphilis
http://www.labtestsonline.org/understanding/analytes/syphilis/test.html

Disease Watch: Syphilis
http://www.who.int/tdr/dw/syphilis2004.htm

Understanding the Disease
http://www.nlm.nih.gov/medlineplus/syphilis.html

Syphilis in the HIV Era
http://www.cdc.gov/ncidod/eid/vol10no8/03-1107.htm

What is Syphilis?
http://familydoctor.org/380.xml

Azithromycin Treatment Failures
http://www.cdc.gov/mmwr/preview/mmwrhtml/mm5309a4.htm

Health Politics Online

For Original Health Politics Programs and Slides:

Syphilis: Historic, Ancient, and on the Rebound
http://www.healthpolitics.com/program_info.asp?p=prog_66
Slide Briefing
http://www.healthpolitics.com/media/prog_66/brief_prog_66.pdf

CHAPTER 3.6

SARS

LESSONS LEARNED

While the focus over the past two years has been on bioterrorism, infectious diseases are an increasing worldwide threat, with or without the help of terrorists. As we learned from Severe Acute Respiratory Syndrome, or SARS, new and inventive viruses and bacteria travel on the backs of innocent victims far and wide, reaching into unsuspecting and often unprepared populations. In 2004, SARS once again emerged as a headline issue.

In an Institute of Medicine report in March of 2003, titled "Microbial Threats to Health: Emergence, Detection, and Response," the authors warn that we have become too complacent and cite dual risks: first, an increase in animal-borne diseases, and second, bioterrorism.[1]

The timeline of SARS illustrates that in a world filled with migrating populations, high-speed travel and urban mass crowding, infectious agents predictably spread worldwide at lightning speed. With SARS, a single ill physician from Guangdong Province in China arrived in Hong Kong on February 21, 2003.[2] By the next day, 12 guests had become infected and within a week an epidemic was off and running in Hong Kong, Vietnam, Singapore and Canada.

It could have been much worse than it was, were there not vigilant, trained public health professionals on the ground. Dr. James Hughes of the National Center for Infectious Disease at the Centers for Disease Control and Prevention cites one example in an editorial in the *Journal of the American Medical Association*: "One of the first persons to recognize the potential gravity of the situation was Carlo Urbani, an infectious disease physician working for the [World Health Organization] in Hanoi. Urbani observed that a patient who had recently arrived from Hong Kong had a highly transmissible form of atypical pneumonia, and he promptly alerted WHO officials." He goes on, "Tragically, his heroic actions exposed him to the disease that claimed his life."[3]

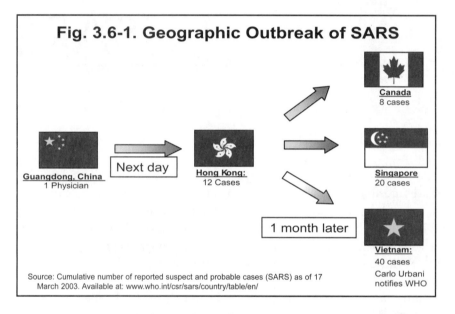

Fig. 3.6-1. Geographic Outbreak of SARS

Guandong, China
1 Physician

Next day

Hong Kong:
12 Cases

1 month later

Canada
8 cases

Singapore
20 cases

Vietnam:
40 cases
Carlo Urbani
notifies WHO

Source: Cumulative number of reported suspect and probable cases (SARS) as of 17 March 2003. Available at: www.who.int/csr/sars/country/table/en/

What Carlo Urbani unleashed was a series of highly successful public health strategies, including isolation of suspected cases, contact tracing, quarantine of potentially exposed individuals, use of protective equipment, emphasis on respiratory and hand hygiene, special training for health care workers and enhanced global communications.[4]

His call engaged the WHO early. On March 12, the organization responded with a Global Alert recommending that patients with atypical pneumonia be isolated and that all suspected cases be reported. In response, Toronto reported four cases and two deaths by March 14.[5] And on March 15th the WHO took the unusual step of issuing a travel advisory for the affected areas, a step not without economic consequences for the areas named, but crucial to gaining an upper hand on the disease.[6]

Expert teams were rapidly mobilized. A global network of laboratories was organized. And worldwide information sharing though a common data repository was implemented. Within a relatively short period of time, the disease was contained.

Studies now reveal that there is a high likelihood that SARS comes from an animal reservoir in southern China, but the original source of the disease remains unknown.[7,8] What we do know, thanks to three collaborating laboratories, is that SARS is a coronavirus, and thanks to two other labs, its genome structure has been entirely mapped. We know where it originated — southern China — but don't know its natural animal host.[3]

Recurrence of SARS and the emergence of new natural threats is a near certainty. These challenges require scientific leadership, planning and readiness. Clinicians, laboratory specialists, public health experts, epidemiologists and veterinary specialists all need to be on the same page. Future spread may be through reintroduction from an animal reservoir, as an occupational infection of a health care worker or researcher, or as a secondary infection transmitted from a persistently infected primary individual.[3]

But if it were not SARS, it would certainly be something else. As Dr. Hughes of the CDC counsels, "...newly recognized pathogens will continue to emerge, requiring preparedness, planning, a vigilant health system, a commitment to timely reporting of disease, and strong interdisciplinary partnerships to contain their spread."[3]

ONE YEAR LATER

Toronto is the capital of Ontario, Canada. It is Canada's largest city and home to more than 2.5 million people of diverse backgrounds and origins. Toronto is also the site of North America's largest outbreak of SARS. Between February and July 2003, in response to the SARS crisis, Toronto fielded more than 316,000 hotline calls, quarantined 23,000 people, investigated more than 2,000 potential cases, confirmed 358 of them as SARS, and suffered 38 deaths.[9]

The human and financial impact of this outbreak on the city was enormous. Of the 358 people confirmed to have SARS in the Toronto area, 225 were Toronto residents. Of these, 24 percent required placement in an intensive care unit, 83 percent survived, and 17 percent died. The financial impact, fueled by the disease itself and a travel advisory from the World Health Organization, was significant. The province of Ontario estimated total losses at 1.13 billion in Canadian dollars, with the tourist industry suffering a decline of 260 million in Canadian dollars. And 11 percent of Toronto's tourism-related businesses initiated layoffs.[10,11]

How did this happen? It began with a single index case — a Toronto resident returning home ill from a visit to Hong Kong. On March 5, 2003, she died at home. On March 7, her son was admitted to the hospital, critically ill. Six days later, he died. The following day, March 14, four other family members were admitted with the illness. Within one week, the first cases in hospital staff began to appear, and four days later, the hospital was closed. The closure necessitated the transfer of patients to other Toronto hospitals. There are a total of 19 acute-care hospitals serving the city, and, ultimately, 11 of them were drawn into the epidemic. This occurred as the infection spread rapidly through the hospitals, primarily through mucus secretions and respiratory droplets. Before it was over, staff, patients, family, and friends would be affected, and the city paralyzed.[9]

Seventy percent of the people infected with SARS were exposed to it in hospitals. Outside hospitals, the most common sites of exposure included work and school, which accounted for nearly 20 percent of the cases.[9]

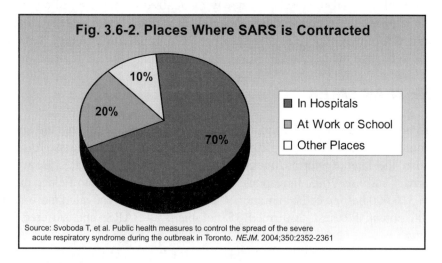

Fig. 3.6-2. Places Where SARS is Contracted

- 10%
- 20%
- 70%

- ■ In Hospitals
- ▨ At Work or School
- ☐ Other Places

Source: Svoboda T, et al. Public health measures to control the spread of the severe acute respiratory syndrome during the outbreak in Toronto. *NEJM*. 2004;350:2352-2361

As bad as the situation was, it could have been a great deal worse had it not been for Toronto's strong public health response. All hospitals with SARS cases were evaluated by expert public-health teams, which worked in unison with medical and nursing staffs. All non-essential hospital employees were immediately barred from the facilities. All elective surgery cases and outpatient visits were cancelled. All staff, patients and visitors were screened for SARS. Universal precautions were implemented and N95 super screener respirators were used for protection by caregivers. All contacts of those infected were vigorously pursued, identified and evaluated. All close contacts were quarantined at home for 10 days, with careful instruction and monitoring to avoid family cross infection. And, in two cases, when there was a resurgence of the infection, the causes were quickly identified and addressed.[9]

What lessons should we take away from this event? Clearly, it doesn't take much in the modern world to create an epidemic. One individual, intentionally or unintentionally, can get the ball rolling for a population that is unaware. SARS spread because it was initially unrecognized, not because it was untreatable or impossible to contain.

Once recognized, infection-control strategies worked. These included aggressive pursuit of contacts, shutting down the sources, quarantining potential future cases, and effectively interfacing public health specialty teams with clinical hospital leadership. For the future, we now know that team readiness, a high index of suspicion, close monitoring, good planning, and vigilance are key to controlling outbreaks like the one Toronto endured.[9]

REFERENCES

1. Smolinski MS, ed, Hamburg MA, ed, Lederberg J, ed, for the Committee on Emerging Microbial Threats to Health in the 21st Century, Board on Global Health, Institute of Medicine. Microbial Threats to Health: Emergence, Detection, and Response. Washington, DC: National Academies Press; 2003. Quoted in Hughes JM. The SARS response: Building and assessing an evidence-based approach to future global microbial threats. *JAMA*. 2003;290:3251-3253.
2. Centers for Disease Control and Prevention. Update: outbreak of severe acute respiratory syndrome-worldwide, 2003. *MMWR Morb Mortal Wkly Rep*. 2003;52:241-248. Quoted in Hughes.
3. Hughes JM. The SARS response: Building and assessing an evidence-based approach to future global microbial threats. *JAMA*. 2003;290:3251-3253.
4. Pang X, Zhu Z, Xu F, et al. Evaluation of control measures implemented in the severe acute respiratory syndrome outbreak in Beijing, 2003. *JAMA*. 2003;290:3215-3221. Quoted in Hughes.
5. WHO issues global alert about cases of atypical pneumonia [press release]. Geneva, Switzerland: World Health Organization; March 12, 2003. Available at:

http://www.who.int/csr/sars/archive/2003_03_12/en/. Quoted in Hughes.

6. World Health Organization issues emergency travel advisory [press release]. Geneva, Switzerland: World Health Organization; March 15, 2003. Available at: http://www.who.int/csr/sars/archive/2003_03_15/en/. Quoted in Hughes.

7. Guan Y, Zheng BJ, He YQ, et al. Isolation and characterization of viruses related to the coronavirus from animals in southern China. *Science*. 2003;302:276-278. Quoted in Hughes.

8. Martina BE, Haagmans BL, Kuiken T, et al. SARS virus infection of cats and ferrets. *Nature*. 2003;425:915. Quoted in Hughes.

9. Svoboda T, Henry B, Shulman L, et al. Public health measures to control the spread of the severe acute respiratory syndrome during the outbreak in Toronto. *NEJM*. 2004;350:2352-2361.

10. The impact of SARS on Toronto's business community: a survey of Toronto employers. Toronto: Toronto Board of Trade; May 2003. Cited in Svoboda T, Henry B, Shulman L, et al.

11. Toronto tourism revenue loss exceeds quarter of a billion [press release]. Toronto: KPMG Canada; July 2, 2003. Cited in Svoboda T, Henry B, Shulman L, et al.

TEACHING TOOLS

Policy Premises

1. SARS landing in Toronto was the luck of the draw.
2. The impact affected the city on multiple serious levels.
3. Cases were primarily hospital- or home-spread.
4. The strong public health response was essential for success.
5. We must absorb the lessons of SARS since we will face similar challenges in the future.

Review

1. What are two important sources of risk for an infectious disease outbreak?
2. What factors contributed to the rapid spread of SARS?
3. What steps did WHO take to contain SARS?
4. What do we understand about the SARS virus today?
5. How can we best be prepared for future outbreaks of infectious disease?
6. How many people were confirmed to have SARS in Toronto?
7. How did the epidemic start?
8. Where were most of the people infected with SARS in Toronto exposed to it?
9. Why did SARS spread?
10. What were the city's infection-control strategies?

Online Resources

 Access online resources with this book's CD.

Update 3: Announcement of Suspected SARS Case in Southern China; Investigation of Source of Infection for Confirmed Case Begins Tomorrow
http://www.who.int/csr/don/2004_01_08/en/

What Everyone Should Know About SARS
http://www.cdc.gov/ncidod/sars/basics.htm

Preventing the Spread of Severe Acute Respiratory Syndrome (SARS)
http://www.wml.com/video_lib/special/who_sars.jsp

Severe Acute Respiratory Syndrome: The U.S. Experience
http://www.who.int/csr/sars/conference/june_2003/materials/presentations/en/sarsusa170603.pdf

SARS: A to Z
http://www.who.int/csr/sars/sarsfaq/en/

Public Health Precautions
http://www.city.toronto.on.ca/health/sars/index.htm

SARS Vaccine Tests Show Promise
http://news.bbc.co.uk/2/hi/health/3291791.stm

China's Recent SARS Outbreak
http://www.wpro.who.int/sars/docs/update/update_07022004.asp

Health Canada
http://www.hc-sc.gc.ca/english/diseases/sars-sras_e.html

What Everyone Should Know
http://www.cdc.gov/ncidod/sars/basics.htm

Health Politics Online

For Original Health Politics Programs and Slides:

Lessons Learned From SARS
http://www.healthpolitics.com/program_info.asp?p=prog_36
Slide Briefing
http://www.healthpolitics.com/media/prog_36/brief_prog_36.pdf

Toronto's SARS Outbreak: One Year Later
http://www.healthpolitics.com/program_info.asp?p=prog_57
Slide Briefing
http://www.healthpolitics.com/media/prog_57/brief_prog_57.pdf

CHAPTER 3.7

The Politics of Vaccines

THE NEED FOR NATIONAL LEADERSHIP

The development of vaccines to control infectious diseases has been rightly viewed as one of 20th century medicine's greatest achievements.[1] And as the annual flu outbreaks, SARS and Anthrax scares remind us, the need for new vaccines will likely continue to increase.[2]

While the number of vaccine producers has declined over the past decade, the output of vaccines and demand for these products stands at an all-time high.[3] According to the Centers for Disease Control and Prevention (CDC), some 200 million doses of vaccine were supplied to Americans in 2001. This included 18.4 million doses of DTP, or Diphtheria, Tetanus and Pertussis vaccine; 18.1 million doses of polio vaccine; 11.6 million doses of MMR, or Measles, Mumps and Rubella vaccine; and 78 million doses of flu vaccine. The costs were covered by a mix of public and private funds. Federal, state and local governments provided 57 percent of the funding, and private payers provided 43 percent.[4]

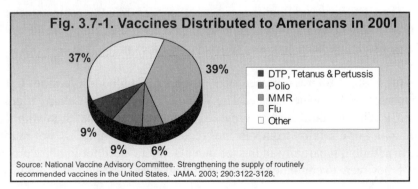

Fig. 3.7-1. Vaccines Distributed to Americans in 2001

- 37%
- 39%
- 9%
- 9%
- 6%

Legend:
- DTP, Tetanus & Pertussis
- Polio
- MMR
- Flu
- Other

Source: National Vaccine Advisory Committee. Strengthening the supply of routinely recommended vaccines in the United States. JAMA. 2003; 290:3122-3128.

In spite of the well-documented benefits of vaccines, they tend to be undervalued by the American public. The reality is that the vast majority of our citizens have not directly experienced the diseases that vaccines are designed to prevent. What they have experienced is a wide range of negative coverage in traditional and electronic media that often overstates the risks of vaccines.[5,6,7]

Yet government's voice on appropriate vaccination as a cornerstone of public health has been clear and direct. The Health and Human Services National Vaccine Advisory Committee outlined three primary goals in 2002: first, to maintain a predictable and safe supply of essential vaccines; second, to ensure availability of vaccines to all eligible children and adults; and third, to stimulate the development of new vaccines to address the challenges of the future.[4]

While these goals are noteworthy and on the mark, none is easily attainable. To begin with, vaccines are difficult to produce in a timely manner. They are produced from living organisms which literally must be grown to begin the production process. Once produced, the actual vaccine must be separated out from the growth media through a purification process. Finally, each lot, or batch, of vaccine requires a separate quality check for composition and potency.[4]

The challenges in production have contributed to a chronic problem of shortages of our most widely utilized vaccines. Tracking government action on vaccines reveals points of recurring weakness. In 1976, the assistant secretary of Health requested advice from public and private sources on how best to strengthen vaccine supply. A follow up report in 1977 warned of "a steady attrition of specific pharmaceutical manufacturers from the entire field of biologics."[4]

The CDC requested funds to accomplish a six-month vaccine stockpile in 1982, and received a $4.6 million appropriation for this purpose in 1983.[8] This stockpile has been activated at least nine times in the past 20 years.[4]

In 1986, Congress passed the National Childhood Vaccine Injury Compensation Act, which created The Vaccine Injury Compensation Program, or VICP. This no-fault system provided compensation to children who suffered injury or disability from vaccines recommended by the CDC for routine use. In addition, it partially addressed manufacturers' need for liability protection if they were to continue to discover and produce these complex products.[9]

By 1994 Health and Human Services commissioned a full study of vaccine economics and the need for expansion of cross-sector partnerships to address future challenges with creative solutions.[4] But beginning in 2000, shortages reappeared. In fact, between 2000 and 2002 the country experienced significant shortages of 8 of 11 childhood vaccines and the American Academy of Pediatrics and American Academy of Family Practice were forced to recommend deferral of some vaccines in order to prioritize and ration a dwindling supply.[10, 11, 12, 13]

Today, managing the vaccine stockpile and managing vaccine liability remain twin challenges. Stockpile issues include forecasting the need and funding of vaccines; having the vaccines properly packaged, labeled and ready to ship; managing the process of purchase, storage, regulation and activation of the stockpile; managing the time lag between discovery and production and between defined need and supply; and finally, addressing the special needs associated with bio-terrorism.[4]

On the liability side, the 1986 Vaccine Injury Compensation Program (VICP) provided no-fault compensation for children using CDC-recommended vaccines. But a wide range of other issues remain that discourage private investment in vaccines, leading the National Vaccine Advisory Committee to recommend in 2003 that "VICP be maintained and strengthened" and that "coverage of vaccines by the VICP should define a vaccine as including the active ingredient as well as preservatives, additives" and other ingredients.[4]

Now, more than ever, national leadership is required. Recommendations in 2003 advise fully funding the national vaccine stockpile, supporting governmental research and advisory bodies, ensuring that companies provide advance notice of vaccine product withdrawals, improving cross-sector partnerships, ensuring adequate financial incentives, and consumer education through a national campaign promoting appropriate vaccine use.[4]

After years of defining the problem, we must rise to the challenge of creating together an appropriate response.

REFERENCES

1. Centers for Disease Control and Prevention. Ten great public health achievements - United States, 1900-1999. Morbidity and Mortality Weekly Report. 1999;48:241-243. Quoted in National Vaccine Advisory Committee. Strengthening the supply of routinely recommended vaccines in the United States. *JAMA*. 2003;290:3122-3128.
2. U.S. General Accounting Office, Childhood Vaccines: Ensuring an Adequate Supply Poses Continuing Challenges. Washington, DC: US General Accounting Office; 2002. Quoted in National Vaccine Advisory Committee.
3. Barker LE, Luman ET. Changes in vaccination coverage estimates among children aged 19-35 months in the United States, 1996-1999. *American Journal of Preventive Medicine*. 2001;20:28-31. Quoted in National Vaccine Advisory Committee.
4. National Vaccine Advisory Committee. Strengthening the supply of routinely recommended vaccines in the United States. *JAMA*. 2003;290:3122-3128.
5. Davis MM, Kemper AR. Valuing childhood vaccines. Journal of *Pediatrics*. 2003;143:283-284. Quoted in National Vaccine Advisory Committee.
6. Davies P, Chapman S, Leask J. Antivaccination activists on the World Wide Web. *Archives of Disease in Childhood*. 2002;87:22-25. Quoted in National Vaccine Advisory Committee.
7. Wolfe RM, Sharp LK, Lipsky MS. Content and design attributes of antivaccination web sites. *JAMA*. 2002;287:3245-3248. Quoted in National Vaccine Advisory Committee.
8. Pauly M, ed, Robinson CA, ed, Sepe SJ, ed, Sing M, ed, William MK, ed. Supplying Vaccine: An Economic Analysis of Critical Issues. Washington, DC: IOS Press; 1996. Quoted in National Vaccine Advisory Committee.
9. Health Resources and Services Administration. Information about the National Vaccine Injury Compensation Program. Available at: http://www.hrsa.gov/osp/vicp/. Accessed September 24, 2003. Quoted in National Vaccine Advisory Committee.
10. Centers for Disease Control and Prevention. Shortage of varicella and measles, mumps, and rubella vaccines and interim recommendations from the Advisory Committee on Immunization Practices. *Morbidity and Mortality Weekly Report*. 2002;51:190-191. Quoted in National Vaccine Advisory Committee.

11. Centers for Disease Control and Prevention. Deferral of routine booster doses of tetanus and diphtheria toxoids for adolescents and adults. *Morbidity and Mortality Weekly Report.* 2001;50:418. Quoted in National Vaccine Advisory Committee.

12. Centers for Disease Control and Prevention. Update: Supply of diphtheria and tetanus toxoids and acellular pertussis vaccine. *Morbidity and Mortality Weekly Report.* 2002;50:1159. Quoted in National Vaccine Advisory Committee.

13. Centers for Disease Control and Prevention. Updated: Recommendations on the use of pneumococcal conjugate vaccine in a setting of vaccine shortage -- Advisory Committee on Immunization Practices. *Morbidity and Mortality Weekly Report.*2001;50:1140-1142. Quoted in National Vaccine Advisory Committee.

TEACHING TOOLS

Policy Premises

1. The development of vaccines to control infectious diseases has been one of 20th century medicine's greatest achievements.
2. Vaccines are undervalued by the public because most have not experienced the disease they prevent, and the risks of vaccines are over-represented in media.
3. Vaccines are difficult to produce in a timely manner.
4. Shortages of vaccines have been a recurring issue.
5. Managing the vaccine stockpile and vaccine liability are both critically important.
6. Now, more than ever, national leadership in vaccine development, distribution and promotion is essential.

Review

1. Why does the American public undervalue vaccines?
2. What factors contribute to the shortage of vaccines?
3. What are three primary government goals for the vaccine supply?
4. What strategies have government agencies used to attempt to meet these goals?
5. What can we do to ensure our need for vaccines will continue to be met?

Online Resources

Access online resources with this book's CD.

Influence of Insurance Status and Vaccine Cost on Physicians' Administration of Pneumococcal Conjugate Vaccine - Abstract
http://pediatrics.aappublications.org/cgi/content/abstract/112/3/521

**Estimating Costs for Budgeting and Cost-Effectiveness
Analysis Related to New Vaccine Introduction: Review of Draft
Guidelines**
http://www.who.int/vaccinesaccess/vacman/technet21/tc21_kou.pdf

**Statement to the National Vaccine Advisory Committee on
Reimbursement for Vaccine Administrations**
http://www.acponline.org/hpp/reimbursement.htm

**Improved Vaccine Affordability and Availability Act - Letter to
Senator First**
http://www.acponline.org/hpp/vaccine_afford.htm

Health Politics Online

For Original Health Politics Programs and Slides:

The Politics of Vaccines
http://www.healthpolitics.com/program_info.asp?p=prog_34
Slide Briefing
http://www.healthpolitics.com/media/prog_34/brief_prog_34.pdf

CHAPTER 4

Chronic
Diseases

"In the absence of policy actions, consumption of tobacco, alcohol, and foods high in fat and sugar increases with gross national product, followed by associated increases in chronic diseases later. This contrasts with infectious diseases, which generally decline with economic growth."

— K.S. REDDY
New England Journal of
Medicine, 2004

"The rising tide of cardiovascular risks like obesity...is affecting more and more of the younger segments, as well as the older segments of our population. We have to stem the rising tide to prevent the next wave of cardiovascular events, heart attack, and stroke from happening."

— PETER LIBBY
Chief, Cardiovascular Division
Harvard Medical School

CHAPTER 4.1

Cardiovascular Disease

STILL NO. 1

Only six in 10 Americans believe that cardiovascular disease, in the form of heart attacks and strokes, remains the leading cause of death in the United States.[1] This is surprising, since the 2003 facts on cardiovascular disease are eye-catching. Forty percent of all deaths are cardiovascular.[2] Seventeen million Americans currently live with a cardiovascular disease diagnosis.[3] This year there were over one million heart attacks in our country, and if you are searching for the leading cause of disability in the U.S., you don't have to look far. It is cardiovascular disease.[4]

As bad as the facts are, they're better than they used to be. In fact, death rates from heart attack and stroke have declined by more than 50 percent since 1950.[5] A variety of factors have contributed to the decline, including decreased cigarette smoking, decreases in our nation's mean blood pressure, and decreases in cholesterol. So why the concern?

The concern is that the positive trends are showing signs of reversing. Dr. Peter Libby, chief of the Cardiovascular Division at Harvard Medical School, said: "The rising tide of cardiovascular risks like obesity...is affecting more and more of the younger segments, as well as the older segments of our population. We have to stem that rising tide to prevent the next wave of cardiovascular events, heart attack and stroke from happening."[6]

Just over the horizon, cardiovascular trouble is clearly brewing. The rate of decrease in cardiovascular death is slowing. Cases of heart failure and stroke are on the rise. Fewer young people have healthy lifestyles, with two-thirds of Americans at 40 now showing some blockage of their coronary arteries by plaque. And then there are the "boomers," a large demographic surge of Americans, poised together to enter the senior ranks.[3]

The risk factors associated with cardiovascular disease are becoming increasingly clear, thanks to the participation of some 10,000 citizens of Framingham, Massachusetts, a community 20 miles west of Boston.[7] These citizens have continuously participated in the Framingham Heart Study, which began in 1948. By tracking their progress over the past 50 years, our understanding of cardiovascular disease and how to address this disease has made considerable progress.

In fact, the connection between risk factors, disease and death has never been clearer. In the U.S. population today, there are some 11 million Americans with diabetes. Fifty million citizens have high blood pressure. Sixty-one million are obese, with weights 20 percent or more above average. One-hundred and five million have total cholesterol levels that exceed 200.[2,3] If one looks in the aggregate, 22 percent of American men and 27 percent of American women have three or more risk factors for cardiovascular disease.[8] And this at-risk population accounts for 75 percent of all heart attacks.[9]

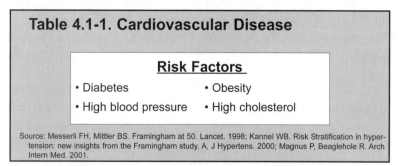

Table 4.1-1. Cardiovascular Disease

Risk Factors

• Diabetes   • Obesity

• High blood pressure   • High cholesterol

Source: Messerli FH, Mittler BS. Framingham at 50. Lancet. 1998; Kannel WB. Risk Stratification in hypertension: new insights from the Framingham study. A, J Hypertens. 2000; Magnus P, Beaglehole R. Arch Intern Med. 2001.

The truth is that Americans have become amazingly complacent about heart disease and stroke, considering the risks and damage involved. Recent studies clearly show that we overestimate, by a large degree, our cardiovascular health. Seventy-six percent say they try to maintain a healthy weight, but only 36 percent do. Sixty-eight percent say they try to exercise regularly, but only 19 percent do. And more than 60 percent say they try to avoid high fat, high cholesterol foods, but only 10 percent follow national nutrition guidelines.[1]

What's clear is that we're in cardiovascular denial. Fifty-seven percent do not believe they're at "much risk" for cardiovascular disease, and 59 percent do not believe it's our number one killer, even though the disease is responsible for 40 percent of all mortality and the majority of morbidity and disability in the United States.[1]

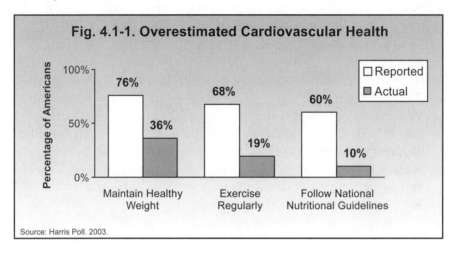

Fig. 4.1-1. Overestimated Cardiovascular Health

Source: Harris Poll. 2003.

Fifty-one years ago, the famous preventative cardiologist, Dr. Paul Dudley White, said: "Heart disease before 80: It's man's fault, not God or Nature's will."[6] He was right then. He's still right today. What do the experts advise doctors and nurses who are working with patients to do in order to help patients change their own behaviors? First, start in the waiting room, with highly visible promotional materials from the American Heart Association or others. Second, keep track of the numbers and make the cardiovascular risk assessment part of the medical record. Third, reward positive behavior. Find ways to root for and with the patient. Fourth, make it a team effort, taking advantage of including pharmacists, dieticians, therapists, web managers and self-help groups. And finally, involve the family, with group visits to define family-wide strategies.

With cardiovascular disease, we've made great progress. It would be unfortunate to let those gains slip away.

REFERENCES

1. Harris Poll. The Pfizer Journal Survey on Preventative Cardiovascular Health. www.pfizerjournal.com. 2003
2. CDC. Chronic diseases and their risk factors. 12/99. At: www.cdc.gov. Accessed 06/02/03.

3. US HHS. A Public Health Action Plan to Prevent Heart Disease and Stroke. Atlanta, GA: CDC: 2003.

4. American Heart Association (AHA). Heart Disease and Stroke Statistics-2003 Update. Dallas TX: AHA: 2002.

5. CDC. Achievements in public health. 1990-1999: decline in deaths from heart disease and stroke-US, 1990-1999. *MMWR*. 1999:48:649-656.

6. Heart Disease: An All Out Attack on Risk. *The Pfizer Journal*. Volume VII: 4: 2003. p.5

7. Messerli FH, Mittler BS. Framingham at 50. *Lancet*. 1998;352:1006.

8. Kannel WB. Risk Stratification in hypertension: new insights from the Framingham study. A, *J Hypertens*. 2000;13:3S-10S.

9. Magnus P, Beaglehole R. The real contribution of the major risk factors to the coronary epidemics: time to end the "only-50%" myth. *Arch Intern Med*. 2001:161:2657-2660.

TEACHING TOOLS

Policy Premises

1. Cardiovascular disease, in the form of heart attacks and strokes, remains the leading cause of death in the United States.
2. As bad as cardiovascular disease is, it is better than it was.
3. But postive trends are showing signs of reversing.
4. Risk factors have been known for many years.
5. The connection between risk factors, disease and death has become more and more clear.
6. Americans have become complacent about cardiovascular disease, and overestimate their cardiovascular health.

Review

1. Approximately what percentage of yearly deaths can be attributed to cardiovascular disease?
2. Is cardiovascular health improving in the United States?
3. What is the percentage of American men and women with three or more risk factors for cardiovascular disease?
4. How do Americans generally feel about their risk for heart disease and stroke?
5. What do experts suggest doctors and nurses can do to help patients reduce their cardiovascular risk?

Online Resources

 Access online resources with this book's CD.

The Framingham Study: historical insight on the impact of cardiovascular risk factors in men versus women
http://www.ncbi.nlm.nih.gov/entrez/query.fcgi?cmd=Retrieve&db=PubMed&list_uids=11974672&dopt=Abstract

Cardiovascular Health
http://www.cdc.gov/cvh/index.htm

Interventions to Reduce Cardiovascular Risk Factors in Children and Adolescents
http://www.aafp.org/afp/990415ap/2211.html

Heart Disease and Stroke Statistics - 2004 Update
http://www.americanheart.org/downloadable/heart/1072969766940
HSStats2004Update.pdf

Framingham Heart Study
http://www.nhlbi.nih.gov/about/framingham/index.html

Health Politics Online

For Original Health Politics Programs and Slides:

Cardiovascular Disease: Still #1
http://www.healthpolitics.com/program_info.asp?p=prog_35
Slide Briefing
http://www.healthpolitics.com/media/prog_35/brief_prog_35.pdf

CHAPTER 4.2

Diabetes

THE GROWTH OF DIABETES AND WHAT TO DO ABOUT IT

Diabetes is now the fifth deadliest disease in the United States, and its prevalence is continuing to increase.[1] Between 1990 and 1999, the disease grew by more than 40 percent, affecting 4.9 percent of the population in the beginning of the decade and 6.9 percent by the end. Future projections offer little encouragement. For those born in the year 2000, roughly 1 in 3 males and 2 in 5 females will suffer from diabetes in their lifetime. For minority groups, the outlook is particularly grim. Trends show that African Americans and Hispanics will continue to be disproportionately affected if the diabetes epidemic is not addressed head-on.[2,3,4]

How serious is diabetes? Let's put it in these terms: diabetes is somewhat predictable when it comes to its effect on both lifespan and quality of life. If you are a male, diagnosed with diabetes at age 40, your life, on average, will be shortened by 11 to 13 years. When you consider both numbers of years and quality of life during those years, the impact is greater. Males with diabetes lose 18 to 20 quality-adjusted life years. Females fare worse, losing 12 to 17 years of life and 21 to 24 quality-adjusted life years.[2]

The financial impact of diabetes on our nation is also staggering. With a total cost of health care of $865 billion in 2002, diabetes accounted for about $132 billion of that. Direct medical expenditures totaled $92 billion, including $23 billion for diabetes care, $25 billion for chronic diabetes-related complications, and $44 billion for excess prevalence of general medical conditions. More than $40 billion worth of indirect costs were attributable to lost workdays, restricted activity days, mortality, and permanent disability due to diabetes. [1]

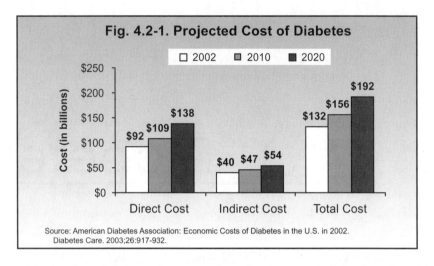

Fig. 4.2-1. Projected Cost of Diabetes

Source: American Diabetes Association: Economic Costs of Diabetes in the U.S. in 2002. Diabetes Care. 2003;26:917-932.

The burden of diabetes is greater for minority populations than the white population in the United States. Diabetes affects 10.8 percent of African Americans and 10.6 percent of Hispanics, compared with 6.2 percent of whites.[5] Approximately 2.7 million, or 11.4 percent, of African Americans aged 20 years or older have diabetes — a rate that is 60 percent higher than in whites. Thus, they experience higher rates of at least four serious complications of diabetes: cardiovascular disease, blindness, amputation, and kidney failure. For example, among people with diabetes, African Americans are twice as likely to suffer from lower-limb amputations and twice as likely to suffer from diabetes-related blindness.[3]

Hispanics are in a similar situation. Two million, or 8.2 percent, of Hispanics aged 20 or older, are affected by diabetes — a rate that is 50 percent higher than in whites. As for complication rates, 35 percent of Mexican Americans are plagued by eye complications, and, among people with diabetes, Mexican Americans are 5 times more likely to suffer from kidney failure.[4]

Considering these risks that are associated with poor management of diabetes, it's remarkable how many diabetics, in every population, neglect their condition. Eighteen percent of diabetics have poor control of their blood sugar. Thirty-seven percent have had no eye exam in the past year, and almost half have had no foot exam.[6]

When we add all this together, it's obvious that we have a large-scale health problem on our hands — one in which women and minorities are particularly vulnerable. How can we ever begin to address such a massive challenge?

To start with, we need leadership from the medical community. And the scale of our response needs to match the scale of the problem. That's why a new effort by the California Academy of Family Physicians is particularly impressive. CAFP has launched an ambitious project called "New Directions in Diabetes Care" to help physicians optimize the care of patients with diabetes in office practice. According to the group's president, Eric Ramos, M.D., "The over-arching strategy is directed at inducing organizational changes in physicians' offices to better accommodate disease management systems and streamline patient care to lead to improved efficiency and greater provider and patient satisfaction."[7]

In partnership with Lumetra, the Medicare quality improvement organization for the State of California, and the University of California at San Francisco Department of Family and Community Medicine and its Collaborative Research Network, two streams of work have been outlined. First, clinical education will be expanded through the use of traditional and electronic platforms, expanded treatment guidelines, outcome measures, patient education with a focus on self-management, public awareness and legislative linkages to issues such as school nutrition.[7]

The second focus is on comprehensive practice redesign, including family member involvement in the health care team, disease registries, group office visits, open access scheduling, electronic health records, and leveraging technology to improve surveillance and outcomes.[7]

The CAFP initiative illustrates that effectively addressing a complex disease such as diabetes requires a strategic plan that reforms daily care practices in the office, in the community, and in the home.

It will take measures such as this to get our country's diabetes epidemic under control.

REFERENCES

1. American Diabetes Association: Economic Costs of Diabetes in the U.S. in 2002. *Diabetes Care*. 2003;26:917-932.
2. Venkat Narayan KM, Boyle JP, Thompson TJ, Sorensen SW,

Williamson DF. Lifetime risk of diabetes mellitus in the United States. *JAMA*. 2003;290:1884-1890.

3. American Diabetes Association: Diabetes Statistics for African Americans. Available at: www.diabetes.org/diabetes-statistics/african-americans.jsp. Accessed March 14, 2005.

4. American Diabetes Association: Diabetes Statistics for Latinos. Available at: www.diabetes.org/diabetes-statistics/latinos.jsp. Accessed March 14, 2005.

5. Mokdad AH, Ford ES, Bowman BA, et al. Diabetes trends in the U.S.: 1990-1998. *Diabetes Care*. 2000;23:1278-1283.

6. Saddine JB, Engelfau MM, Beckles GL, et al. A diabetes report card for the United States: quality of care in the 1990s. *Ann Intern Med*. 2002;136:565-74.

7. Personal Communication. California Academy of Family Physicians, 2005.

TEACHING TOOLS

Policy Premises

1. Diabetes, the fifth deadliest disease in the United States, is growing and carries with it huge human and financial costs.
2. The financial burden of diabetes includes direct and indirect costs.
3. The burden of diabetes is unequally borne by women and minorities in the United States.
4. Diabetes translates risk factors into an array of many disabling complications.
5. Considering the risks that flow from poor management of diabetes, care systems are deficient on multiple counts.
6. Progress in management of diabetes requires improved clinical education, fundamental redesign of office practice, and family inclusion in the health care team.

Review

1. What is the diabetes outlook for individuals born in the year 2000?
2. How does diabetes affect lifespan and quality of life?
3. How much does diabetes cost the United States each year?
4. What are some of the medical complications associated with the disease?
5. What is the California Academy of Family Physicians doing to address the diabetes epidemic?

Online Resources

Access online resources with this book's CD.

All About Diabetes
http://www.diabetes.org/about-diabetes.jsp

Diabetes Prevention
http://my.webmd.com/content/article/101/106220.htm?z=1685_810
00_5050_f1_05

Diabetes Detection Initiative: Finding the Undiagnosed
http://www.ndep.nih.gov/ddi/

California Academy of Family Physicians
http://www.familydocs.org/

Diabetes in Hispanic Americans
http://diabetes.niddk.nih.gov/dm/pubs/hispanicamerican/

Diabetes in African Americans
http://diabetes.niddk.nih.gov/dm/pubs/africanamerican/index.htm

National Diabetes Education Program
http://www.cdc.gov/diabetes/ndep/index.htm

Paso a Paso (Step by Step)
http://www.ndep.nih.gov/campaigns/PasoaPaso/Paso_a_Paso.htm

Effects of Diabetes
http://www.cdc.gov/diabetes/faq/concerns.htm

Pre-Diabetes: A Serious Health Threat
http://health.discovery.com/encyclopedias/3394.html

Do You Know Your Blood Glucose Level?
http://www.diabetes.org/for-media/2004-press-releases/03-23-04.jsp

Health Politics Online

For Original Health Politics Programs and Slides:

The Growth of Diabetes and What to Do About It
http://www.healthpolitics.com/program_info.asp?p=diabetes
Slide Briefing
http://www.healthpolitics.com/media/diabetes/brief_diabetes.pdf

Osteoporosis

A TICKING TIME BOMB

Most of us have heard about osteoporosis, but we're about to start hearing a lot more. That's because the incidence of osteoporosis is sharply rising as populations age — in the United States and around the world. This growing epidemic will have major implications for our society — especially in homes where older women act as caregivers.[1]

The condition is serious enough that the U.S. Surgeon General's office issued a major report on osteoporosis on Oct. 14, 2004, noting that many people are unaware that their bone health is in jeopardy.

The good news is that osteoporosis is a treatable condition, and some organizations are already taking action. Groups such as the internationally based Bone and Joint Decade and the U.S.-based National Osteoporosis Foundation and National Women's Health Resource Center are stepping up to shed light on this painful and disabling problem that disproportionately affects women.[2]

Osteoporosis is a progressive skeletal disease characterized by low bone mass and micro-architectural deterioration, with a consequent increase in bone fragility and susceptibility to fracture.[2] It currently affects more than 75 million people in Europe, Japan and the United States alone. But what is especially alarming about osteoporosis is its projected growth worldwide. In the past decade, the number of osteoporotic hip fractures has quadrupled. By 2040, the number of people over age 65 is expected to double, so the number of hip fractures will certainly continue to skyrocket as well.[1,2]

Osteoporosis is especially common in white and Asian women over 50. Fifty-two percent have early bone mass loss, and 20 percent have clinical osteoporosis. Hispanic women have a slightly lower incidence rate, while Black women are less often affected. White and Asian men demonstrate early bone mass loss 35 percent of the time, and 7 percent suffer clinical osteoporosis. Again, Hispanic and Black men are less vulnerable.[3]

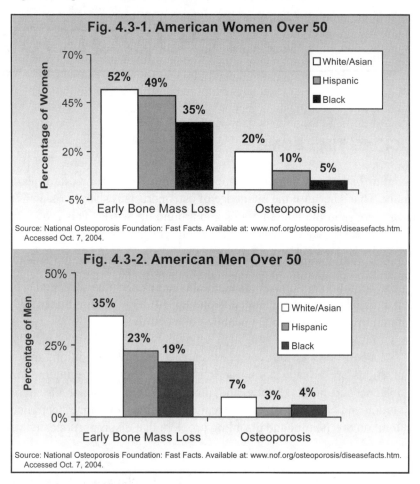

Fig. 4.3-1. American Women Over 50

Source: National Osteoporosis Foundation: Fast Facts. Available at: www.nof.org/osteoporosis/diseasefacts.htm. Accessed Oct. 7, 2004.

Fig. 4.3-2. American Men Over 50

Source: National Osteoporosis Foundation: Fast Facts. Available at: www.nof.org/osteoporosis/diseasefacts.htm. Accessed Oct. 7, 2004.

The risk factors for osteoporosis are well known. They include being female, over 50, having low estrogen, being thin with a body mass index of less than 19 kg/m^2, having low bone mass, having a history of fragility fractures in yourself or a family member, having poor nutrition with deficient calcium and vitamin D intake, smoking, excessive use of alcohol, having an inactive lifestyle, or having taken steroids or anti-convulsant drugs.[1,3]

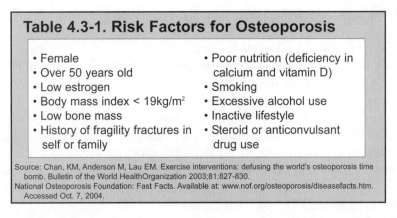

Table 4.3-1. Risk Factors for Osteoporosis

- Female
- Over 50 years old
- Low estrogen
- Body mass index < 19kg/m²
- Low bone mass
- History of fragility fractures in self or family

- Poor nutrition (deficiency in calcium and vitamin D)
- Smoking
- Excessive alcohol use
- Inactive lifestyle
- Steroid or anticonvulsant drug use

Source: Chan, KM, Anderson M, Lau EM. Exercise interventions: defusing the world's osteoporosis time bomb. Bulletin of the World HealthOrganization 2003;81:827-830.
National Osteoporosis Foundation: Fast Facts. Available at: www.nof.org/osteoporosis/diseasefacts.htm. Accessed Oct. 7, 2004.

Of these, being a female over 50 presents an important area of concern. Statistics show that women in this age group continue to play an important role as caregivers for aging parents, ill spouses and others.[4]

As Amy Niles, President and CEO of the National Women's Health Resource Center, puts it, "The harmful effects of osteoporosis can add an enormous burden to the already daunting task of family caregiving. Many women are at risk."

Osteoporotic fractures caused by falls is another key area that needs our attention. Because their bones are weaker, people with osteoporosis are at a greater risk of injuring themselves when they fall. By 2050, it is expected that 6.3 million people will suffer hip fractures worldwide.[1]

Symptoms of osteoporosis are often silent, and the disease may not be recognized until a fracture occurs. There are approximately 1.5 million osteoporotic fractures in the United States each year, including 300,000 hip fractures, 700,000 vertebral fractures, and 250,000 wrist fractures. In 2001, the cost of care was estimated at $17 billion per year or $47 million per day. Only 15 percent of hip fracture patients walk unaided at six months, and 25 percent require long-term care, usually by female caregivers whose average age is 60. Multiple fractures are common, leading to disability, loss of height, and stooping posture.[2,3]

Many of the hip, back, and wrist fractures among Americans over age 50 are related to osteoporosis. Forty-four million people are vulnerable right now — 10 million have the disease, and 34 million have low bone mass. One in every two women, and one in every four men, will suffer a fragility fracture in their lifetime. And if you have one fracture, you're twice as likely to have a second.[3]

When people are admitted to the hospital for care of a fragility fracture, they are usually not evaluated for osteoporosis. In fact, 90 to 95 percent will go home without a bone density test.[2]

The Bone and Joint Decade believes physicians should do much more on behalf of their patients with fractures. According to Professor Lars Lidgren, chairman of the organization: "Orthopedic surgeons are missing a major opportunity to prevent future fractures by not providing appropriate investigation of fragility fracture patients themselves or initiating appropriate protocols of care to be provided by their colleagues."

The Bone and Joint Decade, which calls osteoporosis a "ticking time bomb," has launched a major action initiative, including an international osteoporosis survey and a joint health awareness project with the World Health Organization.

Clearly, osteoporosis is manageable, and fractures are avoidable — but we should be much more proactive in addressing the problem. First, we must realize that sound bones are established early in life. By age 20, 98 percent of a woman's skeletal mass is established.[3] Therefore, it's crucial to have proper early nutrition, high intake of calcium and vitamin D, and plenty of weight-bearing exercise. Second, healthy adult lifestyles including exercise, excluding smoking, and practicing modest alcohol use are preventative. Third, if you're 50 and a woman with risk factors, you need a bone density scan. Fourth, if you suffer a hip, wrist or back fracture, you require a complete evaluation for osteoporosis, and you likely will benefit from strategies to increase bone formation and decrease bone resorption. Finally, more research and education is essential.

Osteoporosis has been out of sight and out of mind for too long. It's time to get it under control.

REFERENCES

1. Chan, KM, Anderson M, Lau EM. Exercise interventions: defusing the world's osteoporosis time bomb. Bulletin of the World Health Organization 2003;81:827-830.
2. Dreinhofer MD, Feron JM, Herrera A, et al. Orthopaedic surgeons and

fragility fractures: a survey by the Bone and Joint Decade and the International Osteoporosis Foundation. *The Journal of Bone and Joint Surgery.* 2004;86:958-961.

3. National Osteoporosis Foundation: Fast Facts. Available at: www.nof.org/osteoporosis/diseasefacts.htm. Accessed Oct. 7, 2004.

4. U.S. Department of Health and Human Services. Frequently Asked Questions: Family Caregiving. Available at: http://aspe.hhs.gov/daltcp/CaregiverEvent/faq.htm. Accessed Oct. 7, 2004.

TEACHING TOOLS

Policy Premises

1. Osteoporosis is a silent killer, increasing as populations age, and affecting the elderly and their caregivers.
2. Osteoporosis is especially common in white and Asian women over 50.
3. The risk factors for osteoporosis are well known.
4. The majority of wrist, hip and vertebral fractures are related to osteoporosis.
5. Fracture follow-up infrequently includes work-up for osteoporosis or treatment.
6. Osteoporosis is both preventable and highly treatable.

Review

1. How many people are currently affected by osteoporosis?
2. What are the risk factors for the disease?
3. When do many people first realize they have osteoporosis?
4. When should a bone density scan be performed?
5. What steps can help prevent osteoporosis?

Online Resources

Access online resources with this book's CD.

Fall Prevention
http://www.nof.org/patientinfo/fall_prevention.htm

Bone Mass Measurement
http://www.osteo.org/newfile.asp?doc=r209i&doctitle=Bone+Mass +Measurement%3A+What+the+Numbers+Mean&doctype=HTML +Fact+Sheet

Bone Health and Osteoporosis: A Surgeon General's Report
http://www.surgeongeneral.gov/library/bonehealth/

Boning Up On Osteoporosis
http://www.fda.gov/fdac/features/796_bone.html

Osteoporosis in Men
http://www.osteo.org/newfile.asp?doc=r615i&doctitle=Osteoporosi
s+in+Men&doctype=HTML+Fact+Sheet

Put Your Bones to the Test
http://www.nos.org.uk/quiz.asp

Osteoporosis in Children
http://www.hmc.psu.edu/childrens/healthinfo/o/osteoporosis.htm

Medications and Osteoporosis
http://www.nof.org/patientinfo/medications.htm

Health Politics Online

For Original Health Politics Programs and Slides:

Osteoporosis: A Ticking Time Bomb
http://www.healthpolitics.com/program_info.asp?p=prog_68
Slide Briefing
http://www.healthpolitics.com/media/prog_68/brief_prog_68.pdf

CHAPTER 4.4

Lung Cancer

AN EPIDEMIC AMONG AMERICAN WOMEN

Lung cancer in American women has now reached epidemic proportions. Yet for the American public, it remains under the radar and out of sight. This is surprising when you look at the numbers. Between 1930 and 1997, women's death rate from lung cancer has increased sixfold.[1,2] In just the last 13 years, between 1990 and 2003, there has been a 60 percent increase in the incidence of lung cancer among women.[3]

Part of the fuel behind the epidemic is that smoking cessation efforts have been less successful with women. Smoking rates among men have decreased by nearly one-half over the past four decades, while women's smoking rates have decreased by only one-quarter. This is clearly a critical factor since nine out of ten lung cancer patients have a history of smoking.[4] As women have continued to smoke, their rates of lung cancer deaths have continued to rise. In 1930, lung cancer was only the seventh leading cause of cancer death among women. Today it's a clear number one.[5]

The causes of smoking's prevalence among women are complex and multifactorial. Addictive properties certainly play a role, but as important has been Big Tobacco's ability to target the vulnerable, especially young girls. Those most at risk include teens seeking independence and equality, and teens actively dieting. Teens who do not complete a high school education are a special case. Their smoking rates are three times those of college-educated women.[1] In 2000, 30 percent of American high school senior girls reported having smoked in the previous month.[6]

Deaths from lung cancer among women now exceed deaths from breast cancer by a wide margin. This is not unexpected. In 1987, lung cancer risk took the lead, and the gap grows every year. In 2003, there were 20,000 more deaths among women from lung cancer than from breast cancer.[1] The fact that one-quarter of American women continue to smoke, factored against the significant success of breast cancer awareness, prevention, and early treatment programs, means that the trend lines for these two diseases will likely continue to diverge.[7]

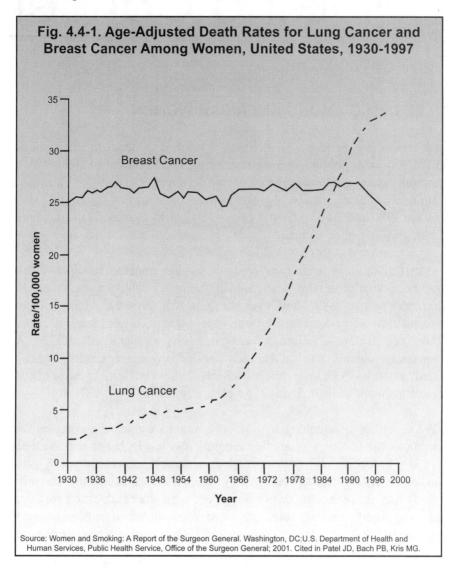

Fig. 4.4-1. Age-Adjusted Death Rates for Lung Cancer and Breast Cancer Among Women, United States, 1930-1997

Source: Women and Smoking: A Report of the Surgeon General. Washington, DC:U.S. Department of Health and Human Services, Public Health Service, Office of the Surgeon General; 2001. Cited in Patel JD, Bach PB, Kris MG.

The trend lines are not only worrisome in the United States, but internationally as well. In the United States, rates of lung cancer deaths among women have been flat for the past five years, but that may change, since the age group with the highest rates of smoking has not yet reached lung cancer age.[5] Outside the United States, women are responding to aggressive targeted marketing and joining the ranks of smokers every day. In China alone, 20 million women have become addicted since the 1990s.[8] And in Japan, smoking among women has doubled over a five-year period — from 9 percent to 18 percent of Japanese women.[9]

What can be done? Clearly we need to learn from the success of breast cancer prevention. Holistic, aggressive, women-to-women, straight-talk campaigns can greatly expand awareness as they inform and empower. These campaigns must address the social factors that make our young girls so vulnerable to tobacco marketers, including body image issues, tobacco and dieting, and the desire for independence and equality. Campaigns by women for women should advance and promote positive role models and individual responsibility. Issues of personal health and achieving one's full potential are important. So is a woman's unique role as a mother. An estimated 13 to 22 percent of all pregnant women in the United States continue to smoke cigarettes.[2] Finally, a "Women Against Big Tobacco" campaign, with a large and active role for young girls, could effectively counter subtle and not-so-subtle target marketing while converting the passive high school culture into an active, energized preventive force.

Lung cancer in women deserves all our attention.

REFERENCES

1. Patel JD, Bach PB, Kris MG. Lung cancer in U.S. women: a contemporary epidemic. *JAMA*. 2004;291:1763-1768.
2. Women and Smoking: A Report of the Surgeon General. Washington, DC: U.S. Department of Health and Human Services, Public Health Service, Office of the Surgeon General; 2001. Cited in Patel JD, Bach PB, Kris MG.
3. Patel JD, Kris MG, Venkatraman E, et al. Collateral damage from the lung cancer explosion in American women: has sex migration replaced stage migration as a confounding factor in lung cancer trials? *Proc Int Assoc Study Lung Cancer*. 2003;41(suppl 2):S61. Cited in Patel JD, Bach PB, Kris MG.

4. Giovino GA. Epidemiology of tobacco use in the United States. *Oncogene.* 2002;21:7326-7340. Cited in Patel JD, Bach PB, Kris MG.

5. Jemal A, Murray T, Samuels A, Ghafoor A, Ward E, Thun MJ. Cancer statistics, 2003. *CA Cancer J Clin.* 2004;54:8-29. Cited in Patel JD, Bach PB, Kris MG.

6. Johnston LD, Bachman JG, O'Malley PM. Monitoring the Future: Questionnaire Responses From the Nation's High School Seniors, 1997. Ann Arbor: Institute for Social Research, University of Michigan; 2001.

7. Prevalence of Current Cigarette Smoking Among Adults and Changes in Prevalence of Current and Some Day Smoking-United States, 1996-2001. *MMWR Highlights.* 2003:52:303-307. Centers for Disease Control and Prevention. Available at: http://www.cdc.gov/mmwr/preview/mmwrhtml/mm5214a2.htm. Cited in Patel JD, Bach PB, Kris MG.

8. Tomlinson R. Smoking death toll shifts to Third World. *BMJ.* 1997;315:565. Cited in Patel JD, Bach PB, Kris MG.

9. Chaloupka FJ, Laixuthai A. Cigarette smoking in Pacific Rim countries: the impact of U.S. trade policy: National Bureau for Economic Research. In: Program and abstracts of the WEA International 1996 Pacific Rim Allied Economic Organizations Conference; January 10-15, 1996; Hong Kong. Working Paper No. 5543. Cited in Patel JD, Bach PB, Kris MG.

TEACHING TOOLS

Policy Premises

1. The incidence of lung cancer in American women has reached epidemic proportions.
2. Smoking cessation in women has lagged behind cessation rates in men.
3. The causes of women smoking are complex and multifactorial.
4. Death from lung cancer exceeds death from breast cancer by a wide margin.
5. The trend lines for cancer in women in the United States and internationally are worrisome.
6. New concerted preventive campaigns to address lung cancer in women are long overdue.

Review

1. How much did the incidence of lung cancer among American women increase between 1930 and 1997?
2. Has smoking among women declined as sharply as among men in the past four decades?
3. How many Chinese women have become smokers since the 1990s?
4. What could anti-tobacco campaigners learn from the tactics of breast cancer prevention campaigners?
5. What are some of the social factors contributing to smoking's prevalence among women?

Online Resources

 Access online resources with this book's CD.

Women and Lung Cancer
http://www.lungcancer.org/patients/fs_pc_women.htm

Women, Cigarettes, and Death
http://msnbc.msn.com/id/4880289

What Is Lung Cancer?
http://www.cancer.org/docroot/cri/content/cri_2_4_1x_what_is_lun
g_cancer_26.asp

Lung Cancer in Women Neglected Epidemic
http://www.womensenews.org/article.cfm/dyn/aid/1665/context/arc
hive

Women's Lung Cancer Epidemic
http://www.ncpa.org/iss/hea/2004/pd041404b.html

**From Social Taboo to "Torch of Freedom": The Marketing of
Cigarettes to Women**
http://tc.bmjjournals.com/cgi/reprint/9/1/3

What Are the Key Statistics for Lung Cancer?
http://www.cancer.org/docroot/cri/content/cri_2_4_1x_what_are_th
e_key_statistics_for_lung_cancer_26.asp

Health Politics Online

For Original Health Politics Programs and Slides:

Women and Lung Cancer
http://www.healthpolitics.com/program_info.asp?p=prog_49
Slide Briefing
http://www.healthpolitics.com/media/prog_49/brief_prog_49.pdf

Colorectal Cancer

PREVENTION IS POSSIBLE — WHAT ARE WE WAITING FOR?

Colorectal cancer is the second leading cancer killer in the United States.[1] Some 90 million Americans are at risk of developing the disease — most from a slow process that changes silent, asymptomatic colon polyps into deadly cancers. About 145,000 Americans will be diagnosed with colorectal cancer in 2005, and 57,000 are expected to die. Of those stricken with the disease, 58 percent are men, and 42 percent are women. Sadly, many of the cancerous tumors are discovered too late, mainly because screening was not taken seriously.[2,3,4]

The fact is, screening can prevent many cases of this disease because most colorectal cancers evolve from benign adenomatous polyps that develop during a 10-year silent window. A single colonoscopy exam, using fiberoptics to visualize the entire large bowel from the inside through a tube inserted through the rectum, can remove polyps when they are still harmless and decrease the life-long risk of colon cancer death by 31 percent.[3,4] And that's just one exam. Repeating the exam every 10 years does much more. Early diagnosis of colon cancer carries an excellent five-year survival rate of 90 percent with treatment. But late diagnosis, after the tumor has already spread, lowers the five-year survival rate to 10 percent.[2]

Certain populations are at greater risk. These include men and women over 50; those with a family history of colon cancer; those with a history of colon polyps or ulcerative colitis; smokers; and those who are obese. But even without these risk factors, rates of the precursor colon polyps are quite high.

In one study, 30 percent of asymptomatic patients undergoing colonoscopy had polyps, and removal of the polyps decreased the cancer risk of these growths by more than 90 percent.[2,4]

Relatively few people, however, are properly screened for colon cancer. While roughly 80 percent of U.S. women are screened for breast cancer with mammography, fewer than 20 percent of Americans over age 50 have even had the least invasive colon cancer screening test in the past 5 years. This is the fecal occult blood test where a stool smear from a rectal exam is tested for blood.[1] Between 20 and 30 percent of Americans over 50 have had a sigmoidoscopy or a colonoscopy in the last five years. A sigmoidoscopy is a partial exam of the lower portion of the colon and rectum, and a colonoscopy is a complete examination of the entire large bowel.[1] If we separate out individuals between ages 50 and 64, the prevalence rates of these tests are lower, and they're particularly lower among individuals who are non-white, female, have fewer years of education, lack health care coverage, and are recent immigrants.[1]

Of the various screenings available, only one is thorough, diagnostic and therapeutic — colonoscopy. Preparation involves taking medicine 24 hours before the procedure to clear the colon of stool. On the day of the procedure, the patient is usually put under light anesthesia, and the exam is performed by physicians with special training. The exam directly visualizes the inside of the bowel all the way from the rectum up to the point where the small bowel meets the large bowel, a junction called the cecum. During the procedure, if a polyp or small tumor is seen, it can be removed and sent for pathologic examination. Sigmoidoscopy has some similarities, but it is often done by general physicians and it can only visualize the rectum and the most distal portion of the colon, called the sigmoid colon.

Considering where colon cancers occur in the body, several points about screening become obvious. One study comparing whites, blacks and Asians demonstrated that 55 percent, 47 percent, and 66 percent of tumors, respectively, appeared in the rectum or sigmoid colon. This means that 45 percent of the tumors in whites, 53 percent in blacks, and 34 percent in Asians would be missed by a sigmoidoscopy.[5,6] Most protocols say if you find a tumor with sigmoidoscopy, it should be followed by a complete exam with colonoscopy. But here's the problem. Seventy percent to 80 percent of patients with tumors in the cecum, ascending colon, transverse colon or descending colon do not have polyps or tumors in the sigmoid colon or rectum. As a result, those with negative sigmoidoscopy who have a silent tumor farther upstream never get the more complete exam. As a result, those with cancers in the first parts of the large bowel are often diagnosed too late and end up suffering from aggressive, high-stage cancers that are difficult to treat.[7]

The barriers to proper screening for colon cancer involve misperceptions, money, manpower and mindset. The misperceptions include the thought that this disease only strikes older men. The reality is, if you are male or female, age 50 or older, you're well within striking distance.[1] Another misperception is that screening for colon cancer is terribly painful and uncomfortable. The reality is the bowel prep is somewhat annoying but quite manageable at home, and colonoscopy with light sedation is painless. The expense of the tests can be a roadblock, but insurance companies are coming on board, as they should, because colonoscopy to screen for this cancer has been proven to be as cost effective as mammography for breast cancer.[8] Manpower issues exist since more training is required to do colonoscopy than sigmoidoscopy, and a specially designed setting, equipment and sedation are all required, but ease and efficiency have greatly increased in the past decade. Finally, because of the situations I just mentioned, health care leaders have often sent confusing mixed messages that seem to equate the value of fecal occult blood testing and sigmoidoscopy with colonoscopy because the simpler exams were more realistically achievable, but the numbers do not support this. In actuality, they require more frequent interventions that all end in colonoscopy, should there be a positive result.[1,7]

While new approaches are being pursued, including virtual colonoscopy involving CT and MRI scanning, they still require bowel prep, as well as a rectal tube to carry gas or air into the colon and the results are significantly less reliable than colonoscopy, which has only a 6 percent error rate for tumors 1 cm or greater.[7]

Rather than delay further, we need to actively address this curable disease. The first step? Focus on baseline colonoscopy for everyone over age 50.[9,10] If a polyp or tumor is detected, it can be addressed early and directly. If your exam is clean, you are good for 10 years. All in all, it seems a relatively small price to pay. There aren't many bad cancers that allow a 10-year window for detection before they steal your life away. Fewer, still, have relatively painless detection technology and skilled clinicians already in place to ensure success. Let's get on with it.

REFERENCES

1. American Cancer Society. Colorectal Cancer: Facts and Figures. Special Edition 2005. Available at: http://www.cancer.org/docroot/STT/stt_0.asp. Accessed March 21, 2005.
2. American Cancer Society. Frequently Asked Questions About Colon Cancer. Available at: http://www.cancer.org/docroot/cri/content/CRI_2_6x_Frequently_Ask ed_Questions_About_Colon_Cancer.asp. Accessed March 21, 2005.
3. Gorman C. Everything You Need to Know about Colon Cancer and How to Prevent it. Time Europe. 2000;155:Cover.
4. Foxhall LE. Colorectal Cancer Screening: Article. American Academy of Family Physicians. Available at: http://www.aafp.org/x21003.xml. Accessed March 21, 2005.
5. Wu X, Chen VW, Martin J, Roffers S, Groves FD, Correa CN, Hamilton-Byrd E, Jemal A. Subsite-specific colorectal cancer incidence rates and stage distributions among Asians and pacific islanders in the United States, 1995 to 1999. *Cancer Epidemiol Biomarkers*. 2004;13:1215-1222.
6. Nelson RL, Dollear T, Freels S, Persky V. The relation of age, race, and gender to the subsite location of colorectal carcinoma. Science Writers' Seminar of the American Cancer Society, San Francisco. March 26, 1996.
7. Walsh JME, Terdiman JP. Colorectal cancer screening: scientific review. *JAMA*. 2003;289:1288-1296.
8. Frazier AL, Colditz GA, Fuchs CS, Kuntz KM. Cost-effectiveness of screening for colorectal cancer in the general population. *JAMA*. 2000;284:1954-1961.
9. Podolsky DK. Going the distance – the case for true colorectal cancer screening. *NEJM*. 2000;343:207-208.
10. Sonnenberg A, Delco I. Cost-effectiveness of a single colonoscopy in screening for colorectal cancer. *Arch Intern Med*. 2002;162:163-168.

TEACHING TOOLS

Policy Premises

1. Colorectal cancer is the second leading cancer killer in the United States.
2. Theoretically, colon cancer is largely preventable.
3. Relatively few people are properly screened for colon cancer.
4. Of the various screenings available, only one — colonoscopy — is thorough, diagnostic and therapeutic.
5. The barriers to proper screening involve misperceptions, money, manpower and mindset.
6. While new approaches are being pursued, baseline colonoscopy should become standard for all patients over 50.

Review

1. How many Americans are at risk of developing colorectal cancer?
2. How many Americans are expected to die from the disease in 2005?
3. What is the difference between colonoscopy and other colorectal cancer screening procedures?
4. What are some of the barriers to proper screening for this disease?
5. What is the first step to actively addressing colorectal cancer?

Online Resources

Access online resources with this book's CD.

What is Colonoscopy?
http://www.gastro.org/clinicalRes/brochures/colonoscopy.html

Truths and Myths
http://www.askasge.org/pages/tentruths.cfm

Risk Factors
http://www.mayoclinic.com/invoke.cfm?objectid=13D504C5-40A0-40DA-9F61138EEAAE162F&dsection=4

Virtual Colonoscopy
http://digestive.niddk.nih.gov/ddiseases/pubs/virtualcolonoscopy/index.htm

Colorectal Cancer Screening
http://cis.nci.nih.gov/fact/5_31.htm

Facing the Cold, Hard Facts of Colon Cancer
http://msnbc.msn.com/id/4625211/

African Americans and Colorectal Cancer
http://www.preventcancer.org/colorectal/aboutcolorectal/minorities.cfm

Colorectal Cancer Screenings and Medicare
http://www.medicare.gov/health/awareness.asp

Colorectal Cancer Glossary of Terms
http://www.cdc.gov/cancer/screenforlife/terms.htm

Health Politics Online

For Original Health Politics Programs and Slides:

Colorectal Cancer Prevention: What are we waiting for?
http://www.healthpolitics.com/program_info.asp?p=colorectal_cancer
Slide Briefing
http://www.healthpolitics.com/media/colorectal_cancer/brief_colorectal_cancer.pdf

CHAPTER 4.6

Depression and Suicide

AN UNFORTUNATE LINK

Depression is an extraordinarily common and serious disorder, which all too often leads directly to death by suicide. Turn on the TV any morning and you're confronted by homicides in the United States. But suicide reporting occurs relatively infrequently. That's surprising when you consider that suicides in America are actually almost twice as common as homicides.[1]

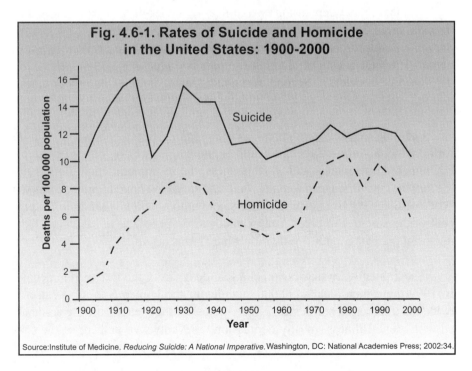

Fig. 4.6-1. Rates of Suicide and Homicide in the United States: 1900-2000

Source: Institute of Medicine. *Reducing Suicide: A National Imperative.* Washington, DC: National Academies Press; 2002:34.

In the United States, approximately 16 percent of our population will encounter depression in their lifetime. In any 12-month period, some 6 percent of our citizens suffer from depression.[2] Worldwide, depression is on the rise. It currently affects an estimated 1 percent to 6 percent of individuals in all populations. By 2020 it is expected to be the second leading cause of world-wide disability and the number one disabling condition in the developing world.[3] And the cost of the disease is staggering. In the United States in 2002, the cost was estimated at $44 billion.[4]

We think of depression as a condition of the brain, but newer evidence reveals it is a brain and body disorder of remarkable complexity. For example, if you suffer from depression and happen to have a heart attack, you are three-and-a-half times more likely to die of that heart attack than if you didn't suffer from depression.[5] In fact, the risk is as great as if you previously had heart damage. Those with depression are more vulnerable to suffering from stroke, diabetes and osteoporosis.[6] And what is truly remarkable is that if you effectively treat depression in a diabetic patient, the anti-depression therapy actually improves control of the diabetes.[7] So we know that the functions of the brain and other bodily organs affect each other. We just don't know how — yet.

The fact is that depression is significantly under-diagnosed in this country even though it's relatively easy to screen for. In fact, the U.S. Preventive Services Taskforce has designed a two-question screen to be used by care-givers. The first question: "During the past two weeks have you felt down, depressed or hopeless?" Second question: "During the past two weeks, have you felt little interest or pleasure in doing things?"[8]

Learning to recognize depression is one thing. Helping people to be more forthcoming about their mental health is another. There are lots of obstacles. Feelings of hopelessness and worthlessness, the stigma of mental illness, and the fact that this disease is often chronic and recurring have together created a "code of silence."[9] But keeping silent is not without risk. For example, 75 percent of the suicides in older Americans occur in people who have seen their doctor in the past month.[10] Why didn't the alarms go off?

The link between depression and suicide is direct and not open to debate. In 1999 there were nearly 30,000 suicides in the United States — close to twice the number of homicides. Ninety percent of the suicides were associated with mental illness, mostly depression.[11] Seventy-five percent of the successful suicides on a repeat attempt occurred in patients receiving no mental health therapy at the time of the suicide.[12] The breeding ground for suicide is broad and deep when one considers that only 25 percent of our citizens with depression receive adequate therapy.

Even so, when we do make a diagnosis, our success in treating depression actually exceeds our success in understanding it. Specific biomarkers and tests for depression do not currently exist. We don't know yet the specific gene or genes that make one more likely to suffer depression. We don't know how nerves affect our moods. And we don't understand how stress changes the function of our brain and body. But we do know that 70 percent of the patients treated for depression see significant decline in their symptoms. We know the medications we use increase the chemical neurotransmitter levels that allow nerves in the brain to communicate with each other. And we know that psychotherapy for less severe non-psychotic patients can be effective.[13]

More knowledge is needed, and research into depression could yield incredible benefits. The National Institute of Mental Health has pointed us all in the right direction with its Strategic Plan for Mood Disorders. It recommends we concentrate on these seven key areas: First, identify the genes that make us vulnerable to depression. Second, explain how nerves affect our moods. Third, define which life factors or experiences increase the risk of depression. Fourth, develop new medicines for the disease. Fifth, as knowledge grows, make certain our caregivers absorb it and use it more effectively to diagnose and treat early. Sixth, explore the connection between depression and other disease, and break the link between the two. And finally, reduce our rate of suicide, which is a national disgrace.

REFERENCES

1. Institute of Medicine. Reducing Suicide: A National Imperative. Washington, DC: National Academies Press; 2002:33. Quoted in Insel TR, Charney DS. Research on major depression: Strategies and priorities. *JAMA*. 2003;289:3167-3168.
2. Kessler RC, Berglund P, Demler O, et al. The epidemiology of major depressive disorder: results from the National Comorbidity Survey Replication. *JAMA*. 2003;289:3095-3105. Quoted in Glass RM. Awareness about depression: Important for all physicians. *JAMA*. 2003:289:3169-3170.
3. Weissman MM, Bland RC, Canino GJ, et al. Cross-national epidemiology of major depression and bipolar disorder. *JAMA*. 1996;276:293-

299. Quoted in Glass RM.
4. Stewart WF, Ricci JA, Chee E, et al. Cost of lost productive work time among US workers with depression. *JAMA*. 2003;289:3135-3144. Quoted in Glass RM.
5. Frasure-Smith N, Lespérance F, Talajic M. Depression following myocardial infarction: impact on 6-month survival. *JAMA*. 1993;270:1819-1825. Quoted in Insel TR, Charney DS.
6. Krishnan KR, Delong M, Kraemer H, et al. Comorbidity of depression with other medical diseases in the elderly. *Biol Psychiatry*. 2002;52:559-588. Quoted in Insel TR, Charney DS.
7. Lustman PJ, Clouse RE. Treatment of depression in diabetes: impact on mood and medical outcome. *J Psychosom Res*. 2002;53:917-924. Quoted in Insel TR, Charney DS.
8. US Preventive Services Task Force. Screening for depression: recommendations and rationale. *Ann Intern Med*. 2002;136:760-764. Quoted in Glass RM.
9. Glass RM. Awareness about depression: Important for all physicians. *JAMA*. 2003:289:3169-3170.
10. Conwell Y. Suicide in later life: a review and recommendations for prevention. *Suicide Life Threat Behav*. 2001;31(suppl):32-47. Quoted in Insel TR, Charney DS.
11. Institute of Medicine. Reducing Suicide: A National Imperative. Washington, DC: *National Academies Press*; 2002:99. Quoted in Insel TR, Charney DS.
12. Hawton K, Houston K, Shepperd R. Suicide in young people: study of 174 cases, aged under 25 years, based on coroners' and medical records. *Br J Psychiatry*. 1999;175:271-276. Quoted in Insel TR, Charney DS.
13. Insel TR, Charney DS. Research on major depression: Strategies and priorities. *JAMA*. 2003;289:3167-3168.

TEACHING TOOLS

Policy Premises

1. Depression is considered a common and serious disease, often leading to suicide.
2. Depression is a multisystem disorder with high direct and indirect costs.
3. Depression is significantly underdiagnosed but relatively easy to screen for. Effective treatments exist.
4. Failure to identify and treat depression can be, and often is, fatal.
5. Specific biomarkers and tests for depression do not currently exist.
6. Research into all aspects of depression is an extraordinarily wise investment.

Review

1. How common is suicide in America?
2. How strong is the link between suicide and depression?
3. What is the cost of depression to our economy?
4. Are depression sufferers receiving the therapy they need?
5. How effective is treatment for depression?

Online Resources

Access online resources with this book's CD.

Help Stop Suicide
http://www.mentalhealth.samhsa.gov/suicideprevention/surveil-lance.asp

Anatomy of a Killer
http://www.nlm.nih.gov/medlineplus/depression.html

National Institute of Mental Health: Suicide
http://www.nimh.nih.gov/suicideprevention/index.cfm

Mental Health: A Report of the Surgeon General
http://www.surgeongeneral.gov/library/mentalhealth/summary.html

Older Adults: Depression and Suicide Facts
http://www.medicalmoment.org/_content/risks/dec03/187856.asp

Stanford Researchers Test Drug to Fight Depression Faster in Elderly
http://mednews.stanford.edu/releases/2002/october/fight_depression_faster.html

National Institute on Aging: Depression increases your risk of physical disabilities
http://www.defeatdepression.org/pdf/old_bp.pdf

Health Politics Online

For Original Health Politics Programs and Slides:

Depression and Suicide
http://www.healthpolitics.com/program_info.asp?p=prog_39
Slide Briefing
http://www.healthpolitics.com/media/prog_39/brief_prog_39.pdf

CHAPTER 4.7

Organa Transplants

A SUPPLY AND DEMAND CRISIS

In spite of a serious focus by government, academic, and patient support groups, the waiting list for organ transplants in the United States continues to grow. As of March 15, 2004, there were 83,985 Americans awaiting a transplant. In 2003, nearly 6,000 people died while waiting for a transplant.[1,2,3] A look at the waiting time for a kidney transplant helps explain why — more than 1,000 days, on average.[4]

The issue is classic supply and demand. In 2003, the demands of nearly 84,000 citizens were only marginally matched by the donor supply. There were 13,263 donors overall, who provided 25,448 total organs. A slight increase in the level of organ donation resulted in about 550 more transplantations than the preceding year — a gain in supply, which was, sadly, more than offset by the growth of demand. During the same period, the number of patients on the waiting list grew by more than 4,000.[1,2,4]

Over the past 15 years we have more than doubled the number of organs donated and implanted, from 12,618 in 1988 to 25,448 in 2003.[5] Nearly half of these organs have come from dead or dying patients.[1] If one looks at the supply from non-living patients, the challenge is obvious. Significant portions of these patients are ineligible as donors because of infectious diseases like HIV, hepatitis, or cancer throughout the body, or organs that are already poorly functioning. Of those who are eligible, statistics show that 16 percent of patients and families are never approached by health care workers. Of the 84 percent approached, the current 52 percent consent rate knocks us down to only about 44 percent of eligible patients saying yes.[3,4]

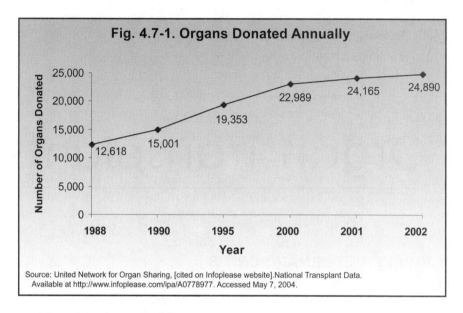

Fig. 4.7-1. Organs Donated Annually

Source: United Network for Organ Sharing, [cited on Infoplease website].National Transplant Data. Available at http://www.infoplease.com/ipa/A0778977. Accessed May 7, 2004.

There have been significant attempts over the past three years to improve the numbers of organ donors in the United States. In 2001, the Department of Health and Human Services announced its Gift of Life Donation Initiative to "raise awareness about the vital importance of organ and tissue donation." Two years later, the same department announced the Organ Donation Breakthrough Collaborative to "generate significant, measurable increases in organ donation by helping the national community of organ procurement organizations and hospitals to quickly identify, learn, adapt, replicate and cel-ebrate 'breakthrough practices' that are associated with higher donation rates." A stated goal is to move the conversion rate for non-living donors from 43 per-cent to 75 percent.[6,7]

The focus has been on re-engineering processes and adopting the prac-tices of stellar performers in the OPTN, or Organ Procurement and Transplantation Network. The OPTN is operated under a contract from the Department of Health and Human Services, and exists to collect transplant data, facilitate organ matching, and "bring together medical professionals, transplant recipients and donor families to develop organ transplantation pol-icy."[8]

Helping them out in the breakthrough project is the Institute for Healthcare Improvement, or IHI, of Boston, populated with well-known qual-ity improvement professionals and veterans in process re-engineering. So far they have engaged 98 hospitals and 43 organ procurement programs in the effort. The focus is on big, high-volume hospitals since 90 percent of donated organs come from just 850 hospitals. But even if they were to meet their goal of 75 percent consent, the gains in eligible non-living donors would be just a few thousand, not much of a dent in the nearly 84,000 left waiting.[3,4,6,7,9]

The issues behind the meager supply are real, and deal with safety and ethics. There are multiple strategies at work to increase supply. These include simplified registration, as with donor's driver's licenses. More aggressive outreach inside and outside our hospitals may help some. Financial incentives have been proposed, though the current consensus is that funds should be provided primarily to cover travel and funeral expenses. Advance directives that clearly define a person's wishes and inform family members are now available online. Some have encouraged legislation to allow surrogates to approve donation by individuals who are in persistent vegetative states, though this remains highly controversial and problematic since it is difficult to exclude the rare case of unpredicted recovery. For example, in one study of 166 patients removed from their respirators to die naturally, four percent went on to recover. Finally, some have recommended adopting a broader legal definition of death (as loss of cerebral cortex function) to expand the pool of potential donors.[9]

Counterbalancing these strategies are a variety of issues that trouble a portion of patients, families, and physicians. These include a general fear of death in our society that works against advance planning. Some distrust the system. Others' belief in afterlife complicates the decision to donate an organ. In spite of advance directives, almost all doctors and major hospitals refuse to proceed with organ harvesting without family consent. And finally, the tragic deaths of live donors in the past four years have raised questions regarding donor safety and resulted in a decline of live donors, from 506 in 2001 to 264 in 2003.[1,4,9]

Dr. Francis Delmonico, head of kidney transplants at the Massachusetts General Hospital in Boston, sounded the alarm when he said that a living donor is "not just a client or a commodity."[10]

The solution to the problems facing organ transplantation, then, cannot be reached with supply-side strategies alone. The demand is too large, and, with aging, will likely grow. That said, slow, steady increases in non-living donors, and growth in living donors — if we focus on safety — may modestly increase supply.

But the real gains — largely overlooked — are to be found on the demand side.[3,9] First, increased prevention, with early diagnosis and consistent treatment of chronic progressive diseases, could markedly decrease the need and demand for organs.

Second, increased organ graft survival and decreased rates of retransplantation could be accomplished with improved immunosuppressive drugs, better infectious disease prophylaxis, and improved donor and recipient selections.

Finally, and most important, HHS could reverse its stand on stem cells and send an unambiguous message to the National Institutes of Health and the biotechnology and pharmaceutical industries. The message is this: the real hope for organ failure patients does not lie in finding more solid organs, but rather in harvesting and directing pluripotential cells to non-invasively rebuild organ capacity from the inside out.

REFERENCES

1. 2003 deceased organ donation at highest rate in five years. [news release on UNOS website.]. March 24, 2004. Available at: http://www.unos.org/news/newsDetail.asp?id=313. Accessed May 7, 2004.
2. Organ Procurement and Transplantation Network (OPTN), Scientific Registry of Transplant Recipients (SRTR). 2003 OPTN/SRTR Annual Report. Available at: http://www.optn.org/AR2003/default.htm. Accessed May 7, 2004.
3. OPTN data reports page. Available at: http://www.optn.org/data/. Accessed March 15, 2004.
4. Langone AJ, Helderman JH. Disparity between solid-organ supply and demand. *NEJM.* 2003;349:704-706.
5. United Network for Organ Sharing, [cited on Infoplease website].National Transplant Data. Available at http://www.info-please.com/ipa/A0778977. Accessed May 7, 2004.
6. Organ Donation Breakthrough Collaborative homepage. Available at: http://organdonation.iqsolutions.com. Accessed May 7, 2004.
7. Breakthrough collaborative met with enthusiasm. [news release on OPTN website]. January 30, 2004. Available at: http://www.optn.org/news/newsDetail.asp?id=307. Accessed May 7, 2004.

8. UNOS. Who we are. Available at: http://www.unos.org/whoWeAre/. Accessed May 7, 2004.

9. Wendler D, Emanuel E. Assessing the ethical and practical wisdom of surrogate consent for living organ donation. *JAMA*. 2004;291:732-735.

10. Vastag B. Living-donor transplants reexamined: experts cite growing concerns about the safety of donors. *JAMA*. 2003;290:181-182.

TEACHING TOOLS

Policy Premises

1. The waiting list for organ transplantation in the United States continues to grow.
2. The issue is supply and demand with organization and policy primarily concentrating on supply.
3. In 15 years the number of organs provided has doubled.
4. Attempts to increase donor supply have focused on process re-engineering, collaboration, and donor promotion.
5. Real issues of safety and ethics have arisen.
6. The solution to this challenge requires decreasing demand while increasing supply.

Review

1. How many people are on the waiting list to receive an organ transplant?
2. How many people died last year while waiting for a transplant?
3. How does the rise in organ donation in 2003 compare with the growth of the waiting list in 2003?
4. How has HHS tried to increase the number of organ transplants?
5. How could the crisis also be addressed through tactics focusing on demand?

Online Resources

Access online resources with this book's CD.

Donation Facts
http://www.kidney.org/general/news/factsheet.cfm?id=30

Stem Cell Basics
http://stemcells.nih.gov/info/basics/

HHS Expands Organ and Tissue Donation Initiative, Promotes Living Donation Safety and Awareness
http://www.organdonor.gov/secgrndbrk.htm

HHS Awards $5.2 Million for Research to Increase Organ Donation Rates
http://newsroom.hrsa.gov/releases/2002releases/donorresearch-grants.htm

Organ Transplantation
http://www.nlm.nih.gov/medlineplus/organtransplantation.html

Spreading the Gift of Life: Organ Donation Breakthrough Collaborative
http://www.ihi.org/IHI/Topics/Improvement/ImprovementMethods/Literature/SpreadingtheGiftofLifeOrganDonationBreakthroughColl aborative.htm

U.S. Organ Procurement System
http://www.aei.org/books/bookID.275,projectID.8/book_detail.asp

Health Politics Online

For Original Health Politics Programs and Slides:

Organ Transplantation: A Supply and Demand Crisis
http://www.healthpolitics.com/program_info.asp?p=prog_48
Slide Briefing
http://www.healthpolitics.com/media/prog_48/brief_prog_48.pdf

Chronic Diseases in the Developing World

RETHINKING THE APPROACH

When it comes to health, many policy leaders think of developed and developing countries as two different worlds. The former is seen as having the problems associated with wealth — available money to pay for poor health habits. The latter is seen as having the problems associated with poverty — poor infrastructure and limited access to care, which leads to famine, infections, and limited life span. But the numbers reflect a different reality.

Chronic diseases are now the largest cause of death worldwide in both developed and developing countries.[1] In 2002, 29 million people died of chronic diseases. This included 17 million deaths from cardiovascular disease, 7 million from cancer, and almost 1 million from diabetes. The big risk factors fueling these numbers were tobacco use, poor diet, lack of physical activity, and alcohol use.[2]

Developing countries actually carry a double burden of disease — they have to respond to a mix of acute and chronic conditions that compete for human, financial, and political resources. This competition has a polarizing effect on the public-health community, which traditionally has focused on nutrition, clean water, maternal-fetal health, and communicable diseases; and has also viewed chronic-disease management as primarily the province of the private sector.

The list of the most common causes of death in developing countries in 2001 tells an interesting story. The top four are cardiovascular disease, cancer, injuries and respiratory diseases.[2]

Between 1990 and 2020, deaths from cardiovascular disease are projected to increase by 120 percent in women and 137 percent in men in developing nations. In fact, 80 percent of cardiovascular deaths and 87 percent of cardiovascular-related disability currently occur in low- and middle-income countries.[3] Cancer rates in this same population increased 19 percent between 1990 and 2000.[4] And diabetes, number 11 on the "cause of death in developing countries" list, is projected to grow from 171 million, or 2.8 percent of the population, to 366 million, or 6.5 percent of the developing population, in the next 30 years.[1]

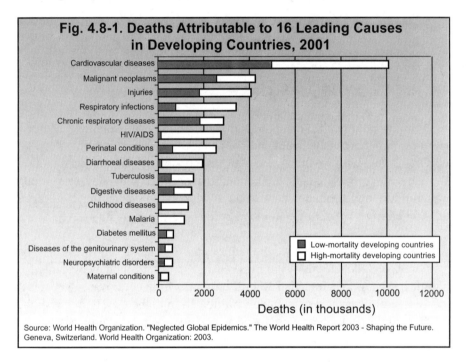

Fig. 4.8-1. Deaths Attributable to 16 Leading Causes in Developing Countries, 2001

Source: World Health Organization. "Neglected Global Epidemics." The World Health Report 2003 - Shaping the Future. Geneva, Switzerland. World Health Organization: 2003.

Why the co-existence of both acute and chronic diseases in developing nations? A summary article on the issue in the *Journal of the American Medical Association* explains it this way: "In the absence of policy actions, consumption of tobacco, alcohol and foods high in fat and sugar increases with Gross National Product, followed by associated increases in chronic diseases later. This contrasts with infectious diseases, which generally decline with economic growth."[5]

The policy challenge, then, is this: How can development be stimulated without increasing the occurrence of chronic diseases? Clearly, putting management of chronic diseases on the agenda of priorities for developing nations is a start. Good information helps as well. For example, we know the percentage of deaths resulting from various risk factors, and we know that risk factors in the poorest nations are generally different than those in the richest. In the poorest nations, more than 30 percent of deaths result from poor nutrition, unsafe sex and unclean water; while in the richest nations, the same conditions lead to fewer than 1 percent of deaths. In contrast, high blood pressure, tobacco, high cholesterol, alcohol and obesity are responsible for nearly 50 percent of deaths in the richest nations and less than 7 percent in the poorest nations. But, as nations begin to move from poorest toward richest, these risk factors merge and create a deadly brew. Tracking risk can aid in health planning and be a marker for health solutions.[6]

Table 4.8-1. National Income Effects on Risk Factors

Deaths from Risk Factors	Low Income Nations	High Income Nations
Poor nutrition	14.9%	—
Unsafe sex	10.2%	0.8%
Poor water	5.5%	—
High blood pressure	2.5%	10.9%
Tobacco use	2.0%	12.2%
Cholesterol	1.9%	7.6%
Alcohol use	—	9.2%
Obesity	—	7.4%

Source: World Health Organization. The World Health Report 2002 – Reducing Risks, Promoting Health Life. Geneva, Switzerland: World Health Organization; 2002. Cited in Yach D et al.

Chronic-disease prevention is fundamentally underfunded and underrepresented in the international public-health area. A World Health Organization study of chronic-disease prevention in 185 countries revealed that only 39 percent had budget lines for this activity, and almost all of those were developed nations.[7] The WHO expends approximately $7.50 per person per death from communicable diseases, and only 50 cents per person per death for chronic diseases.[8] In addition, a review of the core requirements of the curricula of members of the Association of Schools of Public Health revealed that international health course work does not reflect the current global burden of chronic disease.[1]

Chronic disease must be pursued worldwide in parallel with acute-disease prevention, in part because the two overlap. For example, infectious diseases can cause cancer; tobacco use increases death rates from tuberculosis; and the poor, in rapidly growing cities, are at risk regardless of their country.[1]

What to do? First, recognize the obstacles, including lack of up-to-date data, poor understanding of the economics of chronic diseases, and a world-wide bias toward acute interventional care. Second, understand the drivers for growth of chronic diseases in countries emerging from poverty. They include urbanization, free trade, foreign investment and promotional marketing. Third, dispel the myths. Some say chronic diseases affect only the affluent and elderly. The reality is that conditions like cardiovascular disease in developing nations kill as many young and middle-class citizens as HIV/AIDS. Some say chronic diseases are the result of the free choice of risky behaviors. The reality is that international marketing of tobacco, alcohol, unhealthy foods, and unsafe vehicles targets the young and vulnerable. Some say control of chronic diseases is expensive and ineffective. The reality is that a wealth of studies have demonstrated that low-cost prevention and treatment of cardio-vascular disease, hypertension and diabetes can save lives and money.[1]

Our approach to chronic diseases in developing nations needs a fundamental rethinking. If we could harness the non-profit and governmental public-health know-how with the chronic-disease management expertise of industry and academics, we might really have something.

REFERENCES

1. Yach D, Hawkes C, Gould CL, Hoffman KJ. The Global Burden of Chronic Disease: Overcoming impediments to prevention and control. *JAMA*. 2004;291:2616-2622.
2. World Health Organization. The World Health Report 2003 - Shaping the Future. Geneva, Switzerland: World Health Organization; 2003. Cited in Yach D, Hawkes C, Gould CL, Hoffman KJ.
3. Stewart BW, Kleihaus P, eds. World Cancer Report. Lyon, France: IARC Press; 2003. Cited in Yach D, Hawkes C, Gould CL, Hoffman KJ.
4. McKeown T. The Origins of Human Disease. Oxford, England: Basil Blackwell; 1988. Cited in Yach D, Hawkes C, Gould CL, Hoffman KJ.
5. Reddy, KS. Cardiovascular Disease in Non-Western Countries. *NEJM*. 2004;350:2438-2440.
6. World Health Organization. The World Health Report 2002 - Reducing Risks, Promoting Health Life. Geneva, Switzerland: World Health Organization; 2002. Cited in Yach D, Hawkes C, Gould CL, Hoffman KJ.

7. Alwan A, MacLean D, Mandil A. Assessment of National Capacity for Noncommunicable Disease Prevention and Control. Geneva, Switzerland: World Health Organization; 2001. Cited in Yach D, Hawkes C, Gould CL, Hoffman KJ.
8. Financial management report: expenditure on implementation of objectives in programme budget 2002-2003 - all sources of funds, covering the period 1 January 2002-31 December 2002. Geneva, Switzerland: World Health Organization; 2003. Cited in Yach D, Hawkes C, Gould CL, Hoffman KJ.

TEACHING TOOLS

Policy Premises

1. Chronic diseases are now the largest cause of death worldwide.
2. The double burden of disease — acute and chronic — in developing countries has a polarizing effect.
3. The current policy challenge: how do you stimulate development without inheriting chronic diseases?
4. Chronic disease prevention is fundamentally underfunded and underrepresented in public health curricula.
5. Chronic disease management must be pursued worldwide in parallel with acute disease prevention.
6. The obstacles are well-known and must be systematically addressed.

Review

1. How many people die from chronic diseases each year?
2. Why do developing countries carry a double burden of acute and chronic diseases?
3. Can development be stimulated without increasing the occurrences of chronic diseases?
4. What are some of the obstacles to chronic-disease prevention in developing countries?
5. What are some of the myths associated with chronic diseases?

Online Resources

Access online resources with this book's CD.

Risk Factor Awareness
http://www.who.int/dietphysicalactivity/en/

Understanding Chronic Diseases
http://www.ifpri.org/2020/focus/focus05/focus05_08.htm

Warning Signs
http://www.americanheart.org/presenter.jhtml?identifier=3053

Sticking with It
http://www.hivandhepatitis.com/health/070403a.html

Managing Chronic Diseases in Less Developed Countries
http://www.eldis.org/static/DOC11550.htm

Bringing the Global Chronic Disease Epidemic Under Control
http://www.worldheart.org/pdf/press.releases.surf.pdf

Striving for Stability
http://web.worldbank.org/WBSITE/EXTERNAL/EXTDEC/EXTD
ECPROSPECTS/0,,menuPK:476941~pagePK:51084723~piPK:51
084722~theSitePK:476883,00.html

Health Politics Online

For Original Health Politics Programs and Slides:

Attacking Chronic Diseases in Developing Countries
http://www.healthpolitics.com/program_info.asp?p=prog_55
Slide Briefing
http://www.healthpolitics.com/media/prog_55/brief_prog_55.pdf

Fear, Violence and Safety

"Social scientists often consider violence to be a problem caused by a breakdown in social relations. Economists see the underlying economic forces. Those in the justice system see the crime, with a victim and a perpetrator. Health professionals see the biological underpinnings and the medical outcomes. Today, more people see violence as a 'law-and-order' issue than a health issue."

— BO WAGNER SORENSEN
Professor of Anthropology
University of Copenhagen

"Too often, road safety is treated as a transportation issue, not a public health issue, and road traffic injuries are called accidents, though most could be prevented. As a result, many countries put far less effort into understanding and preventing road traffic injuries than they do into understanding and preventing diseases that do less harm."

— LEE JONG-WOOK
Director General
World Health Organization

Fear Management: Post-9/11

THE POST-9/11 REALITY

A random dial telephone survey of 1,000 New Yorkers commissioned by Health Politics and conducted by Quinley Research in April 2004 revealed that the citizens of New York City, while living in relative peace, are increasingly living in fear as well.[1]

Fear is a natural human response to the perception of risk. Fear and risk are complex, according to Dr. Paul Slovic, expert in risk management and Professor of Psychology at the University of Oregon. According to Dr. Slovic, "Risk is socially constructed. Risk assessment is inherently subjective and represents a blending of science and judgment with important psychological, social, cultural, and political factors."[2]

This complexity is reflected in the current reality in New York City. In general, the city is stable, peaceful, and recovering, at least economically. The crime rate has declined steadily every year for the past 15 years — five percent in 2004 and ten percent during the two years prior — while domestic tourism is up five percent.[3,4]

Yet the survey in April 2004, 31 months after 9/11, found that over half of New Yorkers fear they or their families will be the victims of a terrorist attack. More than one-third feel less safe than they did two years earlier. More than one-fifth have seriously considered relocating out of New York City since 9/11 and nearly one-half experienced a flashback to 9/11 during the energy blackout in August 2003.[1]

The 2004 survey clearly demonstrates that fear, absent the ability to contribute in a significant way, creates loss of control, anxiety and despair. While 73 percent of New Yorkers see themselves as more vigilant, careful and alert, fewer than one in five think they could identify a terrorist in their midst. Less than half find color-coded alerts helpful.[1] Residents and workers on Manhattan island are more conscious today that Manhattan is an island than they were on 9/11. Their fears include being trapped, being crowded and congested, being exposed, and lacking information.[5,6]

Fear is an ever-present companion for many New York commuters. More than half of riders fear an attack on the train and ferry; more than one-third fear an attack on the bus.[1] Fear in transit is a large problem in terms of scale. There are 2.4 billion rides taken on New York public transportation each year. That means one out of every three commuter rides and two out of every three train rides in the United States each year occur in New York City. There are an average of 7.7 million passengers using the system each weekday.[3,5]

Fear has disproportionately affected women, blacks and hispanics post-9/11. Five percent more women than men worry that they will become the victims of terrorism. Six percent more women than men feel less safe than they did two years earlier, and 11 percent more women than men feel more at risk for terrorism on the train.[1]

Hispanics are 12 percent more likely than whites, and 10 percent more likely than blacks, to worry that they will become victims of terrorism. While about four in 10 hispanics feel less safe than two years earlier, only about three in 10 whites feel that way. And while concern for safety on the train is present in about six in 10 hispanics and blacks, it is present in only 46 percent of whites.[1]

Table 5.1-1. Fear Disproportionately Affects Minority Populations

	Concerned: Victim of Terrorism	Less Safe Than 2 Years Ago	Unsafe from Terrorism on Train
Men	54%	32%	49%
Women	59%	38%	60%
Blacks	55%	40%	63%
Hispanics	65%	37%	57%
Whites	53%	31%	46%

Source: Quinley Research. *NYC Survey*. Commissioned by Health Politics. April 2004

This pervasive level of fear, overrepresented in minorities and women, has significant corrosive effects on stable, peaceful, civil societies over the long term. Certainly the experience of 9/11 and the associated trauma and fear resulted in highly visible fallout for the city and its people. The changes in physical landscape were more immediately recognizable than were the mental effects. A study of New Yorkers published in the *New England Journal of Medicine* one year after the event revealed that post-traumatic stress disorder was present in 20 percent of the population below Canal Street and 7.5 percent of the population below 110th Street.[7] The survey in April 2004, 31 months post-9/11, found that 35 percent of New Yorkers reported suffering anxiety, depression, or mental illness as a result of 9/11, and 35 percent continue to think about 9/11 "every day or almost every day."[1]

Fear on this level has broad societal implications beyond personal health. It undermines worker productivity, safety and security and the level and tone of civic dialogue as a segment of leaders play to the fear of citizens in pursuit of related or unrelated goals.

Fear management needs to be a major priority in our schools of public health, and public servants need to be especially careful about using fear as currency for short-term objectives. Guidance can be drawn from a wide range of disciplines, including public health, psychology, sociology, philosophy, political science, and medicine. We know a fair amount about what makes an individual feel at risk. Uncertainty in the form of non-observable, new, unknown, delayed or increasing threats, and dread of catastrophic, fatal, random, involuntary, and uncontrollable events trigger fear.[8] The list explains New York's current reality — living in peace, but living in fear as well. We all need to better appreciate that serving our short-term needs for homeland security might inadvertently be undermining our long-term needs for a stable, peaceful, civil and democratic society.

REFERENCES

1. Quinley Research. NYC Survey. Commissioned by Health Politics; April 2004.
2. Slovic P. Assessing and communicating risk and benefits. *The Pfizer Journal*. 2001; 4(5):13. Available at: www.thepfizerjournal.com. Accessed April 29, 2004.
3. Partnership for New York City. Monthly Overview. March 2004.
4. New York Is Nation's Leading Crime Fighter. Available at:

www.nyc.gov/html/nypd/html/crimedown.html. Accessed April 30, 2004.

5. The MTA Network. Available at: www.mta.info/mta/network.htm. Accessed April 30, 2004.

6. Health Preparedness and the Blackout of 2003. Available at: www.healthpolitics.com/program_info.asp?p=prog_10a. Accessed April 30, 2004.

7. Galea S. Psychological sequelae of the September 11 terrorist attacks in New York City. *NEJM.* 2002;346:982-987.

8. Slovic P. *Perception of Risk. Science.* 1987;236:280-285.

TEACHING TOOLS

Policy Premises

1. A survey in April 2004 indicates that while New Yorkers live in relative peace, they also live in fear.
2. Fear, absent the ability to contribute in a significant way, creates anxiety and despair.
3. Fear is ever-present in many New Yorkers' daily travels.
4. Fear, post-9/11, has disproportionately affected blacks, hispanics, and women.
5. Fear has significant corrosive effects on stable, civic, peaceful societies.
6. Fear management needs to become a major priority of public health.

Review

1. According to risk expert Dr. Paul Slovic, what does risk represent?
2. As of April 2004, how many New Yorkers fear they or their families will become victims of a terrorist attack?
3. How many passengers take the New York City public transportation system each year?
4. Compared to men, how safe do women feel?
5. As of April 2004, how many New Yorkers are suffering from some anxiety, depression or mental illness as a result of 9/11?

Online Resources

Access online resources with this book's CD.

Dealing with Fear
http://www.healthink.com/fear/

Mental Health and Primary Care in a Time of Terrorism
http://www.healthtogether.org/healthtogether/facingFear/about.html

Stocks fall on terrorism fear
http://www.detnews.com/2003/business/0311/18/c05-328165.htm

**Terrorism Preparedness Among New York Residents Has
Increased While Overall Fear of Terrorism Has Waned, New
Study Shows**
http://www.nyam.org/news/1744.html

Coping with a National Tragedy
http://www.nasponline.org/NEAT/crisis_0911.html

Threats put nation on edge, but fear doesn't conquer all
http://www.usatoday.com/news/nation/2003-02-13-terror-usat-cover_x.htm

Health Politics Online

For Original Health Politics Programs and Slides:

Fear Management: Post-9/11
http://www.healthpolitics.com/program_info.asp?p=prog_50
Slide Briefing
http://www.healthpolitics.com/media/prog_50/brief_prog_50.pdf

CHAPTER 5.2

Violence as a Public Health Issue

A NEW WAY OF THINKING

Violence has been viewed, historically, as a criminal justice issue because it frequently occurs within the context of crime.[1] The World Health Organization defines violence as "The intentional use of physical force or power, threatened or actual, against another person or against oneself, or a group of people, that results in or has the likelihood of resulting in injury, death, psychological harm, mal-development or deprivation."[1]

Violence, as a social science issue, is enormously complex and affects medicine, politics, economics, justice and human rights. Dr. Bo Wagner Sorensen, professor of anthropology at the University of Copenhagen, says, "Social scientists often consider violence to be a problem caused by a break-down in social relations. Economists see the underlying economic forces. Those in the justice system see the crime, with a victim and a perpetrator. Health professionals see the biological underpinnings and the medical outcomes. Today, more people see violence as a 'law and order' issue than a health issue."[2]

If there is disagreement on what violence is, there is little disagreement on the damage it does. The numbers are staggering. Worldwide, more than two million people a year die as a result of violence. This includes more than one million deaths from suicide, more than 600,000 deaths from homicide, and more than 500,000 deaths from war injuries.[1,3] This, collectively, represents four percent of all deaths worldwide, and 15 percent of all disability.[4] And death and disability is on the rise.[1]

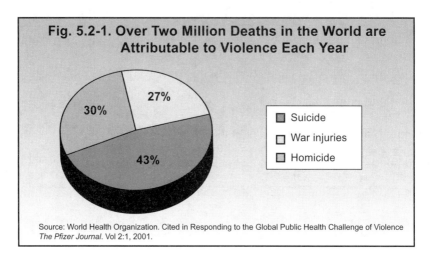

Fig. 5.2-1. Over Two Million Deaths in the World are Attributable to Violence Each Year

27%

30%

43%

- Suicide
- War injuries
- Homicide

Source: World Health Organization. Cited in Responding to the Global Public Health Challenge of Violence *The Pfizer Journal.* Vol 2:1, 2001.

Violence is a serious issue in both developing and developed countries. The percentage of total disability resulting from violence in developed nations is 14.5 percent. In developing nations it's 15.2 percent.[4] In the United States, sadly, violence is epidemic. Each day, 53 people die of homicides, 84 commit suicide, 3,000 attempt suicide, and 18,000 are victims of assaults.[5] Among men 15 to 24, and compared to Canada, France, Germany, Spain, the Netherlands, Switzerland, Finland and the United Kingdom combined, the United States has 10 times the number of homicides annually.[6] Indeed, the United States has the highest suicide and homicide rates among the world's 26 wealthiest nations.[7]

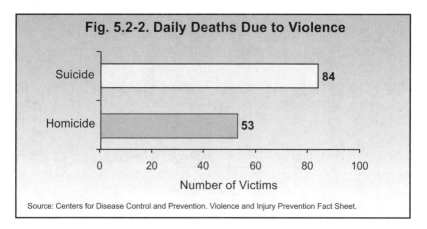

Fig. 5.2-2. Daily Deaths Due to Violence

Suicide   84

Homicide   53

0   20   40   60   80   100

Number of Victims

Source: Centers for Disease Control and Prevention. Violence and Injury Prevention Fact Sheet.

Taking action against violence must begin by moving beyond raw numbers to data analysis. Traditionally we have counted deaths — or mortality, and complications — or morbidity. While these numbers define the comparative extent of the problem, other data is more useful in exploring solutions. Data on risk behaviors, victim demographics, perpetrator demographics, and environmental circumstances are extraordinarily useful and a necessary beginning point.

Dr. Norman Sartorius, former president of the Association of European Psychiatrists, has said, "New attention is focused on the act of violence, sometimes on the perpetrator, sometimes on the victim. But too often, we forget that these people do not act in isolation; the perpetrators have families and friends, and there are often witnesses to the act. There are many ripple effects of one violent episode."[2]

In fact, there are ripples and concentric circles. The individuals have families. The families live in communities with schools and neighborhoods. The communities possess varying cultures and traditions. These circles, then, create a complex web, not only of intersecting risk factors, but also of potential strategies that point toward solutions to the tragedy of violence.[8]

It has been said that the two leading causes of death, throughout human history, are infectious disease and violence.[9] Years ago, we effectively applied a comprehensive public health approach to combating infectious disease. A comprehensive public health methodology is ideally suited for addressing the complexities of violence, as well.

Public health takes a four-step approach encapsulated in the following questions: First, what is the problem? Second, what are the causes? Third, what will prevent these causes? And fourth, how do we implement a plan of action? The emphasis of public health, then, is on understanding, prevention, and problem solving.[10] If we know what the problem is — its definition and extent — we can then address the causes of violence.

REFERENCES

1. Responding to the Global Public Health Challenge of Violence. *The Pfizer Journal*. Vol 2:1, 2001.
2. Buvinic M, Morrison AR. Living in a more violent world. *Foreign Policy*. 2000;118:58-72.
3. Romer C. Global health problems of violence. In: Violence and Health: Proceedings of a WHO global symposium. Kobe, Japan:

WHO Center for Health Development, 2000.

4. WHO. Violence and injury prevention; violence and health.

5. Centers for Disease Control and Prevention. Violence and Injury Prevention [fact sheet].

6. American Academy of Pediatrics. Adolescent assault victim needs: a review of issues and a model protocol. Pediatrics. 1996;98:991-1001.

7. CDC. Rates of homicide, suicide, and firearm-related death among children: 26 industrialized countries. *MMWR Morb Mortal Wkly Rep.* 1997;46:101-105.

8. Hogan MJ. The epidemic of violence in America [editorial]. *Postgrad Med.* 1999;1-5(6).

9. Foege WH. Highway violence and public policy. *N Engl J Med.* 1987;316:1407-1408.

10. Roth JA, Moore MH. Reducing Violent Crimes and International Injuries. Washington, DC: U.S. Department of Justice, October 1995. (Publication NCJ 156089).

TEACHING TOOLS

Policy Premises

1. Violence has been viewed historically as a criminal justice issue since it frequently has occurred within the context of crime.
2. Violence as a social science issue is enormously complex and affects medicine, politics, economics, justice and human rights.
3. The dimensions of violence are staggering.
4. Violence has become a serious issue in both developed and developing countries.
5. Measuring violence must extend beyond counting; it has ripple effects.
6. The public health methodology is ideally suited for addressing the complexities of violence.

Review

1. How does the World Health Organization define violence?
2. How many people in the world die each year as a result of violence?
3. In developing and developed nations, what percentage of total disability results from violence?
4. Of the world's 26 wealthiest nations, which has the highest suicide and homicide rates?
5. What are the ripple effects caused by a violent episode?

Online Resources

Access online resources with this book's CD.

Social Causes of Violence: Crafting a Science Agenda
http://www.asanet.org/pubs/socialcauses.html

The Toll of Global Violence
http://www.ncpa.org/iss/int/2002/pd100302c.html

A public health approach to the violence epidemic in the United States
http://www.preventioninstitute.org/violence.html

Health Politics Online

For Original Health Politics Programs and Slides:

Violence as a Public Health Issue
http://www.healthpolitics.com/program_info.asp?p=prog_19
Slide Briefing
http://www.healthpolitics.com/media/prog_19/brief_prog_19.pdf

Risk Factors
for Violence

LARGELY UNDER HUMAN CONTROL

Experts agree that most violent behavior appears to be learned behavior.[1,2] This growing consensus is leading societies around the world to rethink violence from a public health perspective, including uniform surveillance, identification of causes, thoughtful intervention and prevention.[3]

If violence is learned then perhaps it can be unlearned. Dr. Rodney Hammond, director of the Center for Violence Prevention at the Center for Disease Control notes, "We know that much, probably most, violence is learned behavior. I believe it can be unlearned. Certainly we have learned that the reactive response — arrest and incarceration — does not always work. Fewer resources have been devoted to strategies aimed at preventing violent behavior."

Unlearning violence requires a clear understanding of its causes. Violence lies at the intersection of multiple independent factors, with aggression being the final common pathway. While one factor may not lead consistently to violent behavior, two or more factors can increase the incidence exponentially. This is similar to the case of child mental-health disorders, where having a single risk factor carries with it no increased incidence. However, having two risk factors carries a threefold increase in incidence, while having three risk factors carries a ten-fold increase in incidence.[4]

Risk factors for violence flow from issues arising within the individual, the family, the community and society.[5] Collectively, they create concentric circles of violence that play off one another. To emphasize the complexity of violence, consider some of the factors that have been identified.

On the community level, there is limited social capital, undermining trust and mutual interdependence; diminished economic opportunity, poverty and unemployment; illegal markets; discrimination and inequality; urbanization, collective stress, and migrating transient populations; war and media violence. On the peer and school level, there are negative peer influences, gangs, lack of role models, high tolerance for violence, lack of classroom discipline, crowding, poor teacher performance, low expectations of students and high drop-out rates. Social fragmentation and deprived neighborhoods, regardless of parental income, marital status or educational level, are associated with increases in violent behavior and suicide.[6,7]

Table 5.3-1. Risk Factors of Violence

Community	Peer & School	Family
• Limited social capital; low community development • Diminished economic opportunity; poverty; unemployment • Illegal markets • Urbanization; collective stress; transience • War • Media violence	• Negative peer influences • Gangs • Acceptance of violence • Undisciplined classroom; crowded physical space • High dropout rates • Low expectations	• Chronic abuse • Shame • Humiliation • Neglect • Hostility

Source: WHO Center for Health Development, 2000
J Epidemiol Community Health. 2001; BMJ. 1999

When it comes to violence, families can be significantly preventive or significantly causative.[8] On the negative side, chronic abuse, shame, humiliation, neglect and hostility will, predictably, generate anger, frustration, hopelessness, lack of purpose and impulsiveness, especially in young people. If you add mental disorders or substance abuse to the mix, you see an acceleration in the cycle of violence.[9,10]

On the positive side, loving attention, open communication, modeling constructive behavior, purposefulness and emotional, physical and economic stability are highly preventative. It is easy for circumstances to tip a functional family to dysfunction. Dr. Kocijan-Herigonja, head of psychiatry at

Hospital Dubrau in Croatia, said, "No risk factor exists in isolation from others. With poverty, unemployment and war, you probably also have a dysfunctional family — and everything begins in family. In many societies, poverty and unemployment are common. The stress of these factors can be weathered by a strong family, but tip the balance of a dysfunctional family, and result in aggression."[4]

An awareness of the special vulnerability of young people toward violence is critical. Around the world, the highest rates of homicide and suicide occur in those 15 to 35 years of age.[11] Dr. Hammond notes that, "At a critical developmental stage, where authority figures are being rejected, teens have magical thinking about their vulnerability, and make impulsive choices."[4]

If youthfulness is a significant determinant on the individual level, urbanization is equally important on the societal level. The growth of "mega-cities" presents a special challenge, heightening the risk of violence.[12] It is expected that by 2025, two-thirds of the world's population will reside in cites, accounting for more than five billion people.

Josephine Gilman, executive director of PRISMA, notes that, "Unorganized urban settlements are strongly related to violence. As millions move into newly created cities, creating infrastructure demands beyond that which exists, I envision serious problems with violence, malnutrition, and infectious diseases."[4]

Violence then is a complex web of macro and micro problems, largely under human control, playing off of, and complicating, each other. If these risk factors are constructed of human hands, can they then be dismantled? If the behaviors are learned, can they be unlearned? If we know the causes of violence, can they be prevented?

REFERENCES

1. Roth JA, Moore MH. Reducing Violent Crimes and Intentional Injuries. Washington DC: U.S. Department of Justice, October 1995.
2. Whitley E, Gunnell D, Dorling D, Smith GD. Ecological study of social fragmentation, poverty, and suicide. *BMJ*. 1999;319:1034-1037.
3. Krug E. Proposal: World Report on Violence. Geneva, Switz: WHO; 2000.
4. Annan K. Statement to the General Assembly as he presented his

Millenium Report, "We the Peoples: The Role of the United Nations in the 21st Century." New York, NY: UN; April 3, 2000.

5. Sartorius, N. Responding to the global Public Health challenge of Violence. *The Pfizer Journal.* Vol II: 1, 2001. p.15-16.

6. Romer C. Global Health problems of violence. In: Violence and Health: Proceedings of a WHO global symposium. Kobe, Japan: WHO Center for Health Development, 2000.

7. Kalff AC, Kroes M, Vles JSH, et al. Neighbourhood level and individual level SES effects on child problem behavior: a multilevel analysis. *J Epidemiol Community Health.* 2001;55:246-250.

8. Garbarino, J. Lost Boys: *Why Our Sons Turn Violent and How We Can Save Them.* New York: Free Press; 1999.

9. Markowitz S. An Economic Analysis of Alcohol, Drugs and Violent Crime in the National Crime Victimization Survey. Cambridge, Mass: *NBER*, October 2000. NBER Working Paper No. W7982.

10. Grimes T, Vernberg E, Cathers T. Emotionally disturbed children's reaction to violent media segments. *J Health Community.* 1997;2: 157-168.

11. Buvinic M, Morrison AR. Living in a more violent world. *Foreign Policy.* 2000; 118:58-72.

12. Neilson L. Population dynamics, Structural changes and resource distribution: violence prevention and health development in cities in the next two decades. In: Violence and Health: proceedings of a WHO global symposium. Kobe, Japan: WHO Center for Health Development, 2000.

TEACHING TOOLS

Policy Premises

1. Most violent behavior appears to be learned behavior.
2. Violence lies at the intersection of multiple independent factors with aggression being the final common pathway.
3. Risk factors flow from issues arising within the individual, the family, the community and society.
4. When it comes to violence, families can be significantly preventative or significantly causative.
5. An awareness of the special vulnerability of young people toward violence is critical.
6. The growth of 'mega-cities' presents a special challenge and risk of violence.

Review

1. What does the process of unlearning violence require?
2. How do risk factors leading to violence arise?
3. How can families cause violent behavior?
4. What factors and behaviors have been proven to help prevent violence?
5. What is the relationship between urbanization and violence?

Online Resources

 Access online resources with this book's CD.

Youth Violence
http://www.cdc.gov/ncipc/factsheets/yvfacts.htm#risk

The Effects of Community Violence on Children and Adolescents
http://www.ncptsd.va.gov/facts/specific/fs_child_com_viol.html

Youth Violence: A Report of the Surgeon General
http://www.surgeongeneral.gov/library/youthviolence/summary.ht
m#PublicHealth

Health Politics Online

For Original Health Politics Programs and Slides:

Violence: Part 2 - Risk Factors
http://www.healthpolitics.com/program_info.asp?p=prog_23
Slide Briefing
http://www.healthpolitics.com/media/prog_23/brief_prog_23.pdf

CHAPTER 5.4

Violence
Prevention

A MATTER OF PUBLIC HEALTH

Prevention of violence is a public health imperative. Dr. Rudolf Virchow, one of the early founders of public health, recognized that a health professional's skills could be scaled up to the benefit of populations. In his words, "Medicine is a social science. And politics is simply medicine on a large scale."

Making public policy is largely about setting priorities and wisely allocating resources. Consider the case for public policy and violence. A $1 million investment in prison space will prevent 50 crimes. A $1 million investment in management of juvenile delinquents will prevent 72 crimes. And a $1 million investment in assistance and advocacy for high school graduation will prevent 258 crimes.[1]

Prevention costs money, but so does violence. It has been estimated that, on average, developed countries consume 4 percent of their gross national product (GNP) on violence, while developing countries expend 14 percent of their GNP.[2] One dollar in intervention in the United States saves seven dollars in interdiction.[1] In fact, the annual direct-care costs related to violence in the United States are a staggering $224 billion.[3] Over $12 billion alone is expended to care for children who are physically assaulted.[4] The secondary costs are difficult to even imagine when one considers the cost of the justice system, the loss of tourism, investment and productivity, and the long-term mental health issues for victims and witnesses alike.[2]

Violence is a repetitive, recurrent behavioral disease with a wide array of victims. For a victim of violence, there is a 40 percent chance of a recurrent attack, and 20 percent chance that the attack will result in death.[5] The impact of violence extends to victims, witnesses and perpetrators. Disability extends beyond the physical and includes ongoing fear, anxiety and depression, and often secondary violence to self and others.[6]

That violence is insolvable is a myth. What is true is that violence is too complex to tie to a single solution. Strategies must be tailored.[7] There are a number of ways to subdivide violence prevention to make it more manageable. One can think of categories of prevention, including universal strategies like perinatal care offered to everyone; selective strategies directed at at-risk populations, such as witness-support programs; and indicated programs, such as mental health interventions for victims of rape.

An equally valid approach is to subdivide by location. School-based programs might include conflict-resolution training, violence-prevention counseling, social-competence development, bullying reduction and drug and alcohol education. Family-focused strategies might include parent education, family therapy, preschool programs, home visitation and paid time-off leaves. Community-wide programs might include mentoring, supervised recreation, community policing and surveillance, web-based self-help groups, and proactive programs to address inequality and prejudice.[8]

Table 5.4-1. Violence-Prevention Strategies

School-Based	Family-Focused	Community-Wide
• Conflict-resolution training • Violence-prevention counseling • Social competence development • Bullying reduction • Drug and alcohol education	• Parent education • Family therapy • Pre-school programs • Home visitation • Paid time-off leave	• Mentoring • Supervised recreation • Community policing and surveillance • Web-based self-help groups • Addressing gender inequality and cultural and ethnic prejudice

Source: Roth JA, Moore MH. Reducing Violent Crimes and Intentional Injuries.
U.S. Department of Justice, October 1995.

If violence is complex and multifunctional in nature, it is also cultural in context. The staggeringly out-of-proportion toll of gun-related homicides and suicides in the United States must be examined within the cultural context of the historic right to bear arms, the extraordinary prevalence of violence and fear as central to the nation's media broadcasting and its definition of "entertainment," and an aggressive form of capitalism with dramatic highs and lows.

This is quite different from addressing domestic violence in Ghana, where nearly 50 percent of the population agrees that husbands are justified in beating their wives if the wife uses contraception without the husband's consent.[9] The point is that violence is both complex and contextual, and therefore the solutions must be multifaceted and carefully tailored and targeted by professionals on the ground and in the know.

There is no simple answer to violence. But there are some general interventional principles upon which most experts agree.[4] These include:

- First, raising awareness, through education, the arts, political dialogue, or whatever means are available.

- Second, promote economic development, because people with jobs, and families with financial security, have higher self-esteem and are less aggressive.

- Third, expand social science research so that we might better describe, analyze and address the scope of violent behaviors.

- Fourth, involve health professionals who work at the grassroots level, are well-respected, and readily understand complex, multigenerational issues that touch individual, family, community and society.

- Fifth, support peer-to-peer education (victim-to-victim, witness-to-witness, perpetrator-to-perpetrator), because it has proven to be both effective and cost-effective.

- Sixth, challenge the entitlement to violence. In developed and developing nations, there is an obvious need to raise the level of intolerance of, and revulsion to, violence.

- Seventh, start intervention at age minus one. Parental skill training, including nurturing, nutrition, education, socialization and child discipline, should begin in the prenatal period and continue through the first five years of life.

- Eighth, break the silence. Denial allows destructive behaviors to become regimented and inbred.

- Ninth, support non-violent recreation and immersion in nature. Peace is a product of exposure to goodness.

- And tenth, support victims, not simply because it is right, but to disrupt a cycle of violence that has no end.

Violence prevention is about collective interest, mutually beneficial rules, mutual assistance, shared prosperity, and hope for the future. Violence is always a second choice, when cooperation has failed.

REFERENCES

1. North CS, Nixon SJ, Shariat S, et al. Psychiatric disorders among survivors of the Oklahoma City bombing. *JAMA*. 1999;282:755-762.
2. Kilgour, D. Pathways To Safer Communities: Rethinking Crime Prevention. Available at: www.david-kilgour.com/speeches/crime2.htm. Accessed March 12, 2001.
3. Bonnemaison G. Crime Prevention Digest 1997. International Center for the Prevention of Crime.
4. Healthy People 2010: Understanding and Improving Health. 2nd ed. Washington, DC: U.S. Department of Health and Human Services; November 2000.
5. WHO. WHO recognizes child abuse as a major public health problem [press release.] Geneva, Switz; WHO; April 8, 1999.
6. Goins WA, Thompson J, Simpkins C. Recurrent intentional injury. *J. Natl Med Assoc*. 1992;84:431-435.
7. Roth JA, Moore MH. Reducing Violent Crimes and Intentional Injuries. Washington, DC: U.S. Department of Justice, October 1995. (Publication NCJ 156089).
8. American Academy of Pediatrics. The role of the pediatrician in youth violence prevention in clinical practice and at the community level (RE9832). *Pediatrics*. 1999;103:173-181.
9. UN Population Fund. Ending Violence Against Women and Girls. Available at: http://www.unfpa.org/swp/2000/english/ch03.htm. Accessed March 6, 2001.

TEACHING TOOLS

Policy Premises

1. Prevention of violence is a public health imperative.
2. Prevention costs money but so does violence.
3. Violence is a repetitive, recurrent disease with a wide array of victims.
4. That violence is insolvable is a myth.
5. In addressing violence, cultural context must be considered.
6. There is no simple solution for prevention of violence.

Review

1. What is the annual direct-care cost related to violence in the United States?
2. What percent chance is there of a recurrent attack on a victim of violence?
3. What are some family-focused strategies to combat violence?
4. How is violence cultural in context?
5. What are four interventional principles to address violence?

Online Resources

 Access online resources with this book's CD.

Violence Prevention
http://www.ama-assn.org/ama/pub/category/3242.html

On the Nature of Violence
http://www.americanscientist.org/template/AssetDetail/assetid/14688

National Center for Injury Prevention and Control: Division of Violence Prevention
http://www.cdc.gov/ncipc/dvp/dvp.htm

The Spectrum of Prevention: Developing a Comprehensive Approach to Injury Prevention
http://www.preventioninstitute.org/spectrum_injury.html

Cost and Benefits of Programs to Reduce Crime
http://www.wsipp.wa.gov/

Health Politics Online

For Original Health Politics Programs and Slides:

Violence: Part 3 – Prevention
http://www.healthpolitics.com/program_info.asp?p=prog_24
Slide Briefing
http://www.healthpolitics.com/media/prog_24/brief_prog_24.pdf

CHAPTER 5.5

Bullying

A WORTHWHILE TARGET IN PURSUING PEACE

The creation of peaceful, civil societies requires early investment and reinforcement of nonviolent behavior. Many see peace as the absence of war. But in fact, peace is much more than that. The creation of peaceful citizens is no accident. Citizens choose not to be violent when they possess seven gemstones of peace — mental and physical health, education, opportunity, tolerance, positive conflict resolution, cooperation, and self-esteem. These echo the United Nations' Millennium Development Goals, which were agreed upon in 2000.[1]

One great example of the seven gemstones at work is a program started by the American Medical Association Alliance 10 years ago called SAVE, Stop America's Violence Everywhere. This grassroots program has addressed many forms of violence over the years, but recently it has identified one problem in particular that we all need to pay more attention to: Bullying among children. The AMA Alliance's effort rightly recognizes that our children are the key to a peaceful future. As AMA Alliance President Jean Howard said, "No community is immune to violence. Everyone deserves a safe place to learn and grow. If we want a peaceful society, we must all work together to create an environment of tolerance and peace early in life."[2]

How big a problem is childhood violence? Aggressive violent behavior is pervasive in America's schools. A 2001 study of nearly 16,000 sixth- to 10th- graders in U.S. public and private schools revealed that nearly 9 percent of the children were involved in frequent bullying. Males were more common offenders than females with approximately 13 percent involved, compared with 5 percent of girls. There was very little difference between whites, blacks, and hispanics.[3]

Bullying is a unique form of aggression because it causes long-term damage to both source and target. Both bullies and the bullied often suffer from poor psycho-social functioning. Both show poor academic performance, poor relationship building, and loneliness. Bullies have high rates of discipline problems, usually dislike school, and are more likely to use drugs and alcohol. Bullied kids are more likely to suffer depression and anxiety. By their 20s, former bullies and those who have been bullied are likely to continue to suffer consequences. Bullies have four times the rate of criminal behavior as non-bullies in adulthood, with 60 percent having at least one conviction. Those who were bullied have higher levels of adult depression and poor self-esteem.[4,5]

The rates of bullied children roughly mirror the rates of their tormentors. The behavior is most common in the sixth grade, with rates slowly declining by the 10th grade. Still, in grade 10, nearly 7 percent are bullies and nearly 5 percent are still victimized.[3]

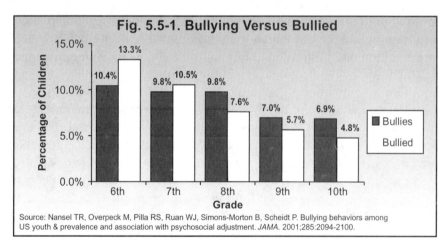

Fig. 5.5-1. Bullying Versus Bullied

Source: Nansel TR, Overpeck M, Pilla RS, Ruan WJ, Simons-Morton B, Scheidt P. Bullying behaviors among US youth & prevalence and association with psychosocial adjustment. *JAMA*. 2001;285:2094-2100.

Both males and females are bullied, but in somewhat different ways. Males are more likely to be physically attacked. They report being physically bullied nearly 18 percent of the time, compared with 11 percent in females. Verbal violence takes multiple forms, including attacking one's looks or speech, attacking religion or race, spreading false rumors, or making sexual comments or gestures — the latter somewhat more common among females.[3]

Bullying is a double-edged sword slicing away at the fabric of society. What can be done to identify those involved and intervene early? Clearly, post-Columbine, most realize that bullying is not just "kids being kids."[2,6] The risk factors for bullies include poverty, overcrowding, disadvantaged schools, difficult childhood temperaments, inadequate parenting, poor socialization skills, and poor school performance. An especially high-risk group exists among those who experience social isolation, difficulties with learning, and a history of problematic behavior. Such individuals often have a history of being, first, bullied, and then becoming bullies. These individuals have been labeled "provocative victims" who exhibit both anxious and aggressive behaviors.[3,5]

What are some of the warning signs? They include unpredictable temper and mood swings; loneliness and depression; vandalism and arson; gun availability and preoccupation with weapons; threats of violence to self, others and animals; gang affiliation; and absence of parental supervision.[3,4]

Table 5.5-1. Identifying Bullying Before It Begins

Risk Factors	Warning Signs
• Poverty • Overcrowding • Disadvantaged schools • Difficult temperaments • Inadequate parenting • Poor socialization skills • Poor school performance	• Temper/mood swings • Loneliness/depression • Vandalism/arson • Gun availability/preoccupation with weapons • Threats of violence to self or others • Gang affiliation • No supervision

Source: SAVE Planning Guide. American Medical Association Alliance. Chicago, 2004.
Nansel TR, Overpeck M, Pilla RS, Ruan WJ, Simons-Morton B, Scheidt P. Bullying behaviors among US youth – prevalence and association with psychosocial adjustment.*JAMA*. 2001;285:2094-2100.
American Medical Association. Report 11 of the Council on Scientific Affairs (I-99). School Violence.

The AMA Alliance's Stop America's Violence Everywhere program reminds us that there is much to be done, and that we all have a role in this society-wide, grassroots effort to assist those who are the source and those who are the victims of childhood violence.[2]

School principals can enforce zero-tolerance policies, devise guidelines on how violence should be handled, and encourage parental involvement. Students can report violence, serve as peer mentors, and participate in violence-prevention programs. Parents can be role models for nonviolence, ensure firearm safety and security if firearms are in their homes, and be accessible to their children. Teachers can work with parents to recognize early warning signs of trouble, report problems when they are still correctable, and practice conflict resolution in their classrooms. Legislators can pass laws to ensure responsible gun control, mandate full health and mental health coverage (that includes children), and fund early intervention and violence-prevention programs. And non-profit organizations, including churches, synagogues and mosques, can together champion social tolerance, community coalitions, and parenting classes.[2]

Peace is not the absence of war. We have to work together for peace and create an environment where tolerance and mutual support are realistic alternatives to hatred and violence.

REFERENCES

1. We the peoples…A Call to Action for the UN Millennium Declaration. New York, World Federation of United Nations Associations (WFUNA), 2002.
2. SAVE Planning Guide. American Medical Association Alliance. Chicago, 2004.
3. Nansel TR, Overpeck M, Pilla RS, Ruan WJ, Simons-Morton B, Scheidt P. Bullying behaviors among US youth - prevalence and association with psychosocial adjustment. *JAMA*. 2001;285:2094-2100.
4. Twemlow SW. Preventing violence in schools. *Psychiatric Times*. 2004;21. Available at: http://www.psychiatrictimes.com/p040461.html. Accessed Oct. 4, 2004.
5. Olweus D. Bullying at school: long-term outcomes for the victims and an effective school-based intervention program. In: Huesmann LR, ed. Aggressive Behavior: Current Perspectives. New York, NY: Plenum Press; 1994:97-130. Cited in Nansel TR, Overpeck M, Pilla RS, Ruan WJ, Simons-Morton B, Scheidt P.
6. American Medical Association. Report 11 of the Council on Scientific Affairs (I-99). School Violence. Available at: http://www.ama-assn.org/ama/pub/article/print/2036-2512.html.

TEACHING TOOLS

Policy Premises

1. Creation of peaceful, civil societies requires early investment and reinforcement of nonviolent behavior.
2. Aggressive, violent behavior is pervasive in America's schools.
3. Bullying is a unique form of aggression causing long-term damage to both the source and the target.
4. Males and females are involved, but in somewhat different ways.
5. Those at risk can be identified and must be helped. Post-Columbine, most realize it's not "kids being kids."
6. There is much that can be done but it requires a society-wide, grassroots effort.

Review

1. What is the purpose of the AMA Alliance's program called "Stop America's Violence Everywhere" (SAVE)?
2. How many children are involved in frequent bullying?
3. What are the differences in the ways males and females bully?
4. What makes bullying such a unique form of aggression?
5. What are the risk factors and warning signs associated with bullies?

Online Resources

Access online resources with this book's CD.

Headed for Trouble
http://www.cnn.com/2003/EDUCATION/09/04/sprj.sch.bullying.prevention.ap/

Tackling Bullying
http://www.dfes.gov.uk/bullying/pdf/Childline%20DP%20Bullying%20(download).pdf

How to Stop Bullying
http://www.education-world.com/a_special/bully.shtml

Intervene Early to Prevent Bullying Behavior
http://www.aacap.org/publications/factsFam/80.htm

Understanding Violent Behavior in Children and Adolescents
http://www.aacap.org/publications/factsFam/behavior.htm

Bully Busting
http://ianrpubs.unl.edu/family/nf309.htm

Back to School
http://www.nmha.org/pbedu/backtoschool/bullying.cfm

Bullying and Your Child
http://kidshealth.org/parent/emotions/feelings/bullies.html

Health Politics Online

For Original Health Politics Programs and Slides:

Bullying: A Worthwhile Target for Peace
http://www.healthpolitics.com/program_info.asp?p=prog_67
Slide Briefing
http://www.healthpolitics.com/media/prog_67/brief_prog_67.pdf

CHAPTER 5.6

Guns, Kids and Suicide

STARTING WITH THE HOME

Suicide is a significant threat to adolescents and young adults. In 2002, there were more than 30,000 suicides in the United States, making suicides nearly twice as common as homicides.[1] When we consider how many of these were young people, the numbers become even more powerful. Suicide is the fourth leading cause of death for children age 10 to 14, and the third leading cause of death for young adults age 15 to 24.[2] According to a study from the Centers for Disease Control and Prevention, 27 percent of high school students have thought about suicide and 8 percent have attempted it.[3]

The risk factors for teen suicide are well known. Triggers include divorce, family violence, bullying, breakdown of the family unit, and undue stress to succeed. Fifty percent of all teen suicide victims have a history of drug and alcohol abuse. Many suffer depression with low self-esteem, confusion, personal turmoil, and a perception or reality of lives in chaos. Gender conflicts, especially in males, are a significant contributor. About 5 percent of adolescent males consider themselves gay, and non-heterosexual youth are two-to-seven times more likely to attempt suicide than their heterosexual peers.[4] According to the American Academy of Pediatrics, communication problems between parents and their kids are also a significant contributor. One study found that 90 percent of suicidal adolescents believed their families did not understand them. They felt alone and isolated and believed their parents either denied or ignored their attempts to bridge the communication gap.[5]

On top of all this, it's well known that the presence of guns is also associated with an increased risk of suicide.[5,6] In 2002, more than 1,000 children in the United States, age 20 and younger, died of firearm suicide. When these deaths are analyzed, it is clear that guns were readily available. Seventy-five percent of the guns used were stored in the homes of the children or the home of a friend or relative.[7]

Despite this statistic, guns are exceedingly common in American homes with children. Thirty-five percent of U.S. homes with children under 18 have at least one firearm. Nearly half of these firearms are unlocked and potentially accessible to children.[8] To deal with this, 18 states have enacted Child Access Prevention laws. These laws hold gun owners responsible if they leave guns easily accessible to children, and a child improperly gains access to the weapon. The laws require safe gun storage practices including locking the gun, locking ammunition, keeping guns unloaded, and separating guns and ammunition.[7,9,10]

Safe storage of guns clearly makes gun suicides among children less likely. The National Shooting Sports Foundation has stepped up to the plate with this counsel for families who keep guns in their homes for protection against potential intruders: "Keeping a gun to defend your family makes no sense if that same gun puts your family members or visitors to your home at risk. Many home firearm accidents occur when unauthorized individuals, often visitors, discover loaded firearms that were carelessly left out in the open ... Special lockable cases that can be quickly opened only by authorized individuals are options to consider."[11]

The epicenter for prevention of gun suicides among young people is clearly the home. First, American families need to recognize that childhood, adolescence and the teen years carry with them great turmoil, disassociation, and vulnerability. Active positive engagement, physical presence, and oversight all make sense, along with ongoing communication and guidance.

The American Academy of Pediatrics says parents should watch closely for signs that their teen might be struggling. Has the child's personality changed dramatically? Are there troubles with friends? Is the quality of schoolwork declining? Is she bored and having trouble concentrating? Is he rebelling in an unexplainable or severe way? Has eating and sleeping changed? Has general appearance changed for the worse?[2] Talk with your child, and seek professional help if it's necessary.

And, lastly, if a gun is to be kept in the home, it's the parents' responsibility to make sure it is safe and securely out of grasp of other family members. The studies and statistics I've mentioned have established that if you keep a gun for protection and prefer to keep it within your easy reach, it is also within the reach of your child, and that could be an extraordinarily costly mistake.

REFERENCES

1. Centers for Disease Control and Prevention. National Center for Injury Prevention and Control. Suicide: Fact Sheet. Available at: http://www.cdc.gov/ncipc/factsheets/suifacts.htm. Accessed May 9, 2005.
2. American Academy of Pediatrics. Some Things You Should Know About Preventing Teen Suicide. Available at: www.aap.org/advocacy/childhealthmonth/prevteensuicide.htm. Accessed May 9, 2005.
3. American Academy of Pediatrics. Understanding Teen Suicide. Available at: www.aap.org/pubed/zzzqzubvr7c.htm?&sub_cat=1. Accessed May 9, 2005.
4. American Academy of Pediatrics. Adolescents Should Feel Safe Discussing Sexual Orientation With Their Pediatrician. Available at: www.aap.org/advocacy/releases/juneorientation.htm. Accessed May 9, 2005.
5. Grossman DC, Mueller BA, Riedy C, Dowd MD, Villaveces A, et al. Gun storage practices and risk of youth suicide and unintentional firearm injuries. *JAMA*. 2005;293:707-714.
6. Kellermann A, Rivara F, Somes G, et al. Suicide in the home in relation to gun ownership. *NEJM*. 1992;327:467-472. Cited in Grossman DC, Mueller BA, Riedy C, Dowd MD, Villaveces A, et al.
7. Cole TB, Johnson RM. Storing guns safely in homes with children and adolescents. *JAMA*. 2005;293:740-741.
8. Stennies G, Ideda R, Leadbetter S, Houston B, Sacks J. Firearm storage practices and children in the home, United States, 1994. *Arch Pediatr Adolesc Med*. 1999;153:586-590. Cited in Grossman DC, Mueller BA, Riedy C, Dowd MD, Villaveces A, et al.
9. Webster DW, Vernick JS, Zeoli AM, Manganello JA. Association between youth-focused firearm laws and youth suicide. *JAMA*. 2004;292:594-601. Cited in Cole TB, Johnson RM.
10. American Academy of Pediatrics. Firearms Injury Prevention. Available at: http://www.aap.org/family/tipp-firearms.htm. Accessed

May 9, 2005.

11. National Shooting Sports Foundation. Firearms responsibility in the home. Available at: www.nssf.org/safety/FRH/FRH_3home_security.cfm?Aol=generic. Accessed May 9, 2005.

TEACHING TOOLS

Policy Premises

1. Suicide is a significant threat to adolescents and young adults.
2. Risk factors for teen suicide are well-known.
3. Guns predispose young people to suicide.
4. Guns are common in American homes with children.
5. Many states have laws regulating safe storage of guns in homes.
6. Safe storage of guns makes suicide for children less likely.

Review

1. How common is suicide among teenagers?
2. What are some of the risk factors for teen suicide?
3. How many American homes have guns?
4. How many children and teenagers died from gun suicides in 2002?
5. What should parents do if they think their child is depressed or contemplating suicide?

Online Resources

Access online resources with this book's CD.

Teen Suicide
http://kidshealth.org/teen/your_mind/mental_health/suicide.html

Child Access Prevention Laws
http://www.jhsph.edu/PublicHealthNews/Press_Releases/PR_2004/Webster_youthsuicide.html

Youth Suicide Risk Factors
http://www.safeyouth.org/scripts/faq/suiciderisks.asp

Youth Suicide Prevention: On the State Level
http://www.nga.org/cda/files/0504suicideprevention.pdf

It's OK to Talk About It
http://msnbc.msn.com/id/7394123/

Stop the Trend
http://www.aap.org/advocacy/childhealthmonth/prevteensuicide.htm

National Youth Risk Behavior Survey (YRBS)
http://www.cdc.gov/HealthyYouth/yrbs/pdfs/trends-suicide.pdf

Teens and Depression
http://my.webmd.com/content/article/45/1663_51231.htm?z=1663_00
000_0000_rl_05

Health Politics Online

For Original Health Politics Programs and Slides:

The Connection Between Guns and Teen Suicide
http://www.healthpolitics.com/program_info.asp?p=teen_suici
Slide Briefing
http://www.healthpolitics.com/media/teen_suicide/brief_teen_sui-
cide.pdf

The Hidden Cost of War in Iraq

MENTAL ILLNESS

It has been well-established for some time that post-traumatic stress disorder and other mental health illnesses are a predictable outcome of war. However, a landmark study in the *New England Journal of Medicine* of U.S. troops in Iraq has, for the first time, documented this hidden cost of war in real time and projected a continued price for Americans in the years ahead.[1]

As noted by the authors from the Walter Reed Army Institute of Research, "Research conducted after...military conflicts has shown that deployment stressors and exposure to combat result in considerable risks of mental health problems, including post-traumatic stress disorder (PTSD), major depression, substance abuse, impairment in social functioning and in the ability to work, and the increased use of health care services."[1]

This study, completed in 2004, is unique because it compares rates of mental disorders in soldiers before they were deployed to Iraq with rates of mental disorders in soldiers after they had returned from Iraq. Roughly 2,500 soldiers were studied prior to deployment and 1,709 were studied several months after their return. The percentage of soldiers with mental-health issues prior to war was 9.3 percent, compared with about 16 percent after returning from Iraq.[1]

The demographics of the study participants were very similar to those of the general, deployed, non-officer population in Iraq. Most of the study participants were young males, under 30 years old, with a high school education or less.

According to responses, PTSD is the most prevalent of the mental ill-nesses experienced by soldiers returning from the Iraq war. This is consistent with findings from studies of soldiers involved in past wars. While PTSD occurs in the general population at a rate of 3 percent to 4 percent, past studies have shown that Vietnam veterans were affected at a rate of 15 percent, and veterans of the first Gulf War experienced PTSD 2 percent to 10 percent of the time.[2,3,4]

The incidence of PTSD in U.S. soldiers returning from Iraq was directly related to the intensity of their wartime experience. The greater the number of firefights encountered, the greater the incidence of PTSD. Those unexposed to firefights had a PTSD incidence rate of 4.5 percent, close to that in the general population. That rate more than doubled to 9.3 percent if a soldier saw significant firefighting once or twice. Three to five firefights yielded an incidence of PTSD of 13 percent, and greater than five exposures brought the incidence rate to nearly 20 percent.[1]

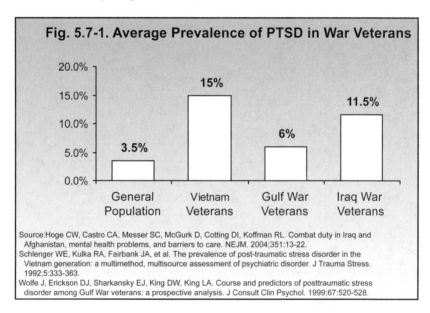

Fig. 5.7-1. Average Prevalence of PTSD in War Veterans

Source:Hoge CW, Castro CA, Messer SC, McGurk D, Cotting DI, Koffman RL. Combat duty in Iraq and Afghanistan, mental health problems, and barriers to care. NEJM. 2004;351:13-22.
Schlenger WE, Kulka RA, Fairbank JA, et al. The prevalence of post-traumatic stress disorder in the Vietnam generation: a multimethod, multisource assessment of psychiatric disorder. J Trauma Stress. 1992;5:333-363.
Wolfe J, Erickson DJ, Sharkansky EJ, King DW, King LA. Course and predictors of posttraumatic stress disorder among Gulf War veterans: a prospective analysis. J Consult Clin Psychol. 1999;67:520-528.

And these numbers, in the opinion of the authors of the study, are likely to be somewhat understated, not only because the prevalence of PTSD may increase during the two years after exposure to trauma, but also because of soldiers' fears of repercussions. Even among soldiers with no mental-health symptoms, general distrust and perceived barriers to seeking mental-health services were obvious. Eighteen percent of these study participants reported they would be too embarrassed to seek mental-health services. Twenty-four percent felt admitting a problem could hurt their careers, and 31 percent felt they would be seen as weak.[1]

Even more striking were the findings related to the soldiers with active mental-health issues. Thirty-eight percent answered that they lack trust in mental-health professionals, 41 percent said they would be embarrassed to seek help, half felt seeking help would damage their careers, and 65 percent feared being labeled as weak.[1]

Together, the incidence of mental illness and the stigma and barriers to treatment create a Catch-22 for today's Iraq war veterans. As stated by Dr. Matthew J. Friedman of the National Center for PTSD at the Department of Veterans Affairs, "The sticking point is skepticism among military personnel that the use of mental-health services can remain confidential."[5]

Nearly 30 percent of male civilians with a mental health disorder seek treatment, but fewer than 20 percent of servicemen with a mental health disorder seek treatment.[5] This is remarkably unfortunate since it is well-established that both cognitive and pharmacologic therapies can help those with PTSD.

PTSD is a price of war. Its cost to everyone involved is chronic in nature. At the least, those affected deserve intensive therapy without fear of reprisal. At the most, those affected should expect that this cost, as well as many others, would be honestly and carefully considered and fully factored in as a part of war before military action is taken and people are placed in harm's way.

REFERENCES

1. Hoge CW, Castro CA, Messer SC, McGurk D, Cotting DI, Koffman RL. Combat duty in Iraq and Afghanistan, mental health problems, and barriers to care. *NEJM*. 2004;351:13-22.
2. Narrow WE, Rae DS, Robins LN, Regier DA. Revised prevalence estimates of mental disorders in the United States: using a clinical significance criterion to reconcile 2 surveys' estimates. *Arch Gen Psychiatry*. 2002;59:115-123. Cited in Hoge CW, Castro CA, Messer SC, McGurk D, Cotting DI, Koffman RL.
3. Schlenger WE, Kulka RA, Fairbank JA, et al. The prevalence of post-traumatic stress disorder in the Vietnam generation: a multimethod, multisource assessment of psychiatric disorder. *J Trauma Stress*.

1992;5:333-363.

4. Wolfe J, Erickson DJ, Sharkansky EJ, King DW, King LA. Course and predictors of posttraumatic stress disorder among Gulf War veterans: a prospective analysis. *J Consult Clin Psychol.* 1999;67:520-528.

5. Friedman MJ. Acknowledging the psychiatric cost of war. *NEJM.* 2004;351:75-77.

TEACHING TOOLS

Policy Premises

1. Post-traumatic stress disorder is a predictable outcome for combatants in war.
2. An assessment of mental-health issues in U.S. soldiers in Iraq was published in 2004.
3. U.S. soldiers in Iraq are predominantly male, non-college educated, and 37 percent non-white.
4. The majority in the study were exposed to significant traumatic events.
5. The incidence of PTSD was linearly related to number of firefights.
6. The majority of soldiers with PTSD are currently resistant to seeking help.

Review

1. According to a recent study, what is the percentage of mental illness in U.S. soldiers before deployment to Iraq, compared with the percentage after they return?
2. Which mental illness is the most prevalent among soldiers returning from Iraq?
3. What intensified soldiers' wartime experience and raised the incidence rate of PTSD?
4. What percentage of soldiers said they felt seeking professional help would damage their careers?
5. What percentage of servicemen with a mental health disorder seek treatment?

Online Resources

Access online resources with this book's CD.

The National Center for PTSD
http://www.ncptsd.va.gov/

Army Uncovers Mental Health Service Gap
http://www.apa.org/monitor/julaug04/army.html

Coping with the Stress of War
http://www.msnbc.msn.com/id/5425543/

Military Families Criticize Mental Health Treatment for Soldiers
http://www.medillnewsdc.com/cgi-bin/ultimatebb.cgi?ubb=get_topic&f=14&t=000207

Army Analyzes GI Suicide Rate
http://www.cbsnews.com/stories/2004/03/25/iraq/main608559.shtml?CMP=ILC-SearchStories

Avoiding PTSD
http://www.apa.org/releases/posttraumastress.html

Health Politics Online

For Original Health Politics Programs and Slides:

Mental Illness: The Hidden Cost of War in Iraq
http://www.healthpolitics.com/program_info.asp?p=prog_60
Slide Briefing
http://www.healthpolitics.com/media/prog_60/brief_prog_60.pdf

CHAPTER 5.8

Road Safety

A PUBLIC HEALTH ISSUE

Some of the greatest opportunity for gains in public health can be found in a surprising place — the world's roadways. Dr. Lee Jong-wook, director general of the World Health Organization, notes that "too often, road safety is treated as a transportation issue, not a public health issue, and road-traffic injuries are called accidents, though most could be prevented. As a result, many countries put far less effort into understanding and preventing road-traffic injuries than they do into understanding and preventing diseases that do less harm."[1]

It is estimated that 140,000 injuries occur on roads worldwide each day. Fifteen thousand people are disabled as a result, and 3,000 die.[1] In the year 2000, 1.26 million people were killed in roadway accidents, accounting for 25 percent of all deaths from injury that year.[2]

Roadway safety is not just a transportation issue. It is a public health issue that is getting worse. In 1990, roadway injuries were the ninth-leading cause of death and disability worldwide. But by 2020, that ranking is projected to shoot to number three, just behind ischemic heart disease and unipolar depression. The change in rank is based on a projection that roadway injuries will increase by 60 percent in 30 years if current trends continue.[3]

The burden of unsafe roads falls most heavily on the most vulnerable. The death rate from road injuries in high-income countries was 12.6 deaths per 100,000 citizens in 2002. The rate in low-income and middle-income countries was 60 percent higher at 20.2 deaths per 100,000 citizens, which accounted for 90 percent of death and disability from roadway injuries in

2002. And children, especially poor children who often use roads as play areas, are at great risk. More than 180,000 children die from roadway injuries every year. In 2002, 96 percent of these deaths occurred in low-income or middle-income countries.[1]

Table 5.8-1. Global Burden of Disease Top 10

1990	2020
1. Lower respiratory infections	1. Ischemic heart disease
2. Diarrheal diseases	2. Unipolar depression
3. Perinatal conditions	**3. Road traffic injuries**
4. Unipolar depression	4. Cerebrovascular disease
5. Ischemic heart disease	5. Chronic obstructive pulmonary
6. Cerebrovascular disease	disease
7. Tuberculosis	6. Lower respiratory infections
8. Measles	7. Tuberculosis
9. Road traffic injuries	8. War injuries
10. Congenital abnormalities	9. Diarrheal diseases
	10. HIV

Source: Murray CJL, Lopez AD, eds. [Table]. The global burden of disease: a comprehensive assessment of mortality and disability from diseases, injuries, and risk factors in 1990 and projected to 2020. Boston, Harvard University Press, 1996.

How roads are used, and by whom, varies widely from country to country. Roads in high-income countries are dominated by cars, while low- and middle-income nations utilize roads as shared space. In this shared space there are large numbers of more vulnerable roadway users, such as pedestrians, bicyclists, and motorbike riders. Intermixed with passenger vans, mini buses, cars, and trucks, these more vulnerable users suffer a rate of injury and death many times greater than drivers of cars, thus contributing to the higher death rates in low-income countries.[1,4]

Thanks, in part, to the leadership of a unique cross-sector health-advocacy group called the Bone and Joint Decade, road safety is emerging as a major focus of the international public-health community. The group has teamed with Dr. Mark Rosenberg, executive director of the United Nations' Task Force for Child Survival and Development, giving their cause a potent catalytic force. They succeeded in getting the topic of road safety on the U.N.'s General Assembly agenda in 2004. Dr. Rosenberg commented, "At the start of this project, we had been told that it would take no less than five years to put road safety on the U.N. agenda; by convening the right players and fostering a successful collaborative effort, we have been able to accomplish this — and more — in less than one year."[5]

The group also captured the imagination of the world health community by declaring "Road Safety is No Accident" as the official slogan of World Health Day 2004. As Kofi Annan, secretary-general of the United Nations, said, "Improving road safety requires strong political will on the part of governments. In a systems approach, not only the driver, but also the environment (infrastructure) and the vehicle are seen as part of the system in which road traffic injuries occur."[2]

As we've seen time and time again, good health makes good financial sense as well. The estimated cost of roadway injuries worldwide is $520 billion per year. In low-income and middle-income countries, roadway injuries cost $65 billion, which is more than developing countries receive in development aid.[1]

The causes of roadway accidents are increasingly clear, as are the solutions. Mixed roadway use and poor road design play a significant role, especially in poor and urban environments. Excessive speed, reckless driving, and poor visibility contribute to the likelihood of disaster. And the lack of reasonable regulation and enforceable laws results in poor vehicle maintenance, failure to use seat belts, air bags, and helmets, and improper handling of hazardous materials. Lastly, the absence of adequate health infrastructure and trauma care maximizes the impact of injury. [1,4,6]

Table 5.8-2. Roadway Accidents

Causes	Solutions

• Mixed road use
• Poor road design
• Excessive speed, reckless driving
• Poor visibility
• Poor vehicle maintenance
• Non-use of seatbelts
• No air bags
• Non-use of helmets
• Hazardous materials
• Lack of infrastructure/trauma care
	• Community and road design
	  — Safe crossings
	  — Road user segregation
	• Public transportation
	• Speed control
	  — Road bumps and round-abouts
	• Better automobile design
	• Enforced automobile safety standards
	• Passenger rules
	  — Seat belt use
	  — Children in rear seats
	  — Helmet use
	  — Cell phone bans
	• Health infrastructure expansion
	• Response capacity

Source: World Health Organization. "Road Safety is No Accident: A Brochure for World Health Day 7 April 2004." Geneva. 2004. Nantulya VM, Reich, MR. Equity dimensions of road traffic injuries in low- and middle-income countries. *Injury control and Safety Promotion.* 2003;10:13-20.
Afukaar FK. Speed control in developing countries: issues, challenges and opportunities in reducing road traffic injuries. *Injury control and Safety Promotion.* 2003;10:77-81.

The solution lies in a highly coordinated, multifaceted planning and execution effort involving governments, public-health leaders, corporations, communities, and citizens. Where to focus? Some high-yield areas include better community and road design with safe crossing zones and deliberate segregation of pedestrians, bikes, small vehicles, and large vehicles. Also, focus should be on maximum use of public transportation; speed control, which can be achieved using road bumps and round-abouts in high-risk areas; better automobile design; and well-enforced automobile safety standards. Passenger rules should be enforced, including seat belt use, placement of children in rear seats only, helmet use, and bans on cell phones while driving.[1,6]

Finally, expanding health infrastructure and capacity to respond to road trauma when it does occur could decrease both deaths and disability for those injured.

REFERENCES

1. World Health Organization. "Road Safety is No Accident: A Brochure for World Health Day 7 April 2004." Geneva, Switzerland; 2004.
2. Ahead of General Assembly, Annan urges commitment to Road Safety. [press release]. Bone and Joint Decade. September 9, 2003. Available at: http://www.boneandjointdecade.org. Accessed May 14, 2004.
3. Murray CJL, Lopez AD, eds. *The global burden of disease: a comprehensive assessment of mortality and disability from diseases, injuries, and risk factors in 1990 and projected to 2020.* Boston, Harvard University Press, 1996.
4. Nantulya VM, Reich, MR. Equity dimensions of road traffic injuries in low- and middle-income countries. *Injury Control and Safety Promotion.* 2003;10:13-20.
5. United Nations moves towards action on Road Traffic Safety following Bone and Joint Decade proposal. [press release]. Bone and Joint Decade. September 16, 2003. Available at: http://www.boneandjoint-decade.org. Accessed May 14, 2004.
6. Afukaar FK. Speed control in developing countries: issues, challenges and opportunities in reducing road traffic injuries. *Injury Control and Safety Promotion.* 2003;10:77-81.

TEACHING TOOLS

Policy Premises

1. Some of the greatest opportunity for gains in public health lies in a surprising place — the world's roadways.
2. Road safety is not a transportation issue. It's a public health issue that is getting worse.
3. The burden of unsafe roads falls heavily on the shoulders of those most vulnerable.
4. How roads are used, and by whom, varies widely from country to country.
5. 'Road Safety is No Accident' was the official slogan for World Health Day 2004.
6. The causes of roadway accidents are increasingly clear, as are the solutions.

Review

1. How many roadway injuries occur worldwide each day?
2. What is the difference in death rates from road injuries in high-income countries versus low- and middle-income countries?
3. What is the estimated cost of roadway injuries each year?
4. What are some common causes of roadway accidents?
5. Who should be involved with implementing solutions?

Online Resources

Access online resources with this book's CD.

Driving Abroad
http://travel.state.gov/travel/tips/safety/safety_1179.html#safety

World Health Day 2004
http://www.who.int/world-health-day/2004/en/

Condition Control
http://www.bts.gov/publications/national_transportation_statistics/2003/html/table_01_26.html

Path to Safer Roads
http://www.who.int/features/2004/road_safety/en/

Global Road Safety Partnership
http://www.grsproadsafety.org/

A Message From the General Assembly President
http://www.un.org/News/Press/docs/2004/gasm342.doc.htm

Health Politics Online

For Original Health Politics Programs and Slides:

Road Safety: A Public Health Issue
http://www.healthpolitics.com/program_info.asp?p=prog_54
Slide Briefing
http://www.healthpolitics.com/media/prog_54/brief_prog_54.pdf

CHAPTER 5.9

Food Safety

THE EFFECTIVENESS OF IRRADIATION

Foodborne illnesses are a significant problem in the United States and around the world. In 1999, there were 76 million cases of foodborne illnesses in the United States that led to 325,000 hospitalizations and 5,000 deaths. The primary causes fell into two categories: the contamination of produce and the improper cooking, handling and storage of meat and poultry.[1]

Many years ago, U.S. policy recognized the value of pasteurized milk, and public acceptance soon followed. Pasteurization is "the critical reduction of pathogens in a substance, especially a liquid, at a temperature and for a period of time that destroys objectionable organisms without major chemical alteration of the substance or the critical reduction of pathogens in perishable food products with radiation."[2]

Irradiation of food has been approved by all government agencies and carries identical objectives as pasteurization. The process does not make food radioactive nor decrease its nutritional content, yet it remains highly controversial and relatively uncommon in the United States. Only 10 percent of herbs and spices, and a miniscule .002 percent of fruits, vegetables, meat and poultry in the US are irradiated for safety.[3]

Irradiation of food is safe and effective. There are three sources of radiation. Two are electrically generated — x-rays and electron beams. One is the result of radionuclide sources, either cobalt-60 or cesium-137. All three generate energy into food but none of the three transfer radioactivity.[2] In addition, the American Dietetic Association, after extensive studies, supports a Food and Drug Administration finding that, "irradiation poses no important risk to any nutrient in the diet."[4]

The concept of irradiating food dates back 100 years. In 1904, Alan B. Green proved that irradiation can inactivate bacteria. One year later, J. Appleby took out a patent citing the use of irradiation to improve food quality. In 1918, David Gillett patented the use of irradiation to preserve organic material. By 1921, the U.S. Department of Agriculture had proved that irradiation could inactivate the parasite causing trichinosis in pork.[5] In 1938, the landmark Food, Drug and Cosmetic Act was passed and 20 years later language defining the use of irradiation in food was added.[2]

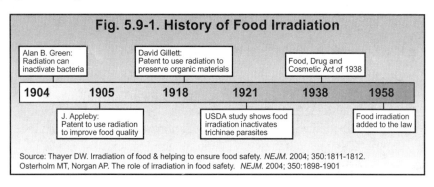

Fig. 5.9-1. History of Food Irradiation

Alan B. Green: Radiation can inactivate bacteria

David Gillett: Patent to use radiation to preserve organic materials

Food, Drug and Cosmetic Act of 1938

| 1904 | 1905 | 1918 | 1921 | 1938 | 1958 |

J. Appleby: Patent to use radiation to improve food quality

USDA study shows food irradiation inactivates trichinae parasites

Food irradiation added to the law

Source: Thayer DW. Irradiation of food & helping to ensure food safety. *NEJM.* 2004; 350:1811-1812. Osterholm MT, Norgan AP. The role of irradiation in food safety. *NEJM.* 2004; 350:1898-1901

In irradiating food, the dose is calibrated to need. The measure of radiation used in food is the kiloGray (kGy). Disinfection of foods to eliminate insects requires less than 1 kGy. Pasteurization can be accomplished with 1 to 10 kGy, while sterilization requires greater than 10 kGy.[6]

While the incidence of food contamination is quite small, the volume can be quite large. Take the case of ground beef. Studies indicate that only .32 percent of U.S. ground beef is contaminated. But we produce 8 billion pounds of U.S. ground beef each year, meaning 26 million pounds are contaminated. The FDA's maximum recommended irradiation dosage for decontaminating ground beef is just 4.5 kGy.[7]

The number of kilogray necessary to kill common food pathogens is well known. Campylobacter requires .48 to .60 kGy, Ecoli .84 to .96 kGy, Listeria 1.26 to 1.44 kGy, Salmonella 1.98 to 2.22 kGy, and Staphylococcus 1.32 to 1.44 kGy.[5]

Irradiating food is not a cure-all. It does not kill all bacterial spores; does not inactivate viruses, toxins or prions; and does not prevent subsequent human contamination.[2] But it does markedly improve food safety, providing an effective critical point of control.

In addition, it increases the shelf life of food, which is part of the reason NASA astronauts and the U.S. military have been dining on irradiated food since 1960. It also decreases the need for use of chemical fumigants and other preservatives. Shelf life and quality are increasingly important in an age of globalization and worldwide food distribution.[2]

Expanding food irradiation to ensure food safety makes good public policy and good sense. The Centers for Disease Control and Prevention says that irradiating 50 percent of our red meat and poultry would prevent 900,000 cases of foodborne illness per year in the U.S. and save 352 lives. The cost? Just 5 cents per pound of meat.[8,9]

Food irradiation for safety has now been approved by the World Health Organization, the European Commission, the Food and Drug Administration, the Centers for Disease Control and Prevention and NASA. The American public's full and undivided support is now long overdue.

REFERENCES

1. Mead PS, Slutsker L, Dietz V, et al. Food-related illness and death in the United States. *Emerg Infect Dis*. 1999;5:607-625. Cited in Osterholm MT, Norgan AP.
2. Osterholm MT, Norgan AP. The role of irradiation in food safety. *NEJM*. 2004; 350:1898-1901.
3. Food irradiation: available research indicates that benefits outweigh risks. Washington, DC: General Accounting Office, August 2000. (GAO/RCED-00-217.) Cited in Osterholm MT, Norgan AP.
4. Wood OB, Bruhn CM. Position of the American Dietetic Association: food irradiation. *J Am Diet Assoc*. 2000; 100:246-253. Cited in Osterholm MT, Norgan AP.
5. Thayer DW. Irradiation of food - helping to ensure food safety. *NEJM*. 2004; 350:1811-1812.
6. Loaharanu P. Irradiated Foods. 5th ed. rev. New York: *American Council on Science and Health*, May 2003. Cited in Osterholm MT, Norgan AP.
7. Roybal J. Beef Industry logs successful week in E. coli O157:H7 battle. BEEF Magazine's Cow-Calf Weekly. September 26, 2003.

Available at www.beef-mag.com/Microsites/Index.asp?pageid=8044&
srid=11116&magazineid=13&siteid=5#a030926_4. Accessed April 8,
2004. Cited in Osterholm MT, Norgan AP.

8. Tauxe RV. Food safety and irradiation: protecting the public from
foodborne infections. *Emerg Infect Dis*. 2001; 7(Suppl)516-521. Cited
in Osterholm MT, Norgan AP.

9. Frenzen PD, Majchowicz A, Buzby JC, Imhoff B. Consumer acceptance of irradiated meat and poultry products. In: Issues in food safety
economics. USDA/ERS agriculture information bulletin no. 757.
Washington, DC: Department of Agriculture, August 2000. Cited in
Osterholm MT, Norgan AP.

TEACHING TOOLS

Policy Premises

1. Foodborne illnesses are a signifcant problem in the United States and around the world.
2. Irradiation of food does not make the food radioactive nor degrade its nutritional content.
3. The concept of food irradiation dates back 100 years.
4. In irradiating food, the dose is calibrated to the need.
5. Irradiating food is not a cure-all.
6. Expanding food irradiation to ensure food safety makes good public policy and good sense.

Review

1. What are the two most common causes of foodborne illnesses?
2. Does the irradiation process decrease a food's nutritional value?
3. What are some common food pathogens?
4. Which U.S. government agencies and worldwide organizations support irradiation of food?
5. How much would it cost to irradiate 50 percent of the red meat and poultry that we consume yearly in the United States?

Online Resources

Access online resources with this book's CD.

Food Irradiation: A Safe Measure
http://www.fda.gov/opacom/catalog/irradbro.html

The "Bad Bug Book"
http://www.cfsan.fda.gov/~mow/intro.html

Frequently Asked Questions About Food Irradiation
http://www.cdc.gov/ncidod/dbmd/diseaseinfo/foodirradiation.htm

Irradiation of Meat and Poultry Products
http://www.fsis.usda.gov/oa/topics/irrmenu.htm

Foodborne Diseases
http://www.niaid.nih.gov/factsheets/foodbornedis.htm

Foodborne Illness: Ten Least Wanted Foodborne Pathogens
http://www.fightbac.org/10least.cfm

Health Politics Online

For Original Health Politics Programs and Slides:

Irradiation of Food and Food Safety
http://www.healthpolitics.com/program_info.asp?p=prog_51
Slide Briefing
http://www.healthpolitics.com/program_info.asp?p=prog_51

CHAPTER 6

Caring for Seniors

"We want life not only to be long but good...This will be one of the central challenges of the 21st century: to make dignity and comfort for the elderly as much a part of our national consciousness as education and safety are for our children."

— DONNA SHALALA
Former Secretary
U.S. Health and Human Services

"We mistakenly define long-term care problems as medical concerns rather than disability concerns. The care needs of most frail older people are primarily supportive: for example, help move from here to there, help them eat and dress, and help them keep track of their medicine."

— JIM FIRMAN
President
National Council on Aging

CHAPTER 6.1

Operating on the Elderly

THE IMPORTANCE OF PLANNING AHEAD AND UNDER-STANDING RISKS

As a large segment of the U.S. population ages in the coming years, operating on the elderly will become increasingly common.[1] In fact, the number of people over age 65 will reach about 70 million by 2030, compared with 35 million people in 2000. And the number of people over age 85 will grow from 4 million to 8.5 million in that same time period.[2]

Even so, today's seniors are quite familiar with the operating suite. Forty percent of all surgical procedures are associated with people over 65, as well as 50 percent of all emergency operations and 75 percent of all surgery-related deaths.[1]

Aging, itself, carries some inherent risks. For example, the skin of elderly patients is slower to heal and generates weaker scars than the skin of younger patients.[3] The heart changes functionally with age as well, not only in the elasticity of the walls, but also in the small vessels that feed the heart muscle and the large vessels through which the heart pushes blood.[4] Similarly, the lungs lose capacity with demonstrated changes in both the upper and lower airways and with the weakening of the respiratory muscles.[5] As for the kidneys, they lose about 10 percent of their filtering capability every decade after age 30.[6]

Progress in medicine and surgery has improved surgical outcomes for all patients. That said, surgery remains riskier for older patients than for younger ones. Surgery-related deaths for patients over 65 occur 5 percent to 10 percent of the time, while younger patients suffer surgery-related deaths at a rate of about 1.5 percent. A particular area of concern for seniors is emergency surgery, where the risk of death is two to four times greater than with elective, planned surgery.[1]

America's surgeons approach operating on seniors with a cautious respect that, at times, converts what could have been an elective case into an emergency. This can eliminate the possibility of preparing for preexisting conditions such as cardiovascular, respiratory, and kidney problems, which increases the risk of complications.[1,7]

While performing surgery on elderly people requires careful evaluation, related decisions will grow increasingly more common as the population ages. Surgeons look at a number of issues beyond patients' chronologic age, including their physiologic age, or how old they look and feel and their level of vitality. Formal evaluation of elderly patients' current functional status should be routine. What is the degree of impairment, if any? How complex is the proposed surgery? What would be an acceptable outcome for the patient, the family, and the surgeon? Are they all in agreement?[1]

While assigning degree of risk is improving, it remains an inexact science that augments, but does not replace, the value of an experienced surgeon with good judgment. Old adages still hold, including "treating the patient, not the disease" and "elderly patients will tolerate an operation, but not the complication."[1]

Table 6.1-1. The American Society of Anesthesiologists' Risk-Classification System

Class 1:	Normal
Class 2:	Controlled medical problem
Class 3:	Medical problem resulting in some functional deficits
Class 4:	Poorly controlled medical problem resulting in life-threatening dysfunction
Class 5:	Critical medical condition that leaves little chance of survival

Source: Richardson JD, Cocanour CS, Kern JA, et al. Perioperative risk assessment in elderly and high-risk patients. *J Am Coll Surg.* 2004;199:133-146

In avoiding the complication, step one is choosing the right patient. The American Society of Anesthesiologists' risk-classification system segments patients into five categories. These are: Class 1 — normal; Class 2 — a controlled medical problem; Class 3 — a medical problem resulting in some functional deficits; Class 4 — a poorly controlled medical problem resulting in life-threatening dysfunction; and Class 5 — a critical medical condition that leaves little chance of survival.

In a study of patients over 80 years old, the surgery-related death rate was less than 1 percent for those in Class 2, but in Class 4 patients, the death rate was 25 percent.[1]

So what does all this mean? First, operating on the elderly will be increasingly common in the coming years. Second, it is generally better to operate on a stable elderly patient electively, even if the patient has medical problems and is at some risk, rather than wait until the problem explodes and requires emergency intervention. Third, careful and thorough evaluation of functional and mental status should be standard practice when an operation on an elderly patient is being considered. This should include realistic expectations and agreement among all concerned on the risks and benefits of surgery.

REFERENCES

1. Richardson JD, Cocanour CS, Kern JA, et al. Perioperative risk assessment in elderly and high-risk patients. *J Am Coll Surg*. 2004;199:133-146.
2. Medical Never-Never Land: Ten Reasons Why America is Not Ready for the Coming Age Boom. Washington, D.C.: Alliance for Aging Research; 2002.
3. Lavker RM, Zheng PS, Dong G. Morphology of aged skin. *Clin Geriatr Med*. 1989;5:53-67. Cited in Richardson JD, Cocanour CS, Kern JA, et al.
4. Lakatta EG. Cardiovascular aging research: the next horizons. *J Am Geriatr Soc*. 1999;47:613-625. Cited in Richardson JD, Cocanour CS, Kern JA, et al.
5. Berry DT, Phillips BA, Cook YR, et al. Sleep disordered breathing in healthy aged persons: possible daytime sequelae. *J Gerontol*. 1987;42:620-626. Cited in Richardson JD, et al.
6. Rowe JW, Andres RA, Tobin FD, et al. The effect of age on creatinine clearance in man: a cross-sectional and longitudinal study. *J Gerontol*. 1976;31:155-163. Cited in Richardson JD, et al.
7. Palmberg S, Hirsjarvi E. Mortality in geriatric surgery: with special reference to the type of surgery, anaesthesia, complicating diseases and prophylaxis of thrombosis. *Gerontology*. 1979;25:103-112.

TEACHING TOOLS

Policy Premises

1. As the population ages, operations on the elderly become more common.
2. Aging carries with it fundamental organ changes that increase operating risk.
3. Surgery-related deaths in the elderly have declined but are still higher than in the young.
4. Fear of operating on the elderly remains common.
5. Surgery in the elderly requires careful evaluation.
6. While there is no perfect system to assess risk of surgery in the elderly, clearly some are at greater risk than others.

Review

1. People over age 65 account for what percentage of surgical procedures?
2. Why is surgery riskier for older patients than for younger ones?
3. What do surgeons take into account when deciding whether or not an elderly patient can withstand surgery?
4. Why should emergency surgery be avoided?
5. What is the first step to help prevent complications during surgery?

Online Resources

Access online resources with this book's CD.

Elderly and Considering Surgery?
http://www.niapublications.org/engagepages/surgery.asp

Elderly Denied Cancer Surgery
http://news.bbc.co.uk/1/hi/health/3223333.stm

What to Expect
http://www.pana.org/My%20geriatric%20parent.htm

Identifying High-Risk Surgical Patients
http://an.hitchcock.org/PatientSafety/Emails/ASA%20Class%20Ide
ntifying%20HIGH%20RISK%20patients%20for%20procedur-
al%20sedation.htm

Effects of Aging
http://orthoinfo.aaos.org/fact/thr_report.cfm?Thread_ID=224&top-
category=Wellness

Health Politics Online

For Original Health Politics Programs and Slides:

Operating on the Elderly
http://www.healthpolitics.com/program_info.asp?p=prog_59
Slide Briefing
http://www.healthpolitics.com/media/prog_59/brief_prog_59.pdf

CHAPTER 6.2

Caring for an Alzheimer's Patient

THE HIDDEN COSTS

The incidence of Alzheimer's disease in the United States is on a steep rise. Over the next 50 years we'll see a 300 percent increase in affected patients. In 2000, there were 4.5 million Americans with the disease. This number will increase to nearly 6 million by 2020, nearly 8 million by 2030, and top 13 million in 2050.[1]

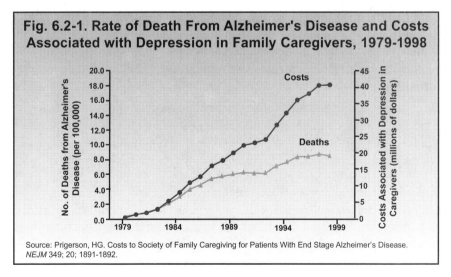

Fig. 6.2-1. Rate of Death From Alzheimer's Disease and Costs Associated with Depression in Family Caregivers, 1979-1998

Source: Prigerson, HG. Costs to Society of Family Caregiving for Patients With End Stage Alzheimer's Disease. *NEJM* 349; 20; 1891-1892.

With the increase in patients comes a predictable increase in costs. Some of those costs are very visible and trackable. For example, it is projected that direct costs to Medicare for Alzheimer's will increase 54 percent to $49 billion in 2010. Medicaid, which carries the burden of nursing home payments, is expected to expend $33 billion an 80 percent increase by 2010 for Alzheimer's patients.[1]

But this only begins to tell the financial story, because the larger burden is hidden in the indirect impact of Alzheimer's.[2,3] For example, it is projected that the annual cost to business this year in indirect outlays related to Alzheimer's patients will top $60 billion with $37 billion tied to lost caregiver productivity.[1] This reflects the reality that the majority of care is provided by family members. In a recent study, the average age of caregivers was 65 while the average age of patients was 81. More than 80 percent of the caregivers were women family members. Of that number, half were children of patients and the other half were spouses of patients.[4]

Caring for patients with significant cognitive impairment is challenging at best. Let's begin with the extraordinary length of the disease — an average of eight years, which can feel like an eternity. During those years, loved ones disappear before your eyes, but they don't go quietly. The level of impairment is extreme, requiring early support with the basics. More than half of caregivers spend an average 11 hours a week on basic activities of daily living and an additional 35 hours a week on instrumental activities of daily living.[4]

The time required to provide care amounts to a full-time job. Over 50 percent in one study averaged 46 hours a week of care. And a similar number felt they were "on-call" 24 hours a day without relief. The impact is rapid and direct, with the clearest evidence being caregivers' abandonment of their regular jobs. Forty-eight percent decrease their regular work hours, and 18 percent resign from their regular jobs.[4]

But that's only what you see. Here's what you don't see. The rates of depression in caregivers are significant. Fully 43 percent of caregivers of Alzheimer's patients in one study were clinically depressed.[4] And only the death of the patient brings lasting relief. Seventeen percent of these caregivers require anti-depressant medicine and 19 percent require anti-anxiety medications. These rates do not decline if the patient is placed in a nursing home, leaving the family caregiver to struggle with the guilt of abandonment, concerns over institutional care, and bereavement for a loved one who is lost but not gone. It is only after a patient dies, with an average of three to 12 months of recovery, that depression levels in family caregivers decline to below the levels of depression that existed when they were active caregivers.[4,5]

So the reality is pretty clear-cut. While unpaid family caregivers of

Alzheimer's patients spare the government direct expenses of institutionalization, they do not come without cost. Equally clear is that patients prefer to be at home, and caregivers receive no mental relief by providing home care. Finally, we know that this complex crisis for the American family will get worse rapidly in our immediate future.

What can be done? The solution lies in better systems for home-based support for patients and caregivers. This has the potential to increase quality of care and decrease cost of care. Experts suggest these services focus on five key areas: Communication techniques, pain control, vigilance or oversight of wandering behavior, counseling and positive reinforcement for caregivers, and team-based long-term support.[6]

If America's health insurers — government and private — are looking for a worthwhile project on which to collaborate, support for the caregivers of Alzheimer's patients might be an excellent place to start.

REFERENCES

1. Prigerson, HG. Costs to Society of Family Caregiving for Patients With End Stage Alzheimer's Disease. *NEJM* 349; 20; 1891-1892.
2. Schultz, R. et al. Psychiatric and physical morbidity effects of dementia caregiving: prevalence, correlates and causes. *Gerontologist* 1995; 35: 771-91.
3. Schultz, R. et al. Caregiving as a risk factor for morbidity. The Caregiver Health Effects Study *JAMA*. 1999: 282, 2215-9.
4. Schultz, R. et al. End-of-Life Care and the Effects of Bereavement on Family Caregivers of Persons with Dementia. *NEJM*, 349; 20: 1936-42.
5. Grant I, et al. Health Consequences of Alzheimer's Caregiving Transitions: Effects of Placement and Bereavement. *Psychosom Med* 2002; 64: 477-86.
6. Ory, MG. Et al. Prevalence and impact of caregiving: a detailed comparison between dementia and non-dementia caregivers. *Gerontologist* 1999; 39: 177-85.

TEACHING TOOLS

Policy Premises

1. The incidence of Alzheimer's disease in the United States is rising steeply, as are the costs.
2. Care for Alzheimer's patients is provided primarily by family members.
3. Caring for patients with significant cognitive impairment is extremely challenging at best.
4. The time required to provide care amounts to a full-time job.
5. The rates of depression in caregivers are higher than expected, and only the death of the patient brings relief.
6. Better systems for home-based care of patients and caregivers could increase quality and decrease the cost of Alzheimer's management.

Review

1. In 2000, how many Americans were afflicted with Alzheimer's disease?
2. What is the average age of Alzheimer's patients and what is the average age of their caretakers?
3. What impact does caring for an Alzheimer's patient have on a caretaker's job?
4. What percentage of Alzheimer's caregivers have been diagnosed with depression?
5. Name three areas that home-based care systems can focus on to build a better support network.

Online Resources

Access online resources with this book's CD.

Caregiving and Depression
http://www.caregiver.org/caregiver/jsp/content_node.jsp?nodeid=393

Work and Eldercare
http://www.caregiver.org/caregiver/jsp/content_node.jsp?nodeid=413

Alzheimer's Disease
http://www.caregiver.org/caregiver/jsp/content_node.jsp?nodeid=567

Caregivers for people with dementia: what is the family physician's role?
http://www.cfpc.ca/cfp/2000/VOL46-2000-
PDFs/Feb00%20PDFs/vol46_feb00_cme_2.pdf

The cultural context of caregiving: a comparison of Alzheimer's caregivers in Shanghai, China and San Diego, California
http://www.hnrc.ucsd.edu/publications_pdf/3351998.pdf

Alzheimer's Disease & Related Dementias: Diagnosis & Management - Caregiving
http://www.une.edu/uhc/bodywise/modules/alzheimer/care.htm

Health Politics Online

For Original Health Politics Programs and Slides:

Hidden Costs of Caring for Alzheimer's Patients
http://www.healthpolitics.com/program_info.asp?p=prog_33
Slide Briefing
http://www.healthpolitics.com/media/prog_33/brief_prog_33.pdf

Long-Distance Caregiving

AN INCREASING REALITY IN THE WORKPLACE

Colliding megatrends are increasingly pitting family loyalties against workplace loyalties. As the U.S. population has aged, families have become more mobile, separated by distance, and occupied by work demands. Large numbers of women have entered the workplace and global competitiveness has placed increasing emphasis on worker retention and productivity. Thus, family caregiving from a distance has become a fact of life for millions of Americans, according to a recent survey commissioned by MetLife Mature Market Institute and the National Alliance for Caregiving.[1]

Approximately 34 million Americans are providing care to older family members. Fifteen percent of these caregivers live an hour or more away from their relative. Nearly one-fourth of these long-distance caregivers are the only or primary care provider, and 80 percent work part or full time, according to the MetLife survey of 1,130 long-distance family care providers.[1,2]

Long-distance caregivers provide a wide array of services at great cost to themselves. According to the survey, they spend an average of $392 per month — about half of this is spent on out-of-pocket purchases and services for the care recipient and half on travel and long-distance communications.[1]

The expenditure in time is no less than the expenditure in dollars. Half of the survey respondents reported spending 13.6 hours a month arranging care services, and half said they spend another 16 hours a month checking on their care recipient or monitoring the care being received. Nearly three-quarters of these long-distance caregivers provide help with Instrumental Activities of

Daily Living (IADLs) such as transportation, shopping, cooking, cleaning, managing finances and medications — for an average of 22 hours per month. And 40 percent are involved in basic Activities of Daily Living (ADLs) such as bathing, dressing, feeding, and toileting, for an average of 12 hours per month.[1]

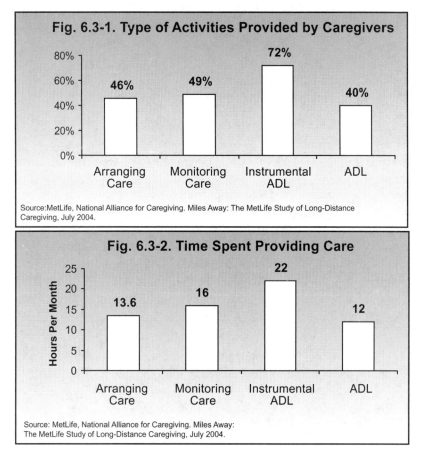

Fig. 6.3-1. Type of Activities Provided by Caregivers

Source:MetLife, National Alliance for Caregiving. Miles Away: The MetLife Study of Long-Distance Caregiving, July 2004.

Fig. 6.3-2. Time Spent Providing Care

Source: MetLife, National Alliance for Caregiving. Miles Away: The MetLife Study of Long-Distance Caregiving, July 2004.

What effect does long-distance caregiving have on professional work schedules? Employed caregivers are often required to make significant adjustments to allow for their caregiving responsibilities. These include coming in late or leaving early, missing days of work, rearranging work schedules, and taking unpaid leave. Twenty-five percent of the surveyed long-distance caregivers had shortened their workday and 36 percent reported missing full days of work. Twelve percent had taken a leave of absence.[1]

Distance, of course, makes a difference in the work accommodations caregivers make. Those caregivers who live closer to the care recipient are more likely to come into work late or leave early, as opposed to missing full workdays.[1]

The forces that have created today's long-distance caregiver realities are unlikely to reverse themselves in the near future. Rather, the challenges and work-balance issues are likely to accelerate. Clearly, long-distance caregiving already impacts retention and productivity. Physical distance is a key determinant in terms of complexity, as is the presence or absence of other relatives in the area. In the absence of "on-the-ground" family support, paid support becomes more critical earlier in the aging cycle.[1,2]

What can an employer do? Certainly, sensitizing line managers to the issue is a reasonable starting point. Adjusting policies to allow job sharing and short-time relief, as well as providing information and help in coordinating eldercare, are definitely worthwhile investments, compared to the cost of attrition and lost productivity. And, since long-distance caregivers have financial burdens as well as time conflicts, programs that offer help with these are beneficial. For example, voluntary pooling of frequent flyer miles for employees who need to travel on family emergencies is an idea worth considering.[1,3]

These tangible expressions of support face the issue head on while reinforcing shared values and joint commitment.

REFERENCES

1. MetLife, National Alliance for Caregiving. Miles Away: The MetLife Study of Long-Distance Caregiving, July 2004.
2. National Alliance for Caregiving, AARP, MetLife. Caregiving in the U.S., April 2004. Cited in MetLife, National Alliance for Caregiving. Miles Away: The MetLife Study of Long-Distance Caregiving, July 2004.
3. Shellenbarger S. When Elderly Loved Ones Live Far Away: The Challenge of Long-Distance Care. *The Wall Street Journal*. July 29, 2004.

TEACHING TOOLS

Policy Premises

1. Colliding megatrends are increasingly pitting loyalty to family against loyalty to one's job.
2. An increasing portion of America's 34 million family caregivers live far away from elderly family members.
3. Long-distance caregivers provide a wide array of services at great cost to themselves.
4. Cared-for family members are often isolated and in fair or poor health.
5. Most long-distance caregivers rely on other relatives on-site for support, but coordination is often weak and jobs and health suffer.
6. Increased workplace support for long-distance caregivers is in the best interest of employers and employees alike.

Review

1. How many Americans are providing care to older family members, and what percentage of these are considered long-distance caregivers?
2. What percentage of long-distance caregivers are employed?
3. What effect does this have on work schedules?
4. What makes long-distance caregiving so complex?
5. How can employers help?

Online Resources

Access online resources with this book's CD.

From a Distance
http://www.aarp.org/life/caregiving/Articles/a2003-10-27-caregiving-longdistance.html

Long-Distance Caregiver's Handbook
http://www.caregiver.org/caregiver/jsp/content/pdfs/op_2003_long
_distance_handbook.pdf

Coordinating Care
http://www.alzheimernyc.org/caregivers/long_distance_caregiv-
ing.htm

Changing America
http://www.cfad.org/html/community_need.html

Staying Informed
http://www.careplanner.org/TopicReq

The Effects of Caregiving on the Workplace
http://www.aarp.org/states/me/me-news/Articles/a2004-02-06-me-
newlook.html

Caring and Connecting: Learn to Be a Better Provider and Caregiver
http://www.caregiving-online.com/

Health Politics Online

For Original Health Politics Programs and Slides:

Long-Distance Caregiving: An Increasing Reality in the Workplace
http://www.healthpolitics.com/program_info.asp?p=prog_72
Slide Briefing
http://www.healthpolitics.com/media/prog_72/brief_prog_72.pdf

Aging and Obesity

MEGATRENDS ON A COLLISION COURSE

Aging and obesity are two intersecting and compounding megatrends. In the United States, 130 million Americans are either overweight or obese. By 2050, the percentage of U.S. citizens over 65 will reach 20 percent. That's up from 12 percent today. But the real story is how these two emerging realities play off of each other. Dr. Martha Daviglus and colleagues from Northwestern University in Chicago recently noted that "...urgent preventive measures are required... to lessen the burden of disease and disability associated with excess weight...and to contain future health care costs incurred by the aging population."[1]

What are the facts on aging and obesity? First, we know that people age 51 to 69 are the most vulnerable in terms of obesity and chronic disease. In this age group, rates of disease in obese people versus non-obese people are remarkable.[2,3] Heart disease is 19 percent in obese seniors and 14 percent in non-obese seniors. Diabetes is 24 percent in obese seniors; 9 percent in non-obese seniors. High blood pressure: 58 percent versus 35 percent, and arthritis: 58 percent versus 45 percent.[4]

Older adults who are obese are more likely to suffer from persistent symptoms of chronic disease, and the impact on daily living is obvious. Twenty-three percent of obese adults over age 51 have severe fatigue, 23 percent have shortness of breath, 15 percent wheeze, and 30 percent experience ankle swelling. Comparative rates are markedly lower among their non-obese counterparts. The same is true of mental health symptoms — obese seniors suffer feelings of worthlessness 8 percent of the time versus 5 percent in non-obese seniors. All of these symptoms, in turn, translate into higher rates of disability. While 3 percent of those over 51 who are not obese need help with three or more Activities of Daily Living, 6 percent of obese seniors are similarly dependent.[4]

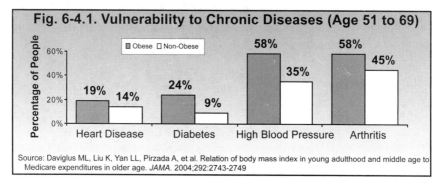

Fig. 6-4.1. Vulnerability to Chronic Diseases (Age 51 to 69)

Source: Daviglus ML, Liu K, Yan LL, Pirzada A, et al. Relation of body mass index in young adulthood and middle age to Medicare expenditures in older age. *JAMA*. 2004;292:2743-2749

Obesity rates in the elderly increase as a function of race, age and income. Those over 51 without a high school education have a 27 percent rate of obesity, while those with a high school education have an incidence rate of 22 percent. Annual incomes of under $20,000 are associated with obesity 26 percent of the time, compared with a 22 percent incidence rate for those with an annual income over $50,000. As for race, the obesity rate among blacks and Hispanics exceeds that of whites by 10 percent and 6 percent, respectively.[4]

The cost of obesity is significant and increases with one's body mass index (BMI). A BMI of less than 25 is considered normal; 25 to 30 is designated as overweight; and more than 30 is obese. In both men and women, minor ECG changes, blood pressure, and total cholesterol rise with rising BMI, and smoking rates decline.[1]

Table 6.4-1. Health Risks Increase With Higher BMI

	BMI	< 25 Normal	25-30 Overweight	> 30 Obese
Men	Minor ECG Changes	6.5%	6.5%	9.5%
	Blood Pressure	134/80	139/82	145/87
	Total Cholesterol	201	211	214
Women	Minor ECG Changes	4.4%	5.5%	7.4%
	Blood Pressure	131/77	137/80	145/85
	Total Cholesterol	213	219	229

Source: Daviglus ML, Liu K, Yan LL, Pirzada A, et al. Relation of body mass index in young adulthood and middle age to Medicare expenditures in older age. *JAMA*. 2004;292:2743-2749

While aging and obesity clearly impact each other in older adults, recent studies strongly reinforce that the damage begins much earlier, in young adulthood and middle age.[1] A landmark study of more than 39,000 Chicago residents over age 18 and from 84 different area organizations has just been completed and published. The participants were first registered for the study between 1967 and 1973. Their overall health status and cost of care was monitored over the following three to four decades. Between 1992 and 2002, nearly 16,000, or 40 percent, of the original study group passed age 65 and received Medicare for more than two years. In this group, annual charges for care of cardiovascular disease and diabetes, in both men and women, revealed a strong positive correlation with their BMI. Men with BMIs higher than 30 had health care costs exceeding non-overweight patients, controlled for age, race, education and smoking, by 42 percent. Women's rates of increase in health care costs were even greater. Those with BMIs higher than 30 had 54 percent higher costs than non-overweight women.[1]

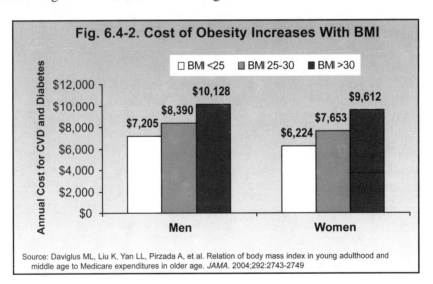

Fig. 6.4-2. Cost of Obesity Increases With BMI

Source: Daviglus ML, Liu K, Yan LL, Pirzada A, et al. Relation of body mass index in young adulthood and middle age to Medicare expenditures in older age. *JAMA*. 2004;292:2743-2749

What, then, is the takeaway? We need to face the facts regarding obesity and aging: First, BMI is a marker for chronic disease, disability, and symptoms of disease. Further, BMI has strong predictive power — it's not only able to point to a future cost in physical distress, altered lifestyle, and need for caregiver support in the later years, but it also signals an escalating expenditure of federal dollars — a burden each citizen will share.[5]

If we as citizens wish to avoid these burdens in our not-too-distant future, we will need to focus heavily on children, young adults, and those of middle age who currently harbor tomorrow's explosive and latent effects of chronic disease.

REFERENCES

1. Daviglus ML, Liu K, Yan LL, Pirzada A, et al. Relation of body mass index in young adulthood and middle age to Medicare expenditures in older age. *JAMA*. 2004;292:2743-2749.
2. Eckel RH, Krauss RM. American Heart Association call to action: obesity as a major risk factor for coronary heart disease. *Circulation*. 1998;97:2099-2100. Cited in Daviglus ML, Liu K, Yan LL, Pirzada A, et al.
3. Shaper AG, Wannamethee SG, Walker M. Body weight implications for the prevention of coronary heart disease, stroke, and diabetes mellitus in a cohort study of middle-aged men. *BMJ*. 1997;314:1311-1317. Cited in Daviglus ML, Liu K, Yan LL, Pirzada A, et al.
4. Obesity Among Older Americans. Center on an Aging Society, Georgetown University. Available at: http://hpi.georgetown.edu/aging-society/pdfs/obesity2.pdf. Accessed February 3, 2005.
5. The Politics of Older Adult Obesity. Panel discussion. Washington, D.C., December 2, 2004.

TEACHING TOOLS

Policy Premises

1. Obesity and aging are two intersecting and compounding mega-trends.
2. Obesity between the ages of 51 and 69 is associated with increased rates of chronic disease.
3. Obesity between the ages of 51 and 69 results in increased symptoms and disability.
4. Obesity rates in the elderly increase as a function of race, age and income.
5. The cost of obesity is significant and increases with BMI.
6. Obesity in young adulthood and middle age leads to increased morbidity, mortality and health care cost in the aged.

Review

1. How many Americans are either overweight or obese?
2. What are the rates of disease in non-obese seniors versus obese seniors?
3. Does obesity affect seniors' mental health?
4. What is the relationship between body mass index and health care costs?
5. How can a disastrous collision of aging and obesity be avoided?

Online Resources

Access online resources with this book's CD.

Do the Math
http://familydoctor.org/x2544.xml

Steps to Healthy Aging
http://www.fiu.edu/~nutreldr/STEPS_Program/STEPS_home.htm

Battle of the Bulge
http://cholesterolmatters.msn.com/article.aspx?aid=5

Senior Health
http://www.cdc.gov/aging/health_issues.htm

Obesity: Its Effects on Your Body
http://www.obesity.org/subs/fastfacts/Health_Effects.shtml

Super-Sized Senior Health Problems
http://seattletimes.nwsource.com/html/nationworld/2002095264_fa
tadults19.html

Height Weight Charts
http://www.a-guide-for-seniors.com/Pages/Healthy_Weight.html

Obesity and Disability: The Shape of Things to Come
http://www.rand.org/publications/RB/RB9043/

Health Politics Online

For Original Health Politics Programs and Slides:

Aging and Obesity: Megatrends on a Collision Course
http://www.healthpolitics.com/program_info.asp?p=agingobesity
Slide Briefing
http://www.healthpolitics.com/media/agingobesity/brief_agingobesi-
ty.pdf

CHAPTER 6.5

Driving Fatalities Among Seniors

HOW CAN THEY BE AVOIDED

More than 40,000 Americans die each year in motor vehicle crashes. Many of the drivers involved in fatal crashes are over age 65, even though seniors account for only about 8 percent of the miles driven each year in the United States. And motor vehicle fatality rates among senior drivers are on the rise, particularly for those 85 or older.[1,2]

According to the Insurance Institute for Highway Safety, "Drivers aged 65 and older...are expected to account for as much as 25 percent of total driver fatalities in 2030, compared to 14 percent currently." As baby boomers age and more seniors get behind the wheel, how can we prevent rising fatalities?[2]

Many states have looked for the answer in stricter license laws for elderly individuals. A comprehensive study of all fatal car crashes involving seniors in the 48 contiguous states between 1990 and 2000 recently appeared in the *Journal of the American Medical Association*. The study analyzes the effects of the following on motor vehicle fatality rates among seniors: frequency of license renewal, whether license renewal must be in-person, and whether vision and road tests are required.[2]

Other general motor vehicle laws that vary from state to state and could affect fatalities among older drivers were also taken into account in the study. These included primary and secondary seatbelt laws, speed limits, blood alcohol level restrictions, and license suspensions.[2]

The study revealed that, of all of these measures, only one showed a definitive preventive impact on senior fatalities — the in-person renewal of motor vehicle licenses. The positive impact primarily affected those over 85.[3]

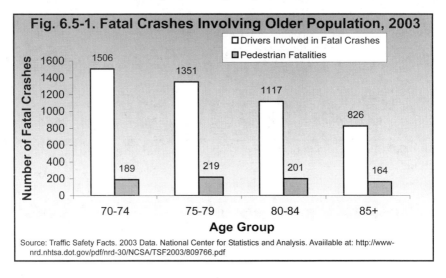

Fig. 6.5-1. Fatal Crashes Involving Older Population, 2003

Source: Traffic Safety Facts. 2003 Data. National Center for Statistics and Analysis. Avaiilable at: http://www-nrd.nhtsa.dot.gov/pdf/nrd-30/NCSA/TSF2003/809766.pdf

Why should auto fatalities among very elderly drivers decline with in-person renewals? Experts have offered two explanations. First, in-person renewal requirements provide an opportunity for license inspectors to either refuse to grant licenses to obviously impaired drivers or to refer them for medical evaluation prior to receiving a new license.[2]

And the second theory suggests that the requirement to appear in person deters some seniors from seeking a renewal. This theory is supported by the common tendency among seniors to impose restrictions on their own driving behavior, including not driving at night, in poor weather, on highways, at rush hour, after having an accident, or after loss of spatial or depth perception. An in-person license renewal requirement might be one more thing that older drivers consider as a reason not to drive.[2,4]

Focusing on motor vehicle safety among seniors makes good sense. First, the elderly population is rapidly growing. Second, the elderly are the most vulnerable — they're more likely to die from crash injuries. And third, solutions are relatively simple and not unduly harsh, such as in-person license renewal requirements for the oldest segment of the senior population.

Establishing sensible guideposts will trigger timely choices that are realistic and can enhance roadway safety for everyone.

REFERENCES

1. Lyman, S, Ferguson, SA, Braver, ER, Williams, AF. Older driver involvement in police reported crashes and fatal crashes: trends and projections. *Inj Prev*. 2002;8:116-120.
2. Grabowski DC, Campbell, CM, Morrisey, M. Elderly licensure laws and motor vehicle fatalities. *JAMA*. 2004;291:2840-2846.
3. Fatality Analysis Reporting System. Department of Transportation, National Highway Safety Administration Web site. Available at http://www-fars.nhtsa.dot.gov. Accessibility verified July 9, 2004. Cited in Grabowski DC, Campbell, CM, Morrisey, M.
4. Ball K, Owsley C, Stalvey B, Roenker DL, Sloane, ME, Graves, M. Driving avoidance and functional impairment in older drivers. *Accid Anal Prev*. 1998;30:313-322. Cited in Grabowski DC, Campbell, CM, Morrisey, M.

TEACHING TOOLS

Policy Premises

1. U.S. motor vehicle fatalities in the elderly are on the rise.
2. A number of deterrents have been identified and tried.
3. Laws impacting traffic safety vary from state to state.
4. In-person renewal of licenses for the elderly decreases fatalities in those over 65.
5. Seniors naturally stop driving as they age. In-person renewal triggers personal assessment.
6. Most states currently do not take advantage of in-person frequent license renewal as a safety strategy for senior drivers.

Review

1. Seniors account for what percentage of miles driven in the United States each year?
2. What are states doing to try to decrease the number of fatalities among senior drivers?
3. Which law shows a definitive preventive impact on senior driving fatalities?
4. Why does this law seem to work?
5. In 2030, seniors are expected to account for what percentage of total driver fatalities?

Online Resources

Access online resources with this book's CD.

Safety and Independence
http://www.asaging.org/webseminars/websem.cfm?EventID=6097

Too Old to Drive?
http://healthinaging.org/public_education/pef/safe_driving_for_sen
iors.php

Senior Drivers
http://www.seniordrivers.org/home/toppage.cfm

Assessing Preventable Injuries
http://www.ama-assn.org/ama/pub/category/10791.html

Health Politics Online

For Original Health Politics Programs and Slides:

Driving Fatalities Among Seniors
http://www.healthpolitics.com/program_info.asp?p=prog_56
Slide Briefing
http://www.healthpolitics.com/media/prog_56/brief_prog_56.pdf

CHAPTER 6.6

Elder Abuse

EXPOSING THE VIOLENCE

The aging of populations carries with it a hidden problem: elder abuse.[1] As Stephanie Lederman, executive director of the American Federation for Aging Research, notes, "A large segment of our population is both dependent and frail. Studies on elder abuse now alert us that seniors are also vulnerable and in need of help."[2]

And the problem is getting worse. According to the most recent study from the National Center on Elder Abuse, the incidence rate of elder abuse increased 150 percent between 1986 and 1996.[3]

How large is the at-risk segment? One study of 2,812 adults over age 65 revealed that 6 percent, or 176, of them were seen by elderly protective services over a nine-year period. Nearly three-quarters of these cases involved self-neglect, but the remaining 27 percent were traced to the actions of others — nearly 6 percent of the elderly people experienced physical abuse, 17 percent had been neglected, and almost 5 percent suffered exploitation.[4]

What is elder abuse? The U.S. National Academy of Sciences defines the problem as "intentional actions that cause harm or create a serious risk of harm to a vulnerable elder by a caregiver or other person who stands in a trust relationship to the elder; or, failure by a caregiver to satisfy the elder's basic needs or to protect the elder from harm."[5]

Elder abuse not only implies that a person has suffered injury or neglect, but also that a specific individual, entrusted to provide care, is responsible.

The abuse may take a variety of forms, including physical abuse, psychological abuse, sexual assault, exploitation of material resources, or neglect.

Studying elder abuse is easier said than done. For example, a simple geriatric study on how to prevent elder fractures due to falls must consider confounding issues such as polypharmacy, visual impairment from cataracts and other conditions, and depression or dementia, to name a few.[6] When one then attempts to decipher naturally occurring injuries from deliberate ones, study design and verification become critical. Was an injury due to loss of balance or assault? Did weight loss occur due to chronic disease and cancer or from neglect? Was under- or over-medicating the result of forgetfulness or malevolence of the caregiver?[1,6]

Risk factors associated with elder abuse are increasingly clear. Most incidences occur in shared living situations where there is prolonged access by a family member, friend or entrusted surrogate. Elder dementia creates both a complex management challenge and an unreliable witness to the abuse, which complicates documentation. Social isolation creates stress that can lead to reactive abuse behavior, as well as a hidden environment to harbor abuse, neglect, or exploitation. The presence of caregiver mental illness, including depression or substance abuse, increases the likelihood of harmful behaviors, as does the use of family-member caregivers who are dependent upon and often resentful of the senior for whom they are charged to provide care.[1,4]

Caring for a frail, dependent and vulnerable senior is challenging under the best circumstances. When abuse is interjected, the consequences are significant, including an increase in mortality rates. One study has documented that the three-year mortality rate for seniors who are exposed to elder abuse was 91 percent, compared with 58 percent in a matched dependent senior population that was not abused.[4]

Dr. Mark Lachs and his colleagues note, "It seems plausible that experiencing elder abuse is an extreme form of negative social support. In the same manner that social integration reduces mortality, it may conversely be the case that the extreme interpersonal stress resulting from elder abuse situations may confer additional death risk."[4]

Screening elders for abuse requires high awareness and good clinical judgment. There is not a clear consensus on routine monitoring or an instrument to be used.[1,4] General concern should be raised when physicians, nurses, and other members of the care team observe a poor social network, poor social functioning, and signs of conflict between a patient and a caregiver. Clinicians should trust their clinical judgment and instincts, do a complete physical assessment with a focus on cognitive function, question the patient in private, and be cautious in discussions with the caregiver, extending empathy while uncovering the individual's mental status and coping skills.[1]

Similarly, families should trust their instincts. Is mom or dad declining without an obvious reason? What is the level of cleanliness of the patient and the home setting? What is the patient being fed, and, under direct viewing, how gentle and effective is the process? Are there unexplained bruises, blisters, or painful areas? Is the senior's mobility rapidly declining? What is being said to the senior, not simply with words, but also with messages and tone? And what do your instincts tell you when you make unannounced visits?

Addressing senior abuse requires a continuum of committed individuals from home to care sites and back home again, providing reliable monitoring, oversight, diagnosis, and intervention when necessary. Such a network must be built, and a good place to begin is with an informed discussion of the issue between family members and their care teams.

REFERENCES

1. Lachs MS, Pillemer K. Elder abuse. *The Lancet*. 2004;364:1263-1272.
2. Lederman S. Private communication, 2005.
3. National Center on Elder Abuse. Reports of Domestic Elder Abuse. Available at: http://www.elderabusecenter.org/pdf/basics/fact1.pdf. Accessed February 28, 2005.
4. Lachs MS, Williams CS, O'Brien S, Pillemer KA, Charlson ME. The mortality of elder abuse. *JAMA*. 1998;280:428-443. Cited in Lachs MS, Pillemer K.
5. National Academies of Sciences. Bonnie R, Wallace R, eds. Elder abuse: abuse, neglect, and exploitation in an aging America. Washington, D.C.: National Academy Press, 2002. Cited in Lachs MS, Pillemer K.
6. Lachs MS, Pillemer K. Abuse and neglect of elderly persons. *NEJM*. 1995;333:437. Cited in Lachs MS, Pillemer K.

TEACHING TOOLS

Policy Premises

1. The aging of populations carries with it a hidden health problem — elder abuse.
2. There is growing consensus on the definition of elder abuse.
3. Studying elder abuse is easier said than done.
4. The risk factors for elder abuse are increasingly clear.
5. Elder abuse is associated with higher mortality rates.
6. Screening of elders for abuse requires high awareness and good clinical judgement.

Review

1. How common is elder abuse?
2. Why is studying elder abuse difficult?
3. What are some of the risk factors associated with elder abuse?
4. What is the difference in the mortality rate of abused elders versus non-abused elders?
5. How should families and physicians screen for elder abuse?

Online Resources

 Access online resources with this book's CD.

Basic Abuse
http://www.elderabusecenter.org/default.cfm?p=basics.cfm

Are You a Caregiver?
http://www.aoa.gov/prof/aoaprog/caregiver/carefam/carefam.asp

Prescription for Abuse
http://www.eurekalert.org/pub_releases/2005-02/uopm-epc020805.php

In Search of Solutions
http://www.apa.org/pi/aging/eldabuse.html

What's Your Role?
http://www.preventelderabuse.org/professionals/professional.html

Crime Against Older People
http://www.niapublications.org/engagepages/crime.asp

States Target Elder Abuse
http://www.stateline.org/live/ViewPage.action?siteNodeId=136&la nguageId=1&contentId=15937

Health Politics Online

For Original Health Politics Programs and Slides:

Elder Abuse
http://www.healthpolitics.com/program_info.asp?p=elderly_abuse
Slide Briefing
http://www.healthpolitics.com/media/elderly_abuse/brief_elderly_a buse.pdf

End-of-Life Care

"Physicians are often reluctant to provide specific information largely out of fear of destroying hope...Dying patients can still have hope for system control, [hope] of resolving personal relationships, and [hope] for a dignified death."

— DAVID WEISSMAN
   Journal of the American Medical Association
   2004

"The medical man who (from ignorance or timidity) withholds hypodermic medicine from a patient afflicted with cancer is...totally without excuse."

— JOHN KENT SPENDER
   1874

CHAPTER 7.1

Discussing Death with Dying Children

SHOULD PARENTS DO IT?

There is nothing more tragic than the loss of a child. And losing a child to cancer is especially challenging — it takes every ounce of a parent's and child's physical, emotional, and spiritual strength. Approximately 1,500 children under age 15 and their parents travel this road each year in the United States.[1] And at the end, despite all the courage and effort, many parents are left to wonder if they made all the right decisions.[2]

One of the most important decisions is whether to discuss death with a dying child. When it comes to children with cancer, the parental bias is to leave no stone unturned, to try anything, within or sometimes outside of reason, to find a cure for their child, to save the great potential of future years, of future life. Therefore, it's sometimes up to the physician to be on the lookout for the fleeting moment that allows him or her to begin to plant the seeds of bereavement, to broach the possibility of the child's death, and to initiate anticipatory grief, even while hope remains, says Dr. Lawrence Wolfe, a pediatric hematology and oncology specialist who has treated terminally ill children for many years.[3]

What is it that parents of dying children fear the most? They fear what dying will feel like to their child. They fear what dying will look like to their family. And they fear what life will be like the moment after their child departs.[3]

Experts, including those from the International Society of Pediatric Oncology, agree it is best for a dying child to discuss death openly.[4] Dr. Wolfe agrees. He notes that, "Even very young children have an understanding that death exists."[3] A dying child may become aware that death is imminent through direct information or by reasoning about his or her health status and experiences. Some children express their awareness; others do not. Those who do may communicate it directly with words, or more indirectly through stories, gestures, or drawings, and, at times, with a silence that begs prompting and interruption to unlock their thoughts.[3]

Just as dying children benefit from discussing death, there is now good evidence that the same is true for their parents. A 2004 study of 561 parents who had lost children to cancer between 1992 and 1997 yielded 429 applicable participants. Nearly 150 of them, or 34 percent, spoke to their terminally ill child about death. None regretted this decision. Out of the 66 percent who did not discuss death with their child, 16 percent experienced regrets, 44 percent did not, and six percent did not say.[2]

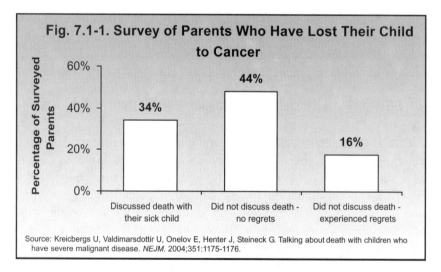

Fig. 7.1-1. Survey of Parents Who Have Lost Their Child to Cancer

Source: Kreicbergs U, Valdimarsdottir U, Onelov E, Henter J, Steineck G. Talking about death with children who have severe malignant disease. *NEJM.* 2004;351:1175-1176.

Those parents with regrets continue to have higher rates of anxiety and depression. What are they anxious or depressed about? They're worried that absent discussion about death, their child was left alone with his or her own thoughts; that their child may have needed the comfort of reassuring words and gestures; or that their child was aware of death but did not communicate it. And now that their child is gone, these parents' decisions to remain quiet cannot be reversed.[2]

Among the parents who chose not to discuss death with their dying child, 33 percent of the women had regrets, versus 20 percent of the men. Thirty-five percent of religious parents versus 19 percent of non-religious parents questioned their decision. And the parents of older children were more regretful that they did not discuss death with their child than the parents of younger children.[2]

What is increasingly clear is that, although parents and children can benefit from a discussion of impending death, it is difficult to arrive at that destination without a guide. Caregivers can and should help. What is their role? According to Dr. Wolfe, it is to "comfort, guide, reassure, and create a presence or a rapport that enables healing before and after the death of a child."[3]

In pursuit of this goal, caring professionals can offer coping skills, help prepare families for grief, identify boundaries of difficult behavior, encourage family cohesiveness, and provide a sense of safety to surviving siblings.[3]

When is the right time to do these things? When death is imminent and confronts those involved in a way they can no longer deny.[3]

REFERENCES

1. American Cancer Society. Cancer Facts and Figures 2003. Available at www.cancer.org/downloads/stt/caff2003pwsecured.pdf. Accessed November 15, 2004.
2. Kreicbergs U, Valdimarsdottir U, Onelov E, Henter J, Steineck G. Talking about death with children who have severe malignant disease. *NEJM.* 2004;351:1175-1176.
3. Wolfe L. Should parents speak with a dying child about impending death? *NEJM.* 2004;351:1251-1253.
4. Nitschke R. Regarding guidelines for assistance to terminally ill children with cancer: report of the SIOP Working Committee on psychosocial issues in pediatric oncology. *Med Pediatr Oncol.* 2000;34:271-273.

TEACHING TOOLS

Policy Premises

1. In children with cancer, the parental bias is to leave no stone unturned.
2. Parents fear discussions of death with their dying children.
3. Experts agree it is best for the children to discuss death openly.
4. Two-thirds of parents of terminally ill children do not talk to their dying child about death; many regret that decision.
5. Failing to do so carries long-term mental health risks for parents.
6. Health care professionals should help facilitate discussion of death and assist in bereavement.

Review

1. What do the parents of dying children fear most?
2. When do children begin to understand death?
3. How might children express their awareness of impending death?
4. When parents don't discuss death with their sick child before he or she dies, what types of regrets do they often experience?
5. What role should caregivers play?

Online Resources

Access online resources with this book's CD.

Young People with Cancer
http://www.cancer.gov/cancerinfo/youngpeople

Do Children Understand Death?
http://www.hospicenet.org/html/understand.html

Discussing Death with Children
http://health.discovery.com/encyclopedias/illnesses.html?article=2690&page=1

Communicating with a Child Who Has Cancer
http://www.cancerwise.org/december_2002/display.cfm?id=4F4C2
EB8-2F20-4885-
80B2B8A58B2AEDBE&method=displayFull&color=green

Approaching Grief
http://www.chionline.org/publications/resources/approaching_grief.
pdf

When Your Child Has Cancer
http://www.cancer.org/docroot/ETO/content/ETO_2_6X_When_Yo
ur_Child_Has_Cancer_7.asp

Health Politics Online

For Original Health Politics Programs and Slides:

Should Parents Discuss Death with Dying Children?
http://www.healthpolitics.com/program_info.asp?p=death_dying_c
hildren
Slide Briefing
http://www.healthpolitics.com/media/death_dying_children/brief_d
eath_dying_children.pdf

Planning a Dignified Death

FACING THE CRITICAL CHALLENGE

Decision-making at the end of life is a critical challenge for the patients, families and physicians involved.[1] In the not-too-distant past, families and physicians were often complicit in hiding information from terminally ill patients. Studies show that this practice is much less frequent today. However, physicians in a 2001 study were found to understate the severity of a terminally ill patient's prognosis 63 percent of the time, and there is general agreement that physicians and health institutions continue to overuse technology and underuse communication when dealing with terminally ill patients.[2] To reinforce this point, an examination of hospital records of 164 patients with significant dementia and terminal metastatic cancer shows that nearly half of the patients received aggressive non-palliative treatments and a quarter received cardiopulmonary resuscitation.[3]

While it's easy in retrospect to critique such behaviors, the reality is that managing the progression toward death is highly complex. The physician is often asked to bridge the chasm between life-saving and life-enhancing care. Guidance must be highly personalized and must consider prognosis, the risks and benefits of various interventions, the patient's symptom burden, the timeline ahead, the age and stage of life of the patient, and the quality of the patient's support system.

Considering all these, the physician, patient, and family are expected to explore all curative options, provide clear and honest communications, invite family input, provide their best recommendations, and ultimately affirm and support a patient's decision.[1]

Walking the road of terminal illness carries special burdens for all involved. For the patient and family, shock gives way to a complex analysis that often intersects with guilt, regret and anger. Fear must be managed and channeled, and loss and its implications for family and loved ones cannot be avoided. On top of this, there are multiple complex decisions that must be addressed within specific time constraints.

Table 7.2-1. Special Burdens of Terminal Illness

Patients/Families	Physicians
• Shock • Guilt, regret, anger • Fear • Loss • Complex, timely decisions	• Complex tasks • Emotional burdens • Accepting responsibility • Balancing hope/truth • Managing grief/depression • Incorporating unique cultures/ spiritual beliefs

Source: McCahill LE, Krouse RS, Chu DZJ, et al. Decision making in palliative surgery. J Am Coll Surg. 2002;195:411-423. Cited in Weissman DE.
Fallowfield LJ, Jenkins VA, Beveridge HA. Truth may hurt by deceit hurts more: communication in palliative care. Palliat Med. 2002;16:297-303. Cited in Weissman DE.

While all this is extremely difficult for patients and families, it's also demanding of physicians.[4,5] The sheer complexity of individualizing and humanizing each passage is complicated by a heavy emotional burden that comes with accepting responsibility for the care of others. Physicians struggle to balance hopefulness with truthfulness. Determining "how much information," "within what space of time," and "with what degree of directness for this particular patient" requires a skillful commitment that matures with age and experience.

Managing both physical and mental health and distinguishing between normal grief and clinical depression add to the challenge.

Finally, incorporating the unique culture and spiritual context that can help define the right course of action for each individual demands a special set of eyes and ears and an ability to reach out and touch.

Studies confirm that 85 percent of terminally ill patients desire as much information as they can get, good or bad. Prognostic information is the most important. Only 7 percent of terminally ill patients seek "good news" exclusively and only 8 percent want no details.[4,5]

When a diagnosis is first made, everyone's focus is on life preservation. But a sharp decline, results of diagnostic studies, or an internal awareness can signal a transition and lead patients and families to recognize that death is approaching. Once acceptance arrives, end-of-life decision-making naturally follows. Denying that death is approaching only compresses the timeline for these decisions, adds anxiety, and undermines the sense of control over one's own destiny.

With acceptance, the goals become quality of life and comfort. Physicians, hospice, family, and other caregivers can focus on assessing physical symptoms, psychological and spiritual needs, quality of support systems, estimation of prognosis, and defining a patient's end-of-life goals.[2] How important might it be for a patient to attend a granddaughter's wedding or see one last Christmas, and are these realistic goals to pursue?

One issue that often gets confused in the process of planning a death with dignity is hope. It is possible to die with hope, with self-control, and with dignity, but it requires some time and planning. Physician participation is critical. End-of-life care expert Dr. David Weissman offers this counsel: "Physicians are often reluctant to provide specific information largely out of fear of destroying hope.... Dying patients can still have hope for system control, of resolving personal relationships, and for a dignified death."[1]

In order to plan a death with dignity, we need to acknowledge death as a part of life — an experience to be embraced rather than ignored when the time comes. Recognizing when that time has arrived is a critical challenge for each of us.

REFERENCES

1. Weissman DE. Decision making at a time of crisis near the end of life. *JAMA*. 2004;292:1738-1743.
2. Lamont EB, Christakis NA. Prognostic disclosure to patients with cancer near the end of life. *Ann Intern Med*. 2001;134:1096-1105. Cited in Weissman DE.
3. Ahronheim JC, Morrison RS, Baskin SA, et al. Treatment of the dying in the acute care hospital. *Arch Intern Med*. 1996;156:2094-2100. Cited in Weissman DE.

4. McCahill LE, Krouse RS, Chu DZJ, et al. Decision making in palliative surgery. *J Am Coll Surg*. 2002;195:411-423. Cited in Weissman DE.

5. Fallowfield LJ, Jenkins VA, Beveridge HA. Truth may hurt but deceit hurts more: communication in palliative care. *Palliat Med*. 2002;16:297-303. Cited in Weissman DE.

TEACHING TOOLS

Policy Premises

1. Decision-making at the end of life is a critical challenge for patients, families, and physicians.
2. The physician is often asked to bridge the chasm between lifesaving and life-enhancing care.
3. Walking the road of terminal illness carries special burdens for all involved.
4. Information, good or bad, is almost always desired by the patient and often incompletely provided by the physician.
5. Once acceptance arrives, end-of-life decision-making naturally follows.
6. It is possible to die with hope, with self-control, and with dignity — but it requires some time and good planning.

Review

1. What is the family's role in the final phase of a loved one's life?
2. What role should the physician play?
3. When a terminal diagnosis is first made, what is often the initial focus?
4. Do most terminally ill patients want truthful prognostic information?
5. With the acceptance of imminent death, how do a patient's goals change?

Online Resources

Access online resources with this book's CD.

End-of-Life Care
http://www.nhpco.org/files/public/NHF_Communicating_Wishes.pdf

The Dying Process
http://www.carefordying.org/mainwebsite_html/dyingProcess/Dying.html

The Importance of Patient-Clinician Communication
http://hab.hrsa.gov/tools/palliative/chap21.html

Culturally Diverse Communities and End-of-Life Care
http://www.apa.org/pi/eol/fsculturallydiverse.pdf

Health Politics Online

For Original Health Politics Programs and Slides:

Planning a Dignified Death
http://www.healthpolitics.com/program_info.asp?p=death_with_dignity
Slide Briefing
http://www.healthpolitics.com/media/death_with_dignity/brief_death_with_dignity.pdf

CHAPTER 7.3

Palliative Care

IMPROVING QUALITY OF LIFE FOR THE CHRONICALLY ILL

As populations age in the United States, chronic illnesses create an uncertain medical future. By 2030, a fifth of the U.S. population will be over 65, and many will face the challenges of managing one or more chronic illnesses for a significant number of years, including physical and psychological distress, functional dependency and frailty, and a need for support.[1]

Traditional care systems are not particularly well-equipped for this situation. For example, our medical system focuses almost exclusively on curing illnesses and prolonging life — goals shaped by the hard-charging interventional past. But in the new order, these two worthwhile goals become hollow if they're not pursued simultaneously with goals of improving quality of life, relieving suffering, and providing physical and emotional comfort.[2]

The palliative care movement addresses this concern. Palliative care, which focuses on supporting the needs of the chronically ill as they approach the final phase of life, is as much a life philosophy and value position as it is a caring revolution. Two leaders of the movement recently noted "The aim of palliative care is to relieve suffering and improve the quality of life for patients with advanced illnesses and their families."[1]

The process of getting there is as important as the goal itself. Palliative care calls for an extraordinarily inclusive team effort with a strong emphasis on planning.

This philosophy of care begins with physicians eliciting the concerns of the patient and loved ones. What is important in the patient's life? What more would he or she like to achieve? Is there something he or she fears worse than death?[3]

Concerns expressed during this conversation help define the patient's value system. Studies have found that patients almost always express the desire for more effective communication with a care team that is comfortable dealing with uncertainty and complexity. It's important for the care team to tailor care to the patient's individual needs.[4]

Palliative care is remarkably focused and pragmatic. If I place myself in an elder patient's shoes — multiple diseases, some compromise in capacity, but an uncertain prognosis — priorities become more obvious. What would I need? What would I ask of my caregivers? First, relieve my suffering. Second, improve the quality of my life. Third, manage my pain and other symptoms effectively over a long span. Fourth, while you are caring for me physically, don't abandon me psychologically or spiritually. Help me grieve my losses. Fifth, be sure to coordinate this as a team effort, remembering that my family and I are part of the team.

At the end of the day, the patient seeks enough comfort to contribute to loved ones' lives, enough resources to not be a burden to family and friends, and enough strength and capacity to control one's own life.[5]

Many people are dealing with these issues with their loved ones now, but it makes good sense to plan ahead for a time when this generation will have multiple medical conditions themselves but will not yet be in the dying process.

Where do hospice services fit in with palliative care? Hospice care has a remarkable track record in supportive, holistic, end-of-life care. In the United States, however, it has been primarily associated with terminal care of cancer patients. Insurance coverage for hospice services requires physician certification that a patient has only six months to live. Such certification in non-cancer chronic diseases is difficult.[6]

But slowly, around the world, care systems are beginning to absorb the teachings of hospice in the form of chronic-disease management, team coordination, and a holistic, patient-centered care approach. When successful outcomes are well-defined, everyone benefits. For example, patients should be able to voice their personal needs and define their long-term and short-term goals. Evaluation should be thorough on the front end and take into account what patients define as an excellent outcome. Care should be well-planned, based on these expectations, and discussions should be summarized in a treatment directive, leaving little to chance. And a trusted health care proxy should be identified, in case the patient becomes incapable of making his or her own health decisions. With this road map, care execution and coordination manage the complexity of the situation, helping to simplify a patient's remaining time.[1]

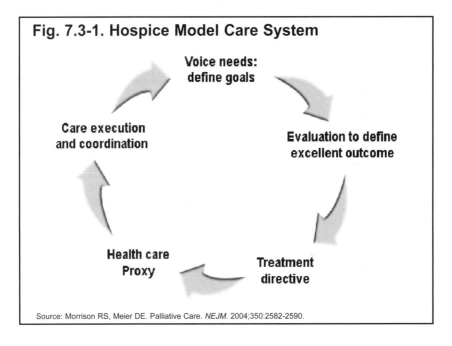

Fig. 7.3-1. Hospice Model Care System

Voice needs: define goals

Evaluation to define excellent outcome

Care execution and coordination

Health care Proxy

Treatment directive

Source: Morrison RS, Meier DE. Palliative Care. *NEJM*. 2004;350:2582-2590.

When palliative care plans are successful, what do we find? More joy and pleasure; less pain and worry. We also find less hospitalization, fewer nursing home placements, greater patient and family satisfaction, greater caregiver health and well-being, and, in the end, a greater likelihood of a peaceful death, surrounded by loved ones, at home.[1]

REFERENCES

1. Morrison RS, Meier DE. Palliative Care. *NEJM*. 2004;350:2582-2590.
2. Field MJ, Cassel CK, eds. Approaching death: improving care at the end of life. Washington, D.C.: National Academy Press, 1997. Cited in Morrison RS, Meier DE.

3. Quill TE, Perspectives on care at the close of life: initiating end-of-life discussions with seriously ill patients: addressing the "elephant in the room." *JAMA*. 2000;284:2502-2507. Cited in Morrison RS, Meier DE.
4. Tulsky JA. Doctor-patient communication. In: Morrison RS, Meier DE, eds. *Geriatric palliative care*. New York: Oxford University Press, 2003:314-331. Cited in Morrison RS, Meier DE.
5. Steinhauser KE, Christakis NA, Clipp EC, McNeilly M, McIntyre L, Tulsky JA. Factors considered important at the end of life by patients, family, physicians, and other care providers. *JAMA*. 2000;284:2476-2482. Cited in Morrison RS, Meier DE.
6. Fox E et al. Evaluation of prognostic criteria for determining hospice eligibility in patients with advanced lung, heart, or liver disease. *JAMA*. 1999;282:1638-1648.

TEACHING TOOLS

Policy Premises

1. As populations age, chronic illnesses create an uncertain medical future.
2. Traditional care systems are not well-suited for managing chronic complex illnesses.
3. Palliative care is a philosophy- and value-driven approach to the care of the chronically ill.
4. Goals of palliative care are focused and pragmatic.
5. Planning and interdisciplinary care coordination are essential.
6. When successful, palliative care outcomes are well-defined and all will benefit.

Review

1. What types of challenges do chronically ill patients often manage?
2. When it comes to chronically ill patients, our medical system currently focuses on which two goals?
3. Is a patient's value system important when determining the type of care he or she needs?
4. Which five points are key to successful palliative care?
5. How does palliative care relate to hospice care?

Online Resources

 Access online resources with this book's CD.

Center to Advance Palliative Care
http://www.capc.org/

Hospice and Palliative Care
http://www.nhpco.org/i4a/pages/index.cfm?pageid=3306&open-page=3306

The National Consensus Project for Quality Palliative Care
http://www.nationalconsensusproject.org/

TIME: Toolkit of Instruments to Measure End-of-Life Care
http://www.chcr.brown.edu/pcoc/toolkit.htm

Palliative Care and HIV/AIDS
http://www.who.int/hiv/topics/palliative/PalliativeCare/en/

Unlikely Way to Cut Costs: Comfort the Dying
http://webreprints.djreprints.com/1036690089843.html

Health Politics Online

For Original Health Politics Programs and Slides:

Palliative Care: Improving Quality of Life for the Chronically Ill
http://www.healthpolitics.com/program_info.asp?p=prog_63
Slide Briefing
http://www.healthpolitics.com/media/prog_63/brief_prog_63.pdf

The Best Place to Die

CONSIDERING HOSPICE

As baby boomers in the United States move en masse toward seniordom, they are beginning to focus as much on dying well as living well. It's not that they are morbid. It's that many of them are seeing the vision of the future in their own parents' reflections.

Twenty-five percent of American households now have family care-givers, mostly women and mostly boomers.[1] And it's the nature of the generation to ramp up expectations and to rebuild them to higher specifications. Currently, they don't like what they see, especially in an age where health care partnerships are replacing paternalism, and health consumers are devouring empowering educational information.[2]

The health community is getting the message and has realized that defining a "good death" requires input from patients and loved ones. The patient is looking for comfort, respect, emotional support, information and well-coordi-nated care. And to no one's surprise, loved ones are looking for the same things.[3]

What is today's deathbed reality? It is that nearly 7 out of 10 of us — some 69 percent — die in institutional settings — such as nursing homes or hospitals. More than 3 in 10, or 31 percent, die at home. Of those who die at home, 36 percent die without any caregiver present, 12 percent have the benefit of some nursing care, and 52 percent are supported by hospice services.[4]

The hospice movement was begun in 1946 with St. Christopher's Hospice in England.[5] It championed a holistic approach to the care of terminally ill patients, primarily those with cancer. Over the years, the approach has been extended to a wide variety of patients with terminal illnesses, and has spread around the globe. In the United States, however, access to insurance coverage for hospice services for terminally ill seniors who do not have cancer remains problematic. It requires certification from two physicians that the patient only has six months to live. Predicting this for chronic disease can be less reliable than for cancer.[6]

The various sites in which people die are associated with different understandings of disease states, different financial circumstances, and different capacities to support the extensive needs of dying patients. They are also associated with different patient groups. For instance, elderly women who are not married are disproportionately represented among nursing home deaths.[4] But is that a problem? After all, what better place to die than in an institution with trained personnel, intravenous medications, and lots of technology?

A recent study surveying loved ones of patients who died indicates that it may be worth the effort to carefully plan where you wish to die. The satisfaction of loved ones with the care of dying family members or friends varies widely by site and staffing. Managing the symptoms of pain and shortness of breath is problematic for a patient dying at home with only some nursing help, but improves if hospice services are in place. Nursing homes are weaker in these areas, while hospitals do well at managing pain, and are the best at managing shortness of breath.[4]

In terms of emotional support and respect for the patient, hospice care is clearly the leader. For example, the study showed that in the judgment of surviving loved ones, only 35 percent of hospice patients lacked adequate emotional support, while 52 percent of hospital patients felt neglected. And while only 4 percent of hospice patients felt respect for them was wanting, 20 percent of hospital patients experienced disrespect.[4]

The study also reveals differences in how the patients' loved ones were treated. Hospice once again markedly outperformed all others. Dissatisfaction with the level of family contact with physicians was only 14 percent in hospice compared with 31 percent in nursing homes and 51 percent in hospitals. Inadequate emotional support for families and loved ones was 21 percent in hospice compared with 36 percent in nursing homes and 38 percent in hospitals, and faulty information support for loved ones was a problem in 29 percent of hospice cases, compared to 44 percent in nursing homes and 50 percent in hospitals.[4]

Overall, looking at the needs of dying patients and the needs of their families and loved ones, it's not just site, but staff, that counts. Less-than-excellent care was noted 29 percent of the time with hospice care, compared with 58 percent of the time with nursing homes and 53 percent with hospitals. But it's not just being at home that makes the difference, because patients dying at home with just some nursing services experienced less-than-excellent care just as frequently as those in hospitals.[4]

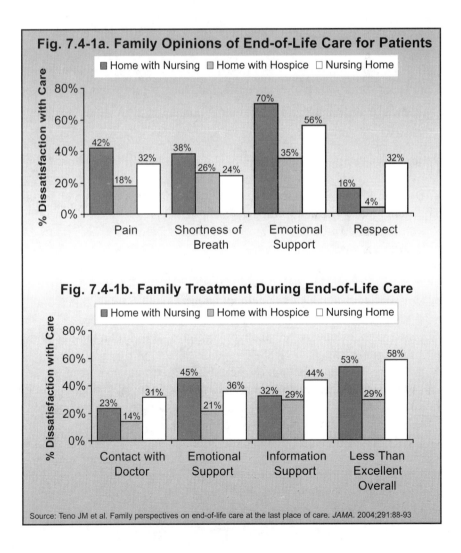

Fig. 7.4-1a. Family Opinions of End-of-Life Care for Patients

■ Home with Nursing ■ Home with Hospice □ Nursing Home

% Dissatisfaction with Care

Fig. 7.4-1b. Family Treatment During End-of-Life Care

■ Home with Nursing ■ Home with Hospice □ Nursing Home

% Dissatisfaction with Care

Source: Teno JM et al. Family perspectives on end-of-life care at the last place of care. *JAMA*. 2004;291:88-93

Careful planning can make a "good death" a more likely outcome for patients and loved ones. In some cases, an institutional setting is the only appropriate choice, as with a patient in extreme pain or respiratory distress. But in general, hospitals and nursing homes appear poorly equipped — with the conflicting demands of acute and chronic care, staffing and budget limitations, and the complexity of operations — to manage the complex and personalized needs of a dying patient and her loved ones to a harmonious conclusion.

Hospice care is not perfect. For example it could improve care of shortness of breath, and emotional support for patients. But the idea of holistic care comes closer to achieving the ideal of a "good death" than any of the current options.

We should build on that ideal of what is necessary for a "good death" — home based, multifaceted care, sustained, and information-rich for both patient and loved one.

REFERENCES

1. Donelan K et al. Challenged to care: Informal caregivers in a changing health system. *Health Affairs.* 2002;21:222-231.
2. Magee M, D'Antonio M. *The Best Medicine.* New York, NY; Saint Martin's Press; 1993.
3. Emanuel EJ, Emanuel LL. The promise of a good death. Lancet. 1998;351(suppl2):S1121-A1129. Quoted in Teno JM et al. Family perspectives on end-of-life care at the last place of care. *JAMA.* 2004;291:88-93.
4. Teno JM et al. Family perspectives on end-of-life care at the last place of care. *JAMA.* 2004;291:88-93.
5. Saunders C. Care of patients suffering from terminal disease at St. Joseph's Hospice, Hackney, London. Nursing Mirror. 1964;vii-x.
6. Fox E et al. Evaluation of prognostic criteria for determining hospice eligibility in patients with advanced lung, heart, or liver disease. *JAMA.* 1999;282:1638-1648.

TEACHING TOOLS

Policy Premises

1. A variety of health megatrends are intersecting on the issues of 'dying well.'
2. Defining a 'good death' requires input from patients and loved ones.
3. Most still die in institutional settings. Certain populations are overly represented.
4. Satisfaction of loved ones with care of the dying patient and support for family varies by site and staffing.
5. Careful planning can make a 'good death' a more likely outcome for patients and loved ones.

Review

1. Where do most Americans die?
2. What type of end-of-life care is rated highest in terms of emotional support?
3. How do we define a "good death"?
4. What type of end-of-life care is most highly rated by patients' loved ones?
5. What areas show room for improvement in all types of end-of-life care?

Online Resources

Access online resources with this book's CD.

How Does Hospice Measure Up?
http://www.nlm.nih.gov/medlineplus/hospicecare.html

Find a Hospice
http://www.hospicefoundation.org/endOfLifeInfo/

New York-Presbyterian: Home Health, Hospice, & Elder Care
http://nyp.org/health/cd_rom_content/adult/homehealth/index.htm

National Hospice and Palliative Care Organization
http://www.nhpco.org/i4a/pages/index.cfm?pageid=3254&open-page=3254

Home Health & Hospice Care
http://www.cdc.gov/mmwr/preview/mmwrhtml/00022103.htm

National Home and Hospice Care Data
http://www.cdc.gov/nchs/about/major/nhhcsd/nhhcsd.htm

What is Hospice Care?
http://www.cancer.org/docroot/ETO/content/ETO_2_5X_What_Is_Hospice_Care.asp?sitearea=ETO

Medicare Hospice Care
http://www.medicarerights.org/maincontenthospice.html

Financing Hospice Care
http://64.85.16.230/educate/content/elements/financinghospice-care.html

Health Politics Online

For Original Health Politics Programs and Slides:

Where is the Best Place to Die?
http://www.healthpolitics.com/program_info.asp?p=prog_40
Slide Briefing
http://www.healthpolitics.com/media/prog_40/brief_prog_40.pdf

Organizing the Dying Process

THE FOUR MANAGEMENT STAGES

I recently experienced two deaths in my family. One, my 50-year-old brother-in-law, married to my younger sister — together, they were the parents of three teenage children. The other, my wife's mother, who suffered from multiple chronic diseases and dementia, who died in her 90th year.

Both deaths involved the complex dynamics of a large family. I am one of 12 children and my wife is one of 10. Both loved ones died at home. Both had the assistance of hospice. And both progressed through a series of stages that taxed the families' management and organizational skills.

Author and psychiatrist Elisabeth Kubler-Ross described the five stages of grief as denial, anger, bargaining, depression and acceptance.[1] Roberta Temes' book, "Living with an Empty Chair" outlines three stages: numbness, disorganization and reorganization.[2] While both have merit, and our families encountered all eight of these stages in varying orders and in differing ways, they do not cover the more predictable organizational stages we encountered, nor do they define the management challenges associated with each stage.

So I have put together what I describe as the four organizational stages of dying: engagement, release, testimony and recovery. The first stage, engagement, focuses on confronting the threat, exploring options for combating it, making decisions about how best to proceed and following through on those decisions. Depending on the threat, time may or may not be an issue. For my brother-in-law, facing an aggressive cancer, time was of the essence. For my mother-in-law, with diabetes and dementia, not so much.

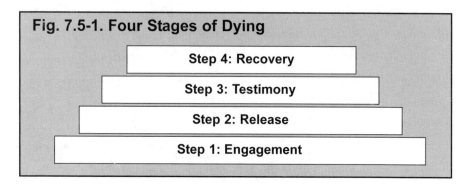

Fig. 7.5-1. Four Stages of Dying

Step 4: Recovery

Step 3: Testimony

Step 2: Release

Step 1: Engagement

During engagement, the patient, family and care team are expected to explore all curative options, provide clear and honest communications, invite family input, provide best recommendations, and ultimately affirm and support the patient's decision. This requires an organizational linkage that may be as uncomplicated as a trusted physician's office, as in my mother-in-law's case, or as complex as dealing with experimental research protocols and interdisciplinary cancer centers, as in my brother-in-law's case. In general, however, engagement translates into five management challenges. First is fact finding through personal research and outreach and through expert opinion and advice, facilitated by the establishment of trust and confidence. Second is decision making, directed at type and course of therapy. Third is intervention, executing the treatment plan, whether long-term or short-term. Fourth is monitoring to assess success and be able to make informed adjustments to the treatment plan. And fifth is active, ongoing reassessment with focus on risks and benefits of each decision point, and consideration not only of life but also quality of life.

The second stage is release. Having engaged and pursued reasonable steps to survive, without success, those involved have to acknowledge that death must now be accepted as a near-term reliability. For my brother-in-law, this reality set in during a third round of chemotherapy, after two previous regimens had failed, and bowel obstruction set in during the fifth of his six months of life following diagnosis. For my mother-in-law, this was a much more subtle and personal transition. She seemed to know when the time was right, almost "choosing her time," and death came 10 days later.

Whether chronic or acute, young or old, when a diagnosis is first made, everyone's focus is on life preservation. But a sharp decline, results of diagnostic studies, loss of control of activities of daily living, or an internal awareness can signal a transition and lead patients and families to recognize that death is approaching. Hopefulness thus collides with truthfulness. And the truth can be harsh and undeniable, especially for the young who haven't had as much time to mentally prepare. But for all ages, stage 2, release, requires acceptance by both the patient and loved ones. Readiness varies, and for progress to occur, there must be alignment and a common vision of what is to come. The focus shifts from life preservation to life enhancement. Quality of remaining life is tied to adjustments in the physical environment (such as moving a bed to the first floor) and ensuring that pain and other symptoms, such as nausea, are effectively managed. Support must be enlisted and resources marshaled.

For my brother-in-law, this meant having one of our sisters, who is a registered nurse, move in for the last two weeks of his life, working in tandem with the family. They also involved hospice and home visits by his doctors. For my mother-in-law, during the last week, it meant that my wife's four sisters joined her and the in-house caregiver who had managed her dementia for many years. They involved hospice to help with pain management and provide support as they accepted the dying process.

Because of the environment, we, as the family, were organized, and because the patients were relatively pain-free but fully conscious, they were able to conduct extensive and enlightened visitations during the closing days. This prepared the families and loved ones for the future and allowed what "needed to be said" to be said. It also created a transcendent atmosphere of great spirit to mix with the seemingly unbearable sorrow and loss. Words were exchanged that we will long remember.

With death, we arrive at the third stage: testimony. How should loved ones be remembered? This is under the control of the living. The obituary, funeral arrangements, family travel, eulogy, burial, and various memorial rituals all require attention. Of the four organizational stages of death, this may be the one most routinely mismanaged. It is critically important, not only in communicating the value and meaning of one's life, and the lives he or she touched, but also in beginning the healing process, and often allowing old wounds to be repaired, and disrupted lives to begin anew. Among the management challenges, first and foremost is inclusion — involvement of as many family members and loved ones as possible. Second is planning, including finances, timing of services, and communication before, during and after the ceremony. Third is performance — readings, eulogies, informal story telling, photo boards, and displays of items important to the individual and the bereaved. Fourth is comforting — coming together to manage those stricken, injured, and weakened by the course of events. And the fifth management challenge is the act of memorializing, which is an opportunity to reinforce goodness, humor, and values that deserve a spotlight. By memorializing, we challenge ourselves to live a better and more complete life.

The final organizational stage of dying is recovery — assisting loved ones in absorbing the loss and remembering in a way that advances the physical, mental and spiritual health of the bereaved.[3] There is not a perfect path or consistent timetable, but the management challenges associated with recovery are somewhat predictable. They include managing shock, confusion and disorientation; accepting the loss; sustaining individual self-worth; pacing recovery; identifying complicated grief if it persists and seeking professional help if it's needed; and, finally, reinvesting in relationships.

Each of these four stages of the dying process have common elements. But each is a unique management challenge in its own right. Similarities include that each stage is complex, requires planning, demands decisions, causes fatigue, and requires team support. That said, true success comes with the insight that each of the four stages is fundamentally different — they involve different missions, players, organizational interfaces, support staff, time pressures, and measures of success.

REFERENCES

1. Elisabeth Kubler-Ross Web site. Available at www.elisabethkubler-ross.com. Accessed May 19, 2005.
2. Cancer Survivors Web site. Available at: http://www.cancersurvivors.org/Coping/end%20term/stages.htm. Accessed May 19, 2005.
3. Prigerson HG, Jacobs SC. Caring for bereaved patients: "all the doctors just suddenly go." *JAMA*. 2001;286:1369-1376.

TEACHING TOOLS

Policy Premises

1. From a family, home-centric perspective, dying with dignity is a four-step process.
2. The first step is engagement: confront the threat, one's options in combating it, and make choices how best to proceed.
3. The second step is release: having pursued reasonable steps to survive, acknowledge that death must now be accepted as a near-term reliability.
4. The third step is testimony: plan a memorial service that captures the meaning and essence of a single life and comforts loved ones who remain.
5. The fourth step is recovery: assisting loved ones in remembering in a way that honors loss while advancing the physical, mental and spiritual health of the bereaved.
6. The four steps of dying with dignity have elements in common, but are each unique as well, and require differing management approaches.

Review

1. What are the patient, family and care team expected to do during the engagement stage of the dying process?
2. During which stage of the dying process should death be accepted as a near-term reliability?
3. What are the fundamental differences between life preservation and life enhancement?
4. Which of the four organizational stages in the dying process is most often mismanaged?
5. What are the similarities and differences of the four stages?

Online Resources

Access online resources with this book's CD.

The Last Days
http://www.mayoclinic.com/invoke.cfm?id=CA00048

Understanding Grief
http://familydoctor.org/079.xml

End-of-Life Care
http://www.nhpco.org/custom/directory/

Coping with Loss
http://www.nmha.org/infoctr/factsheets/42.cfm

Funerals and Memorials: A Part of Recovery
http://www.psych.org/news_room/media_advisories/funerals_mem
recov101601.cfm

Interacting with a Terminally Ill Loved One
http://www.mayoclinic.com/invoke.cfm?id=CA00041

Final Details: A Checklist
http://www.aarp.org/families/grief_loss/a2004-11-15-finalcheck-
list.html

Health Politics Online

For Original Health Politics Programs and Slides:

Organizing the Dying Process — The Four Management Stages
http://www.healthpolitics.com/program_info.asp?p=organizing_dyi
ng_process
Slide Briefing
http://www.healthpolitics.com/media/organizing_dying_process/bri
ef_organizing_dying_process.pdf

The Politics of Pain

APPLYING WHAT WE'VE LEARNED

Pain is a complex problem in our society with a controversial history and a significant social and economic impact. Struggling to understand and deal with pain is literally as old as the human condition. Medical historian Dr. Marcia Meldrum said, "Pain is the central metaphor of Judeo-Christian thought: the test of faith in the story of Job, the sacrificial redemption of the Crucifixion." But at the same time, Dr. Meldrum reminds us that "pain was also a medical problem."[1]

If pain has a philosophic, religious, and medical dimension, it also has an economic one. A recent study found that nearly 13 percent of the U.S. workforce lost time at work during a two-week period as a result of pain. More than 5 percent of the workforce lost time due to headaches; 3.2 percent lost time due to backaches; 2 percent due to arthritis and 2 percent due to other musculoskeletal complaints. The average worker affected by pain lost 4.6 hours of time at work per week, and the overall yearly cost to our nation from pain-related work loss was an impressive $61 billion.[2]

The history of pain management over the past 200 years has been complex and instructive. Opium was first synthesized in 1804 and remains in legitimate and illegitimate use to this day.[3] Morphine was first synthesized in Germany in the 1820s and produced in the United States some 10 years later. For the following 80 years, these medications were loosely regulated, widely available, and frequently suspect due to self-medication.[4]

Anesthesia first appeared on the scene some 160 years ago, a godsend for surgeons and patients alike. Ether was first used by a dentist, William Morton, in 1846, and chloroform was first used for childbirth by James Young Simpson in Britain in 1848.[5] In 1855 came the invention of the hollow hypodermic needle, and within 15 years published reports of a growing American "morphine habit" appeared.[4,6] In 1898 Bayer produced diacetylated morphine (brand name Heroin) as a cough therapy, and in 1899 it introduced aspirin.[7,8]

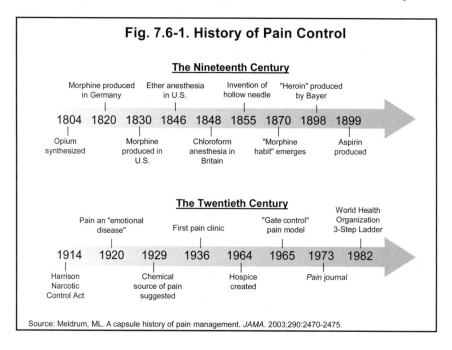

Fig. 7.6-1. History of Pain Control

The Nineteenth Century

Morphine produced in Germany · Ether anesthesia in U.S. · Invention of hollow needle · "Heroin" produced by Bayer

1804 — 1820 — 1830 — 1846 — 1848 — 1855 — 1870 — 1898 — 1899

Opium synthesized · Morphine produced in U.S. · Chloroform anesthesia in Britain · "Morphine habit" emerges · Aspirin produced

The Twentieth Century

Pain an "emotional disease" · First pain clinic · "Gate control" pain model · World Health Organization 3-Step Ladder

1914 — 1920 — 1929 — 1936 — 1964 — 1965 — 1973 — 1982

Harrison Narcotic Control Act · Chemical source of pain suggested · Hospice created · *Pain* journal

Source: Meldrum, ML. A capsule history of pain management. *JAMA.* 2003;290:2470-2475.

Widespread self-medication and abuse led to the Harrison Narcotic Control Act of 1914, drawing legitimate use of pain medication under the wing of physicians.[7] Yet physicians' views of what pain meant and how it should be approached widely varied. In 1920 many physicians considered pain an "emotional disease," and psychoanalytic approaches to therapy of a patient's pain (which appeared often without visible source, and preceded our understanding of the underlying causes of most of today's chronic diseases) created a major disconnect between doctors and patients.[9]

In 1929, a chemical link to pain was first suggested, and in 1936, the first pain clinic was established at Bellevue Hospital in New York City.[10,11] The holistic approach to pain management became firmly established in 1964 as an outflow of the hospice movement at Britain's St. Christopher's Hospital.[12] One year later the gate control model of pain was advanced, stimulating research into the linkages between peripheral sensory stimulation and central pain reception and interpretation by the brain.[13] Pain as a multidisciplinary concern was firmly established with the launching of the medical journal *Pain* in 1973.[14] And nine years later the WHO weighed in with a logical and patient-friendly three-step approach to humane pain management.[15]

So it's been a long and complex road. And the truth is that consistent and effective care for the patient with pain continues to come in conflict with fears of addiction on the left and blaming the victim on the right. The physician John Kent Spender in 1874 said, "[T]he medical man who (from ignorance or timidity) withholds hypodermic medicine from a patient afflicted with cancer is…totally without excuse."[7] But too often now, 130 years later, caregivers struggle with mixed feelings. For some, pain calls for effective therapy, but also brings the risk of substance abuse and long-term addiction, followed by more pain. For others, pain continues to signal weakness and poor character. These judgments can create a sense of powerlessness and hopelessness in patients, which further amplifies their pain.

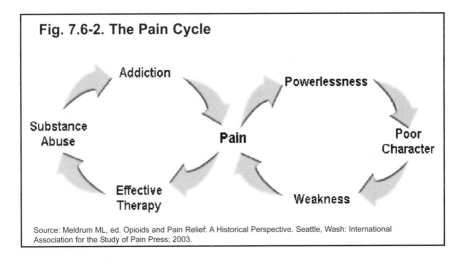

Fig. 7.6-2. The Pain Cycle

Addiction

Powerlessness

Substance Abuse

Pain

Poor Character

Effective Therapy

Weakness

Source: Meldrum ML, ed. Opioids and Pain Relief: A Historical Perspective. Seattle, Wash: International Association for the Study of Pain Press; 2003.

But there are encouraging signs. Pain has emerged as a primary point of focus for clinicians and researchers alike. We now have discriminated between acute pain, the pain of chronic disease, and the suffering of the terminally ill, rather than lumping them all together.[16] We have an International Association for the Study of Pain, founded in 1973, with 6,700 members from 60 disciplines and 100 countries.[1] And we have better science and more structured approaches for pain management.

Some would say the application of rigorous science is long overdue. Harvard pharmacologist Reid Hunt suggested in 1929 that "a thorough study of the morphine molecule might show a possibility of separating the analgesic from the habit-forming property."[17] And if you take that science and place it in context, as was done in 1964, you reach a new level of insight. It was then, according to medical historian Marcia Meldrum, that "[Cicely] Saunders' concept of 'total pain'…compounded physical and mental distress with social, spiritual and emotional concerns…demanding a holistic concept of management."[1]

So what have we learned over the years that must be absorbed by both caregivers and patients with pain? First, pain can be assessed. We know from multiple studies that simple 1-to-10, pictorial and graphic patient self-grading systems accurately define levels of pain and the degree of associated side effects due to treatment for pain.[18,19] We know as well that display of these graphs in the medical record encourages more active and successful pain management.[20] Second, we know that no one treatment works for all patients. Care must be individualized.[21] Third, we know that pain is a multidimensional construct with different sensory outputs, different cortical uptake of stimuli, different cultural expressions of pain consistent with belief systems and mental states, and different levels of impact by depression, malnutrition and shortness of breath.[12] Fourth, we know a three-step approach that modulates therapy for mild, moderate and severe pain is helpful, and that standard therapy can be augmented with anticonvulsants, antidepressants, radiation therapy and other therapies in the most difficult cases.[15,16] And finally, we know that pain is real and treatable, and that there is no merit in suffering.

REFERENCES

1. Meldrum, ML. A capsule history in pain management. *JAMA*. 2003;290:2470-2475.
2. Stewart WF et al. Lost productive time and cost due to common pain conditions in the US workforce. *JAMA*. 2003;290:2443-2454.
3. Schmitz R. Friedrich Wilhelm Sertürner and the discovery of morphine. *Pharm Hist*. 1985;27:61-74. Quoted in Meldrum.
4. Howard-Jones N. A critical study of the origins and early development of hypodermic medication. *J Hist Med Allied Sci*. 1947;2:201-245. Quoted in Meldrum.
5. Pernick MS. A Calculus of Suffering: Pain, Professionalism, and Anesthesia in Nineteenth-Century America. New York, NY: Columbia

University Press; 1985. Quoted in Meldrum.

6. Kerr N. Inebriety, or Narcomania: Its Etiology, Pathology, Treatment and Jurisprudence. London, England: Lewis; 1894. Quoted in Meldrum.

7. Meldrum ML, ed. Opioids and Pain Relief: A Historical Perspective. Seattle, Wash: International Association for the Study of Pain Press; 2003. Quoted in Meldrum.

8. McTavish JR. What's in a name? Aspirin and the American Medical Association. *Bull Hist Med.* 1987;61:343-366. Quoted in Meldrum.

9. Hodgkiss A. From Lesion to Metaphor: Chronic Pain in British, French, and German Medical Writings. Amsterdam, the Netherlands: Rodopi; 2000. Quoted in Meldrum.

10. Acker CJ. Creating the American Junkie: Addiction Research in the Classic Era of Narcotic Control. Baltimore, MD: Johns Hopkins University Press; 2001.

11. Rovenstine EA, Wertheim HM. Therapeutic nerve block. *JAMA.* 1941;117:1599-1603. Quoted in Meldrum.

12. Saunders C. Care of patients suffering from terminal illness at St Joseph's Hospice, Hackney, London. *Nurs Mirror.* 1964;a:vii-x. Quoted in Meldrum.

13. Noordenbos W. *Pain.* Amsterdam, the Netherlands: Elsevier; 1959. Quoted in Meldrum.

14. Liebeskind JC, Meldrum ML, John J. Bonica, world champion of pain. In: Jensen TS, Turner JA, Wiesenfeld-Hallin Z, eds. Proceedings of the Eighth World Congress on Pain: Progress in Pain Research and Management. Vol 8. Seattle, Wash: International Association for the Study of Pain Press; 1997:19-32. Quoted in Meldrum.

15. World Health Organization. Cancer Pain Relief. Geneva, Switzerland: World Health Organization; 1986. Quoted in Meldrum.

16. Bruera E, Kim HN. Cancer Pain. *JAMA.* 2003;290:2476-2479.

17. Eddy NB, May EL. The search for a better analgesic. *Science.* 1973;181:407-414. Quoted in Meldrum.

18. Bruera E, Schoeller T, Wenk R, et al. A prospective multicenter assessment of the Edmonton staging system for cancer pain. *J Pain Symptom Manage.* 1995;10:348-355. Quoted in Bruera E, Kim HN.

19. Bruera E, Neumann C. History and clinical examination of the cancer pain patient: assessment and measurement. In: Rice A, Warfield C, Justin D, Eccleston C, eds. *Clinical Pain Management Cancer Pain.* New York, NY: Oxford University Press; 2003:63-71. Quoted in Bruera E, Kim HN.

20. Guidelines for using the Edmonton Symptom Assessment System

(ESAS). Quoted in Bruera E, Kim HN.

21. Portenoy RK, Foley KM. Chronic use of opioid analgesics in non-malignant pain: report of 38 cases. *Pain*. 1986;25:171-186. Quoted in Meldrum.

TEACHING TOOLS

Policy Premises

1. Pain is a complex problem with significant social and economic impact.
2. Pain has had a controversial history over the past 200 years.
3. Effective therapy continues to fight fears of addiction on the left and blaming the victim on the right.
4. Pain has emerged as a primary medical condition rather than a secondary incidental symptom.
5. Science and structured multidisciplinary approaches are placing pain management on more solid ground.
6. Learnings need to be absorbed by caregivers and reinforced by patients.

Review

1. What is the economic impact of pain?
2. What were the past two centuries' major clinical advances in controlling pain?
3. How has our understanding of pain evolved over time?
4. What are some risks associated with treating pain?
5. What are some of the components of successful pain management?

Online Resources

 Access online resources with this book's CD.

Understanding Pain
http://www.ampainsoc.org/decadeofpain/

Seeking Relief
http://www.library.ucla.edu/libraries/biomed/his/painexhibit/index.html

The National Pain Foundation
http://www.painconnection.org/

Facts About Pain in America
http://www.edc.org/PainLink/plfctr.html

World Medical Association Statement on the Care of Patients with Severe Chronic Pain in Terminal Illness
http://www.wma.net/e/policy/c2.htm

National Pain Awareness
http://www.painconnection.org/NationalPainAwareness/default.asp

Health Politics Online

For Original Health Politics Programs and Slides:

The Politics of Pain
http://www.healthpolitics.com/program_info.asp?p=prog_37
Slide Briefing
http://www.healthpolitics.com/media/prog_37/brief_prog_37.pdf

CHAPTER 8

Science and Society

"The future belongs to science."

— WILLIAM OSLER
1947

"The most important question facing the scientific community in the coming 25 years is: How can it maintain its contact with society to ensure that it has continued license to operate?"

— SIR PAUL NURSE
Nobel Laureate
President, Rockefeller
University, 2003

"The urgency is to re-establish the fundamental position that science plays in helping devise uses of knowledge to resolve social ills."

— JOHN GIBBONS
Science Advisor
Clinton Administration

"Good doctors use both clinical expertise and the best available external evidence, and neither alone is enough. Without clinical expertise, practice risks becoming tyrannized by evidence, for even excellent external evidence may be inapplicable to or inappropriate for an individual patient. Without current best evidence, practice risks becoming rapidly out of date, to the detriment of patients."

— DAVID SACKETT
British Medical Journal
1996

CHAPTER 8.1

Leading With Science

A PATH TO THE FUTURE

What is science? Why should we trust in science? Who is leading us in science? These are all questions more answerable in the past, and hopefully in the future, than they appear to be today. This is somewhat surprising considering the great discoveries on our immediate horizon and the promise of science for our future. But the combination of the bursting of the technology bubble at the end of the past century, the mixing of science and religion, and the leadership pause in anticipation of breakthroughs associated with genomics have all contributed to several years of scientific silence.

That said, science is quietly rediscovering its voice as clinical decision-making is increasingly grounded in treatment guidelines and consensus statements termed "evidence-based medicine." Evidence-based medicine was defined in 1996 by Dr. David Sackett as "the conscientious, explicit, and judicious use of the current best evidence in making decisions about the care of individual patients. The practice of evidence-based medicine means integrating individual clinical expertise with the best available external clinical evidence from systematic research."[1]

Almost all evidence-based medicine flows from clinical research, or scientific trials involving human volunteers. William Osler, a critical figure in the history of medicine, instructed students to "Observe, record, tabulate, communicate."[2] The process to do just that, and to do it in a manner that is reproducible and verifiable, has been slowly evolving over the past 250 years. In 1794, the English physician, William Heberden said, "I please myself with thinking that the method of teaching the art of healing is becoming, everyday, more conformable to what reason and nature require; that the errors introduced by superstition and false philosophy are gradually retreating..."[2] Out of the thinking of the day evolved the clinical trial, a carefully planned experiment designed to expose the benefits and risks of a specific intervention in humans.[3]

While science undeniably has progressed, the process we rely on to separate fact from fiction, the use of randomized, controlled trials that compare a new treatment to a standard treatment or placebo in a matched population, dates back to the 18th century. In 1754, James Lind, a Scottish naval surgeon, studied 12 sailors with scurvy to see if they could be healed by diet. Two were given a quart of cider a day; two sweet oil of vitriol (ether); two vinegar; two seawater; two an herb paste; and two were given oranges and lemons. Within six days, the fruit's effectiveness was obvious. It took another 40 years for the treatment to effectively eliminate scurvy from British ships, and another century before vitamin C was identified as the critical missing nutrient.[4]

Science, traditionally, is directed to where there is a need. The clinical trial process approaches patients with need from three different vantage points. Prevention studies examine treatments or behavioral changes that might prevent illness. Diagnostic studies seek new or improved methods of identifying an illness. Treatment studies test a chemical agent for both safety and effectiveness.

Clinical trials require cooperation among government, academia, industry, health professionals and patients, with a clear understanding and commitment to ethical care. Safety should always be a primary concern. A critical question to answer prior to proceeding: "Is the health problem at issue worth any safety risks involved in developing a treatment?" If the answer is yes, a systematic approach has evolved to limit the inherent risk of clinical trials by staging the study into four phases.[5,6] First, pre-clinical safety assessment, or testing the treatment in animals prior to human studies. Second, pre-approval safety assessment involving a small number of healthy volunteers. Third, safety assessment in large numbers of patients, with FDA reviews. Fourth, ongoing surveillance, post-FDA approval, for side effects.

The success of science, in the global age of health consumer empowerment, is based on broad public confidence in the integrity and utility of scientific research. What is medical science? Medical science is a well-tested, cooperative process of observation, testing and communication, designed to empower patients and caregivers with the best current knowledge to maintain health and prevent and treat disease. Why should we trust science? We should trust science because the process has a strong ethical grounding and a proven process that is transparent and verifiable. Is science perfect? By no means. What we believe we know today may be altered by a new discovery tomorrow. There is much that remains to be learned. That said, science has delivered an increase in the quantity and quality of our lives.

Fifty years ago our physicians barely understood the scientific underpinnings of heart disease, stroke, depression, arthritis, Parkinson's disease, Alzheimer's disease, or the role of cigarettes, diet and exercise in health. And today, this knowledge is commonplace in large segments of our general population. Science created and transferred that knowledge. And with the growing alliance among health consumers, caregivers and scientists, science, with a renewed and stronger voice, could, in the next 10 years, deliver quality of life improvement that would make us all proud. William Osler said, "The future belongs to science."[2] And indeed it does.

REFERENCES

1. McNeill WH. *Plaques and Peoples*. New York, NY: Doubleday; 1989:237.
2. Krentzman BZ. Mayo Clinic Explanation of Clinical Trials.
3. Sackett DL et al. Evidence based medicine: What it is and what it isn't. *BMJ*: 1996:312:71-72.
4. Foege W. A rational health future [keynote address]. At www.hsph.harvard.edu/digest/foege.html. Accessed 12/12/01.
5. Pharmaceutical Research and Manufacturers of America (PhRMA). 2001 Industry Profile. Washington, DC: PhRMA; 2001:24-25.
6. National Institutes of Health (NIH). Clinical Trials.gov. At: www.clinicaltrials.gov. Accessed 4/6/01.

TEACHING TOOLS

Policy Premises

1. Clinical decision making is increasingly grounded in treatment guidelines and consensus statements that have been termed evidence-based medicine.
2. Methods of study to separate fact from fiction and superstition from reason have emerged slowly over the past 250 years.
3. The strongest evidence is data from a randomized, controlled trial, comparing a new treatment with standard treatment or placebo.
4. Science and clinical research trials should be oriented to where there is a need.
5. Clinical trials require cooperation among government, academia, industry, caregivers, and patients who share a clear understanding of goals and a commitment to ethical care.

Review

1. What is evidence-based medicine?
2. Why do we rely on clinical trials?
3. The clinical trial process approaches patients with need from what three vantage points?
4. What are the four staging phases that researchers have adopted to better ensure clinical trial safety?
5. Why should we trust science?

Online Resources

 Access online resources with this book's CD.

Mayo Clinic Explanation of Clinical Trials
http://home.comcast.net/~bkrentzman/meds/clinical.trials.html

Beyond Discovery: The Path from Research to Human Benefit
http://www.beyonddiscovery.org/

Health Politics Online

For Original Health Politics Programs and Slides:

Leading With Science
http://www.healthpolitics.com/program_info.asp?p=prog_15
Slide Briefing
http://www.healthpolitics.com/media/prog_15/brief_prog_15.pdf

CHAPTER 8.2

Does Science Make a Difference?

FINDING ITS PLACE IN A CHANGING WORLD

The voice of science has been remarkably faint over the past few years, raising the age-old question and challenge — does science make a difference? Sir Paul Nurse, president of Rockefeller University and Nobel Prize winner for medicine in 2001, thinks it does, and he says, "The most important question facing the scientific community in the coming 25 years is: How can it maintain its contact with society to ensure that it has a continued license to operate?"[1]

A variety of environmental factors over the past few years have conspired to separate scientists from society and dampen enthusiasm and support for scientific progress. These include the bursting of the technology bubble in the late 90s, the mixing of religion and science in modern politics, the movement toward holistic and homeopathic care, and the explosion of information — some good and some bad — in traditional and electronic media.

We live in an age of health consumer empowerment. Over the past two decades, patients have made considerable progress, largely supported by their physicians, toward educational empowerment.[2] Yet, clearly, scientific enlightenment remains a work in progress. Two-thirds of the American public believe that alternative theories to Darwin's theory of evolution should be taught in public schools.[3]

As a counterbalance, mainstream science has clearly made a positive and undeniable contribution to the human condition. Years of life have been expanded, moving in one century from an average lifespan of approximately

50 years to nearly 80. Between 1950 and 1990, the world's population has nearly doubled and now tops 6 billion. In the last half-century we've made enormous strides in understanding organ function or physiology, and disease processes or pathophysiology. This knowledge, along with a scientific lexicon, is rapidly being transferred to patients, placing them in a position to more actively partner with their caregivers.

As we have gained understanding of disease processes, we have gradually conquered many of them, including infectious diseases, peptic ulcer disease and, increasingly, heart disease. For others, behavioral insights, such as the harmful effects of cigarette smoking and cancer screening and prevention, have made a real difference. Lives have been saved, disability lessened, and all of this has occurred in a moment of time when new worlds have been explored for the first time — ranging from the genome to the outer cosmos, with the help of the Hubble Space Telescope.

And yet, at the same time, science manages to raise a wide variety of troubling questions. Issues of concern include genetic engineering of foods, global warming, human cloning, germ warfare, nuclear power and the use of nuclear weapons. The one underlying, common theme: Will we control science or will it control us? Dr. John Gibbons, science adviser with the Clinton administration, has noted: "People thought of science as a cornucopia of goodies. Now they have to choose between good and bad."[3]

Being a scientist remains a highly prestigious career choice, however, the number of individuals pursuing a career as a scientist is somewhat in decline. A recent Harris poll showed that 57 percent agreed that being a scientist carried very great prestige, above doctors, teachers, nurses, and certainly above lawyers, athletes and actors. And science remains intriguing to the young and bright and inquisitive. Solving riddles, taking pleasure in the craft, craving unique insights all contribute to the allure. When Einstein had the original insight that would underlie his theory of relativity, he said it was the "happiest thought of my life." So, in its simplest terms, science makes scientists happy.

In the global environment however, science is becoming less United States-centric. Some of this may reflect a downward trend in prestige in the U.S. While still at the top at 57 percent, the prestige level for scientists is down from 66 percent in 1977. At the same time, interest in science beyond America's boundaries is increasing. For example, by 1999, the number of foreign students in full-time engineering programs in the United States exceeded the number of U.S. students, according to the National Science Foundation. And more than 25 percent of the U.S. industrial patents are now held by Japan, Taiwan and South Korea.[3] While spending of late has increased in both public and private science sectors in the United States, there is a great need to expand cross-sector cooperation to enhance effectiveness and competitiveness.

Clearly, science is in transition but experts are optimistic. Dr. Gerald Holton, a Harvard professor specializing in the history of science, says: "Science is one of the charismatic activities. This keeps our interest in science at some level even if we are deeply troubled by some aspects of its technical misuse." Noble laureate Dean Lederman adds, "You can smell discovery in the air."

What are the major challenges for science and scientists up ahead? The most dramatic opportunities lie at the intersection of human, environmental and population science. Those science issues in the news include breakthroughs in cancer, AIDS and immunologic diseases, acid rain, environmental toxins, global warming, genetically modified food, sustainable energy and urban city management.

This last item grows in urgency as we move from 3 billion urban dwellers in 2000 to 5 billion in 2005. The only way to manage the predictable issues of waste, water use, congestion, pollution, transportation, and energy are by creating a new science of cities. [4]

Dr. John Gibbons comments, "The urgency is to re-establish the fundamental position that science plays in helping devise uses of knowledge to resolve social ills."[3]

Will science make a difference in tomorrow's world? Probably more than we can even begin to imagine.

REFERENCES

1. Wilford JN. Will we ever find Atlantis? *New York Times*. November 11, 2003.
2. Nash DB. *Connecting with the New Healthcare Consumer*. Aspen Publishers, Gaithersberg, MD 2001.
3. Broad WJ and Glanz J. Does Science Matter. *New York Times*.

November 11, 2003

4. Heiken, G. " Earth Science in the City." American Geophysicial Union, Washington, DC 2002.

TEACHING TOOLS

Policy Premises

1. The voice of science has been remarkably faint over the past few years.
2. Science undeniably has made a positive human contribution.
3. Science has also raised new issues that are troubling.
4. To be a scientist remains highly prestigious but less so than in the past, and alternate theories are on the rise.
5. Leadership in science is shifting overseas.
6. Major challenges for science and scientists lie ahead at the intersection of human, environmental and population science.

Review

1. What environmental factors have led to the separation between science and society in recent years?
2. What are some of the contributions science has made to mankind during the past century?
3. What issues of concern have been raised by science in recent years?
4. How does the public rate the prestige of being a scientist?
5. What major challenges and opportunities are ahead for science and scientists?

Online Resources

Access online resources with this book's CD.

NSF Director Colwell Touts Science's Past, Future in Shannon Lecture
http://www.nih.gov/news/NIH-Record/01_08_2002/story02.htm

'National Academies Keck Futures Initiative' to Transform Interdisciplinary Research
http://www4.nationalacademies.org/news.nsf/isbn/04152003?Open Document

Statement of the Honorable John H. Gibbons, Director, OSTP, before the Committee on Science U.S. House of Representatives
http://clinton1.nara.gov/White_House/EOP/OSTP/other/ts950106.html

Public Perceptions of Scientists
http://www.nsf.gov/sbe/srs/seind02/c7/c7s3.htm#c7s3l2

Public Interest in S&T and Other Issues
http://www.nsf.gov/sbe/srs/seind02/c7/c7s1.htm#c7s1l1

Health Politics Online

For Original Health Politics Programs and Slides:

Does Science Make a Difference?
http://www.healthpolitics.com/program_info.asp?p=prog_31
Slide Briefing
http://www.healthpolitics.com/media/prog_31/brief_prog_31.pdf

Medical
Knowledge

LOST IN TRANSLATION

When we debate issues of health care, we frequently argue over what to cut
and what to add, but infrequently reflect on what we already have that isn't
being utilized. In short, there's a great deal that we lose in the translation.
While most pin their hopes for a healthy future on new discoveries, many fail
to utilize the current knowledge.

Dr. Claude Lenfant from the National Institutes of Health writes,
"Moving the knowledge off the shelves and into practice, making it relevant
and accessible to practitioners and patients, achieving a true marriage of
knowledge with intuition and judgment — all this requires translation."[1]

But the reality is that the eyes of patients and doctors alike are frequently on the future rather than the present. Seventy-two percent of Americans
believe that new scientific and medical breakthroughs are essential for staying
healthy.[2] Yet a 2003 Institute of Medicine report pulls us back to the present
with this comment: "The stark reality is that we spend billions in research to
find appropriate treatments...but we repeatedly fail to translate that knowledge
and capacity into clinical practice."[3]

The truth is, we have trouble moving knowledge off the shelf and down
the "translational highway."[4] This is not surprising when you look at the major
stops along the way. Basic science must give way to clinical research studies.
The studies must weave through the regulatory process to become approved
therapies. The therapies must challenge the status quo to become the new standard of medical practice. And even if clinicians broadly adopt a new approach,

patients must comply to yield positive outcomes.

There is no better example of the chasm between knowledge and practice than cardiovascular disease. "What we know" is frequently not "what we do." We know that beta-blockers used after myocardial infarction save lives. But a study in 1996 — 15 years after this discovery — showed only 62.5 percent of post-MI patients used this medication.[5] We know that all patients post-MI should be screened for cholesterol, but in reality only one-half to three-quarters of them are.[6] We know that aspirin is lifesaving for patients with coronary artery disease and MI, and yet only one-third of them use aspirin.[7] And we know that patients with acute MI should receive clot-dissolving therapy or acute angioplasty, but only one-third of them do.[8]

Establishing and promoting professional standards of care can move the dial. The National Committee for Quality Assurance (NCQA), with its Health Plan Employer Data and Information Set (HEDIS), measures and informs practice in the majority of U.S. health plans. Significant improvement has occurred in NCQA members. For example, beta-blocker use post-MI has risen from 62.5 percent in 1996 to 92.5 percent in 2001. And appropriate use of blood pressure control medication has risen from 39 percent in 1999 to 55.4 percent in 2001.[9]

Patients seem poised to assume greater responsibility as well. A 2001 study revealed that 94 percent of U.S. patients were more involved in health decisions, 92 percent took more control of their own health and 82 percent had more discussions with physicians compared to 10 years ago. That said, patients remain more focused on short-term than long-term benefits, with 93 percent willing to accept the risk of a prescription medicine if it will cure a disease, but only 49 percent willing to comply if it prevents a disease.[10]

Building a successful "translational highway" requires speaking to clinicians and patients simultaneously. Publications are an important first step and fundamental to scientific exchange of ideas.[11] However, there are some 400,000 medical scientific articles published each year, many more than even the most highly motivated clinician can absorb.[12] One strategy to manage this volume and complexity is the consensus conference; one or two days of highly focused discussion yielding consensus on a standard of care. Public education has also proven to be useful. For example, the "Back to Sleep" campaign, encouraging parents to place infants to sleep on their backs to prevent Sudden Infant Death Syndrome (SIDS), resulted in a 43 percent decline in deaths from SIDSfrom 1992 to 1997.[13] Consumer word of mouth, activated by voluntary health organizations, combines education and motivation. Advertising can help provide accurate information, consumer dialogue, and engagement between patients and physicians as we see in many "ask your doctor" campaigns. And finally, leveraging the patient-physician relationship to provide not only clinical support, but also educational support through coordinated teams — especially in the management of chronic disease — can be highly effective.

We're slowly learning how to translate discovery into practice. But with an explosion of discoveries on the horizon and boomer aging just around the corner we need to repave the "translational highway" and add a few lanes while we're at it.

REFERENCES

1. Lenfant C. Clinical research to clinical practice - Lost in translation. *New England Journal of Medicine*. 2003;349:868-74.
2. Belden Russonello & Stewart, for Alliance for Aging Research. Great expectations: Americans' views on aging-Results of a national survey on aging research. Washington, DC: Belden Russonello & Stewart. 2001.
3. Adams K., Corrigan JM, eds. Priority areas for national action: Transforming health care quality. Washington, DC: National Academy Press. 2003.
4. Schwartz K., Vilquin JT. Building the translational highway: Toward new partnerships between academia and the private sector. Nature Medicine. 2003;9:493-5.
5. National Committee for Quality Assurance. The state of managed care quality. Washington, D.C.: National Committee for Quality Assurance. 1997.
6. National Committee for Quality Assurance. The state of managed care quality. Washington, D.C.: National Committee for Quality Assurance. 1999.
7. Awtry EH, Loscalzo J. Aspirin. *Circulation*.2000;101:1206-18.
8. National Registry of Myocardial Infarction. NRMI 4 quarterly data report 2002. San Francisco: Genentech. 2002.
9. National Committee for Quality Assurance. The state of health care quality. Washington, D.C.: National Committee for Quality Assurance. 2002.
10. Magee M. Relationship-based health care in the United States, United

Kingdom, Canada, Germany, South Africa, and Japan: A comparative study of patient and physician perceptions worldwide. Helsinki: Paper presented at World Medical Association General Assembly. 2003

11. Montaner JSG, O'Shaughnessy MV, et al. Industry-sponsored clinical research: A double-edged sword. *Lancet.* 2001;358:1893-1895.

12. Giorganni S, ed. Bench, bedside, and beyond: clinical research at the crossroads. *The Pfizer Journal.* 2002;6:29.

13. United States Senate Joint Economic Committee. 2002. The Benefits of Medical Research and the Role of the NIH. Washington, DC: United States Senate Joint Economic Committee.

TEACHING TOOLS

Policy Premises

1. While most pin their hopes for a healthy future on new discoveries, many fail to utilize current knowledge.
2. Studying it isn't the same as fixing it. We have trouble moving knowledge off the shelves.
3. Treatment of patients with coronary artery disease and myocardial infarction is a case in point.
4. Establishing and promoting professional standards of care can move the dial.
5. Patients are more willing to respond to acute threats to health than to invest in long-term prevention.
6. Building a successful "translational highway" requires speaking to clinicians and patients simultaneously.

Review

1. What are some of the main steps in translating a scientific discovery into clinical practice?
2. What are the roadblocks along the "translational highway"?
3. What does the example of people with coronary artery disease and MI reveal about utilizing medical knowledge?
4. What are ways that organizations and patients can help to better utilize research and treatments?
5. What are some strategies for building a successful "translational highway"?

Online Resources

Access online resources with this book's CD.

Translational Research Initiative
http://ccr.ncifcrf.gov/initiatives/TRI/

Clinical practice guidelines and the translation of knowledge: the science of continuing medical education
http://www.cmaj.ca/cgi/content/full/163/10/1278

Translation of Research Results into Practice
http://www.nhlbi.nih.gov/resources/docs/plan/translat.htm

Knowledge Translation
http://www.cochranemsk.org/professional/knowledge/default.asp?s=1

Health Politics Online

For Original Health Politics Programs and Slides:

Medical Knowledge: Lost In Translation
http://www.healthpolitics.com/program_info.asp?p=prog_29
Slide Briefing
http://www.healthpolitics.com/media/prog_29/brief_prog_29.pdf

CHAPTER 8.4

The Power of Information

BRIDGING GLOBAL HEALTH DISPARITIES

The world's populations are increasingly linked today; our problems increasingly transparent. Populations around the world are increasingly hopeful that knowledge and opportunity can advance our common health and bridge the gaps between rich and poor, between the haves and the have-nots, between those filled with hope and those consumed by despair.[1]

When examining the health priorities that exist, information systems to support the growth of our doctors, nurses and caregivers are often overlooked. This is a mistake. Beyond the obvious benefits of being up-to-date with the latest science and medicine, medical knowledge can be both transformative — motivating growth in a way that advances the standard of care — and energizing — providing the fuel to power groups to overcome what otherwise would appear to be insurmountable obstacles.[2]

A recent *New England Journal of Medicine* editorial on this issue notes, "Warren Stevens of the Medical Research Council Laboratories in Gambia has noted that intellectual isolation represents an important hindrance to the development of world class researchers in African countries. Access to timely, relevant, high-quality scientific information represents a substantial gain for the researchers, students, teachers and policy makers in low-income countries."[3]

Technology can often be the fastest, most efficient and effective way to bridge an economically or geographically based knowledge gap. In 2002, the World Health Organization, in concert with the World Bank and a group of leading biomedical publishers, created HINARI, the Health InterNetwork

Access to Research Initiative.[4]

HINARI's goal was to "improve online access to scientific resources as a way of supporting health professionals, medical researchers and academics in developing countries."[3] What HINARI reveals is that when faced with a compelling societal need, competing medical entities will join hands and collaborate. The technology platform provides an "island of common stewardship" where partners can gather, create and serve together.[5]

The response can be dramatic. The initial offering of HINARI was this: If your country has an annual per capita income of less than $1,000, you can receive access to all biomedical journals electronically for free. If you have an annual per capita income of $1,000 to $3,000, your institution pays only $1,000 per year, and these funds are pooled to support investment in expanding hardware and software in partner countries. The offering has been well-received. Since its inception, 1,043 institutions in 100 of the 113 eligible countries are participants, 69 for free, and 31 for $1,000 per institution per year.[3]

Clearly, information technology solutions require infrastructure. In the past, the needs — from computers to paper, from toner to electric generators, from work stations to Internet access — may have seemed unreachable.[3] But the reality is that these issues can and are being resolved with cooperative investment and improved technology solutions.

It's important to recognize as well that information is clearly only part of the solution. It does not correct in and of itself famine, absence of clean water, infectious disease, absence of shelter, war, political instability, or corruption.[1] But it can enlighten and empower. It can bring people together. It can begin to break the cycle of despair and desperation.

Information technology solutions are transformative and their results are measurable. Take HINARI for instance: In medical institutions in the poorest countries, 56 percent had no subscriptions to international journals, and 21 percent subscribed to an average of two journals. In the next poorest group, 34 percent had five or fewer subscriptions while another 34 percent had none at all.[3]

Yet from January through June of 2003, these very same institutions accessed 34,680 articles from 214 journals. And from July through December they more than doubled their activity, accessing nearly 74,000 articles. Connectivity trumped economics. Several of the largest users — Ethiopia,

Vietnam, and Nepal — were among the poorest countries. HINARI's focus now is on user training.[3]

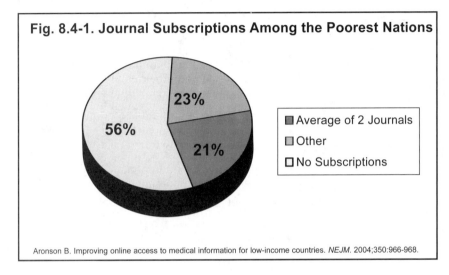

Fig. 8.4-1. Journal Subscriptions Among the Poorest Nations

- Average of 2 Journals
- Other
- No Subscriptions

Aronson B. Improving online access to medical information for low-income countries. *NEJM.* 2004;350:966-968.

So what can we learn from this remarkable "island of common steward-ship"? Three things: First, we must leverage our new information technologies — locally and globally — to our fullest advantage. Second, technology should not be viewed as competitive to more fundamental needs, but rather as a means of expanding access to energy, interest and resources, which may then be applied to a wider range of benefits. Finally, never underestimate the power of knowledge to transform an individual or a society. Where there is hope, there is a future.

REFERENCES

1. The World Health Report 2000: Health Systems: Improving Performance. Geneva, Switzerland: World Health Organization.
2. Healthcare Information and Management Systems Society. Professional Development. Available at: http://www.himss.org/asp/issuesbytopic.asp?topicID=10.
3. Aronson B. Improving online access to medical information for low-income countries. *NEJM.* 2004;350:966-968.
4. HealthInternetwork: HINARI. Available at: http://www.healthinternetwork.org.
5. Magee M. Qualities of Enduring Cross-Sector Partnerships in Public Health. *Amer. J of Surg.* 2003;185:26-29.

TEACHING TOOLS

Policy Premises

1. Limited access to medical information negatively impacts the health of the world's poorest populations.
2. Technology is the fastest, most efficient, and most effective way to bridge an economic or geographic based knowledge gap.
3. Competitive medical organizations will collaborate when faced with a compelling societal need.
4. Information technology solutions require infrastructure that can be built.
5. Information is only part of the solution but an important part.

Review

1. What are some of the benefits of medical knowledge?
2. What is HINARI?
3. How can technology close the gap between developed and developing countries?
4. Has HINARI effectively reached its goal?
5. Can knowledge transform an individual or a society?

Online Resources

Access online resources with this book's CD.

HINARI
www.healthinternetwork.org

HINARI Approaches Major Milestone
http://www.who.int/tdr/publications/tdrnews/news70/hinari.htm

Clear Health Communication Initiative
http://www.pfizerhealthliteracy.com/

The NLM Gateway
http://www.nlm.nih.gov/pubs/factsheets/gateway.html

Guidance for the National Healthcare Disparities Report
http://books.nap.edu/books/0309085195/html/149.html#pagetop

Health Politics Online

For Original Health Politics Programs and Slides:

The Power of Information Technology to Bridge Global Health Disparities
http://www.healthpolitics.com/program_info.asp?p=prog_43
Slide Briefing
http://www.healthpolitics.com/media/prog_43/brief_prog_43.pdf

Stem Cell Research & Policy

UNITED KINGDOM ON THE MOVE

On Feb. 12, 2004, South Korean scientists announced their successful process for somatic cell nuclear transfer — taking the nucleus out of a human egg cell and replacing it with genetic material from an adult cell. With this transfer completed, they were able to stimulate the new cell to divide into a pluripotent stem cell.[1]

Their success was a wake-up call for scientists around the world, but the success did not come easy. In fact, the creation of stem cells occurred on their 176th try.[2] Still, for many American scientists it was concrete progress and bittersweet. Dr. Susan Fisher, co-director of the human stem cell biology program at the University of California at San Francisco, said it feels like she's lost "a lifetime" of research — citing the policy position of the U.S. government as "180 degrees from that of our colleagues in Europe."[3]

The work of the South Korean scientists brought all stem cell scientists one step further along the theory-to-practice timeline. If it's possible to inhabit an enucleated egg cell with a donor nucleus from an individual with a specific disease or genetic disorder, and if the resultant embryo can be stimulated to produce stem cells, then scientists are increasingly becoming convinced that whole new opportunities will appear.[4]

One such innovator is Dr. Douglas Melton, a developmental biologist at Harvard. He recently fleshed out some possibilities, imagining repeating the South Korean scientists' success by using 50 adult Parkinson's patients as nuclear donors. The output of 50 stem cell lines, stimulated to become nerve cells of the type that die in the disease, would be closely observed. Would they die? When and why? In the same way, from the same cause, or were there multiple pathways, processes and agents responsible for Parkinson's disease? Would various drugs have any protective effect?[2,5]

This simple example and line of questioning explains at once why scientific experts in specific conditions or diseases are so focused on stem cell research. It also discounts the recent assertions that placing one's hope on the future of stem cell research is unrealistic.[5]

The debate that currently paralyzes U.S.-based stem cell science — obstructing the flow of federal dollars and undermining U.S.-based cross-sector efforts — was put to rest in the United Kingdom 14 years ago. In 1990, the United Kingdom advanced legislation "specifically allowing embryonic research and technology...in situations related to in-vitro fertilization or screening for genetic defects." This was not an open-ended, careless, or debate-free commitment. Rather, the United Kingdom specified the type of embryos, consent required, project review, and licensure process.[3]

In contrast, six years later, the United States started down an opposite road, quietly approving the Dickey Amendment, authored by U.S. Rep. Jay Dickey, R-Arkansas, as a rider to the Health and Human Services appropriations bill. It prohibited federal support for "the creation of a human embryo or embryos for research purposes; or...research in which a human embryo or embryos are destroyed, discarded or knowingly subject to risk of injury or death."[4]

These contrasting choices have helped define two very contrasting present-day realities. For the United States, the policy announced by President Bush on Aug. 9, 2001, has widened the gap of opportunity between U.S. and non-U.S.-based stem cell scientists. Take the case of the University of California at San Francisco. Following the letter of the policy, which prohibited the use of federal dollars in support of stem cell lines created after Aug. 9, 2001, the stem cell biology program was relocated off-campus — since the campus science buildings were subsidized by federal funding. In the moving process, two or three stem cell lines were lost.[6] The co-director resigned and moved to the United Kingdom, where he saw greater opportunity. And the program, once a cross-sector mix of public and private support and involvement, converted to private support only.[3]

What's currently going on across the ocean? In the same time span, the

United Kingdom has created the first national stem cell bank. Every project is reviewed and licensed by a government board and the fate of each embryo is carefully tracked. Stem cell lines created for therapeutics must be ceded to the national bank to be evaluated and maintained. Transfer of the cells is tightly controlled, requiring application and government approval. The government will soon require that all stem cell lines in the United Kingdom be stored in the stem cell bank and distributed free of charge through this clearinghouse. Reproductive cloning is outlawed — it's a criminal offense punishable with imprisonment.[3]

Initially, $4.7 million in government funding was committed to the creation of this national stem cell bank.[3] In August 2004, the United Kingdom — laser-focused on practical therapies that will evolve from stem cell research — granted its first license for therapeutic cloning, allowing scientists to harvest stem cells that could treat diseases. Advice from U.K. scientists to the U.S. government? Dr. Stephen Minger of King's College London, suggests, "If you're worried about a slippery slope of using embryos, then fine — develop a tightly regulated system like we have."

Adds Dr. Glyn Stacey, director of the U.K. stem cell bank, "We've dealt with a lot of issues and complications of embryonic stem cell research in a straightforward way, and that has put the United Kingdom in a very good position."[3]

HONORING CHRISTOPHER REEVE

On Oct. 10, 2004, we lost the world's most effective voice on behalf of stem cell research — Christopher Reeve. His death, which occurred at the height of the presidential election season, brought into focus once again the serious implications of current U.S. policy on this issue — both for the future of our health care system, and for the health of each of us as individuals.

How can we best honor the life of Christopher Reeve and what he stood for? As with President John Kennedy and the civil rights legislation that was passed following his death, perhaps the best way to honor Christopher Reeve is with legislative action.

There are currently 21 stem cell lines for which the U.S. government will fund research. Around the world, there are 128 new lines that do not qualify for U.S.-funded support because they were created after Aug. 9, 2001, when

President George W. Bush announced the current U.S. policy regarding stem cell research.

The problem is, the 21 federally approved stem cell lines are fundamentally flawed and have limited potential for use in clinical therapy. As Dr. George Daley of Harvard Medical School notes, "All were cultured in contact with mouse cells and bovine serum, which renders them inferior to newer lines, derived under pristine conditions, for potential therapeutic applications. Moreover, given the limited genetic diversity of the lines, transplantation of their products would face the same immune barrier as organ transplantation."[4]

Experts now agree that the most important clinical questions cannot be addressed by the federally approved stem cell lines. Using these lines, one can only explore generic questions about human embryonic stem cells, like what are the optimal culturing conditions; what factors promote growth and differentiation; and how do genes modify and express themselves? The more important questions can only be addressed by means of lines that model specific diseases. Pursuing therapies requires uncontaminated stem cells with lines genetically matched to the specific therapy needs of patients. Such lines already exist, having been created after Aug. 9, 2001, for diseases like neurofibromatosis, Marfan's syndrome, fragile X syndrome, myotonic dystrophy, and Fanconi's anemia.[4]

Who has inherited the platform leadership for stem cell research? First and foremost, other nations.[1] On Feb. 12, 2004, South Korea announced their successful process for somatic cell nuclear transfer.

During this same year, Canada's parliament legalized the use of excess embryos for stem cell research, and Sweden announced support for therapeutic use of stem cells. The United Kingdom authorized development of embryonic stem cells, and Singapore struck a deal with the Juvenile Diabetes Research Foundation, which found that a "more favorable research climate" exists overseas.[7,8] Singapore committed $300 million to a new Biopolis stem cell project. And Spain, Japan, and the United Kingdom are all developing their own stem cell banks. Back in the United States, the NIH awarded $10.6 million in grants in 2002 and $17 million in 2003.[3]

The U.S. states have also recognized the opportunity of stem cell research. Thirty states have generated 78 bills relating to stem cells. Nine have legislation to approve state funding of research, and California, Missouri, New Jersey, and Rhode Island are moving forward with concrete plans.[9,10]

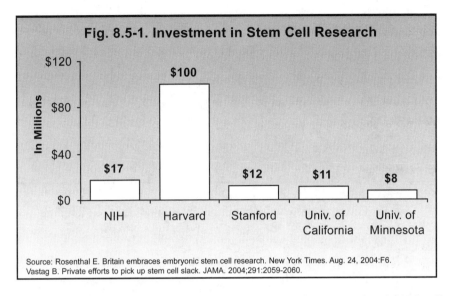

Fig. 8.5-1. Investment in Stem Cell Research

Source: Rosenthal E. Britain embraces embryonic stem cell research. New York Times. Aug. 24, 2004:F6.
Vastag B. Private efforts to pick up stem cell slack. JAMA. 2004;291:2059-2060.

Universities have been active as well. Harvard has committed $100 million in funds; Stanford, $12 million; University of California, $11 million; and the University of Minnesota, $8 million.[10]

These universities and states do so with considerable support from major U.S. medical and scientific organizations, including the American Medical Association, the Association of American Medical Colleges, the Institute of Medicine, the National Academy of Science, and 125 other U.S. medical, science, and patient advocacy organizations that first publicly voiced their support for federal funding of research using human pluripotent stem cells on July 29, 1999.[11,12,13,14,15]

In May 2004, Nancy Reagan, in the final days of President Ronald Reagan's life, publicly encouraged broadening U.S. involvement in stem cell research. One month later, on June 4, 2004, 58 senators came out in support of relaxing federal restrictions.[16]

Dr. George Daley captured what many medical and scientific leaders believe to be our current reality:

First, he says, the current approach "has severely curtailed opportunities for U.S. scientists to study the cell lines that have since been established, many of which have unique attributes or represent invaluable models of human disease." Second, that "as research struggles forward in the absence of federal funding, the number of embryonic stem cell lines will continue to grow, creating ever more valuable tools that are out of the reach for U.S. scientists."[4]

Christopher Reeve never walked after his horseback riding accident in 1995, but that is not to say that his vision for stem cell research and discovery should not fly.

REFERENCES

1. Spar D. The business of stem cells. *NEJM*. 2004;351:211-213.
2. Kolata G. Stem Cells: Promise, in Search of Results. *New York Times*. Aug. 24, 2004:F1.
3. Rosenthal E. Britain Embraces Embryonic Stem Cell Research. New *York Times*. Aug. 24, 2004:F6.
4. Daley GQ. Missed opportunities in embryonic stem-cell research. *NEJM*. 2004;351:627-628.
5. Kennedy R. First Lady Defends Limits On Stem Cell Research. *New York Times*. Aug. 10, 2004:A16.
6. President's decision: transcript of address on federal financing for research with embryonic stem cells. *New York Times*. Aug. 10, 2001:A16.
7. Robeznieks A. Diabetes group looks outside U.S. for stem cell research. *American Medical News*. Nov. 17, 2003.
8. Robeznieks A. States, scientists seek alternate funding for stem cell research. *American Medical News*. March 15, 2004.
9. Murphy K. Embryonic stem cell debate bursts onto state level. Available at: http://www.stateline.org/stateline/?pa=story&sa=showStoryInfo&id=391906&columns=false. Accessed Sept. 15, 2004.
10. Vastag B. Private efforts to pick up stem cell slack. *JAMA*. 2004;291:2059-2060.
11. Report 15 of the Council on Scientific Affairs (I-99): Embryonic/pluripotent stem cell research and funding. American Medical Association.
12. AAMC Applauds Congressional Support for Expanded Stem Cell Funding [news release on AAMC Web site]. April 28, 2004. Available at: http://www.aamc.org/newsroom/pressrel/2004/040428.htm. Accessed on Sept. 15, 2004.

13. Stem Cells and the Future of Regenerative Medicine. Washington, D.C.: *National Academy Press*; 2004.

14. Public Funding of Stem Cell Research Enhances Likelihood of Attaining Medical Breakthroughs [news release on The National Academies Web site]. Sept. 11, 2001. Available at: http://www4.nationalacademies.org/news.nsf/isbn/0309076307?open-document.

15. Letter from the research community to Representative John Porter [March Of Dimes Update on Life Issues Institute, Inc. Web site]. July 29, 1999. Available at: http://www.lifeissues.org/cloningstemcell/escr-letter.html. Accessed on Sept. 15, 2004.

16. Associated Press. Senators ask Bush to relax stem cell restrictions. June 8, 2004. Available at: http://msnbc.msn.com/id/5165300. Accessed Sept. 15, 2004.

TEACHING TOOLS

Policy Premises

1. The field of embryonic stem cell research is only two decades old but moving at the speed of light.
2. Since 2001, there has been tremendous progress in the field, largely out of reach of U.S. scientists.
3. The current federally approved stem cell lines are fundamentally flawed.
4. The most important clinical questions cannot be addressed by NIH-funded studies.
5. Global competitors and state govenments are filling the void created by current federal science policy.

Review

1. Which scientists were first to develop a successful process for somatic cell nuclear transfer?
2. When did the United Kingdom pass the law that allowed embryonic research in certain situations?
3. How did the University of California at San Francisco lose several of its stem cell lines?
4. What are some of the regulations put in place at the new U.K. stem cell bank?
5. What advice does one U.K. scientist have for the U.S. government?
6. How old is the field of embryonic stem cell research?
7. What type of stem cell research is supported by the U.S. government?
8. Are there problems with the federally approved stem cell lines?
9. Who has taken the lead in the field of stem cell research?
10. How many new stem cell lines exist around the world?

Online Resources

Access online resources with this book's CD.

U.K. Stem Cell Bank
http://www.ukstemcellbank.org.uk/

Decision: California
http://ca.lwv.org/lwvc/edfund/elections/2004nov/id/prop71.html

Promoting Stem Cell Research
http://www.isscr.org/

Stem Cell Science: Mirage or Shining City
http://mbbnet.umn.edu/scmap.html

Stem Cell Research
http://www.usatoday.com/tech/science/genetics/2004-09-16-stem-cells_x.htm

California Stem Cell Research and Cures Initiative
http://www.curesforcalifornia.com/

Scientists Clone First Human Embryo
http://my.webmd.com/content/article/82/97161.htm

Reeve's Legacy
http://msnbc.msn.com/id/6224513/

Policy and Politics
http://www.npr.org/templates/story/story.php?storyId=1891207

U.S. Stem Cell Research Lagging
http://www.boston.com/news/science/articles/2004/05/23/us_stem_cell_research_lagging/

What Are Stem Cells?
http://stemcells.nih.gov/index.asp

Government Plans to Open Stem Cell Bank
http://www.msnbc.msn.com/id/5437729/

Christopher Reeve Paralysis Foundation
http://www.crpf.org/index.cfm

Policy Push
http://www.aaas.org/news/releases/2004/0428stemcells.shtml

Monitoring Stem Cell Research
http://www.bioethics.gov/reports/stemcell/chapter2.html

Stem Cells, Alzheimer's Disease, and U.S. Politics
http://www.npr.org/templates/story/story.php?storyId=1964235

Stem Cell Research
http://www.pbs.org/newshour/bb/health/july-dec04/stemcell_8-10.html

Just to Be Clear
http://www.jdrf.org/index.cfm?page_id=100029

Health Politics Online

For Original Health Politics Programs and Slides:

Stem Cell Research: U.K. on the Move
http://www.healthpolitics.com/program_info.asp?p=prog_65
Slide Briefing
http://www.healthpolitics.com/media/prog_65/brief_prog_65.pdf

Stem Cell Policy: Honoring Christopher Reeve
http://www.healthpolitics.com/program_info.asp?p=prog_64
Slide Briefing
http://www.healthpolitics.com/media/prog_64/brief_prog_64.pdf

CHAPTER 8.6

Clinical Research

AT A CRITICAL JUNCTURE

Health care is increasingly reliant on evidence-based medicine. This places an extraordinarily heavy burden on clinical research to provide the knowledge upon which such evidence is based. Meeting that expectation has been, and continues to be, a daunting challenge.

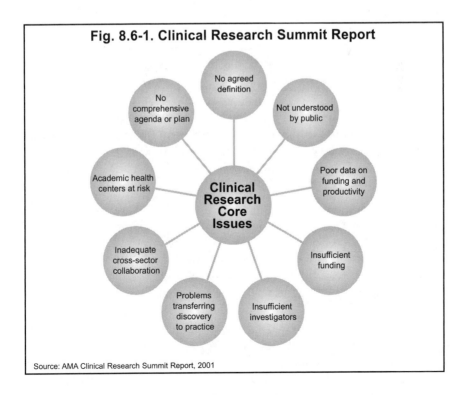

Fig. 8.6-1. Clinical Research Summit Report

No agreed definition

No comprehensive agenda or plan

Not understood by public

Academic health centers at risk

Clinical Research Core Issues

Poor data on funding and productivity

Inadequate cross-sector collaboration

Insufficient funding

Problems transferring discovery to practice

Insufficient investigators

Source: AMA Clinical Research Summit Report, 2001

The AMA's 2001 Clinical Research Summit Report outlined nine core challenges, which included the absence of an agreed-upon definition for clinical research; poor general understanding of clinical research; lack of accurate data on dollars spent and how those dollars are being put to use; insufficient funding; too few clinical investigators; challenges in transferring what has been discovered to clinicians caring for patients; inadequate collaboration between professionals across public and private sectors; the financial instability of academic teaching centers, where much of the research is performed; and finally no comprehensive, agreed upon national agenda or plan.[1]

Clinical research means many things to many people. In 2003, a consensus group noted that "Clinical research lies at the nexus of basic biomedical research and clinical practice, and is the portal through which the future of medicine must pass."[2] If there is confusion on definition, it may be related to the many and diverse outputs that clinical research delivers. Studies on patient populations provide knowledge on the natural history of disease, detection and diagnosis, new therapies, strategies for prevention, and long-term outcomes.[3,4,5,6,7,8,9]

Public funding of clinical research has always lagged behind basic science bench research. The National Institutes of Health were created by the United States Congress in 1930, and for the next 20 years focused primarily on biology and chemistry, preferring small animal studies over human trials.[10] The creation of a 450-bed research hospital in 1953 signaled a change in focus, a shift from mice to men and women.[10] Dr. Norman Topping, the associate director of the NIH at that time, voiced a goal "to carry laboratory findings to clinical evaluations," a chasm he labeled "the great gap."[10] By the 1970s, as the ability to examine cell functions on a molecular level became more refined, the scales began to tip back to bench research. By 1997, the NIH estimated that only 30 percent of its grants were awarded to clinical studies, and only 10 percent to 18 percent were actually centered on patients.[10,11]

That clinical research involves unique challenges is undeniable. There is less public funding available than for basic bench science.[10,11] The work is viewed by some as less scholarly and more variable. It also takes longer and has less predictable outcomes.[12] Refining or adjusting studies means starting from the beginning. Plus, patient safety is a constant concern.[12]

Modern clinical research is no longer the province of the multifaceted solo physician who taught students and treated patients in the morning, and went to the lab late in the afternoon. Today, modern clinical research is a team effort with heavy emphasis on patient safeguards. The team typically includes patients, physicians, basic scientists, research nurses, data managers, statisticians and ethicists. It is primarily funded through private versus public resources.[12]

Safety oversight is a major, multilayered challenge. Institutional review boards, or IRBs, exist on the local level and include non-scientists, as well as scientists not connected to the research. The IRB has the responsibility "to assure that steps are taken to safeguard the rights and welfare of those who agree to be research subjects."[12] They must provide initial approval for a study to proceed and ongoing oversight to ensure patient safety. In addition to the IRB, institutions maintain data and safety monitoring boards. Additional formal oversight and review boards are actively engaged on behalf of corporate partners and government regulatory agencies.[13]

There is no clinical research without patient participation. Participation requires that patients maintain a confidence and trust in the clinical research team and the process. They must see the long-term benefit to themselves and to others. And they must actively choose to partner with the clinicians and scientists in the discovery triad. How do patients learn about clinical trials? Studies show that nearly half learn from their physicians, 35 percent from media, 9 percent from the Internet, and 8 percent from family or friends.[14]

REFERENCES

1. American Medical Association (AMA). Clinical Research Summit Report. Breaking the scientific bottleneck. Clinical research: a national call to action. Jun 7, 2001.
2. Bench, Bedside, and Beyond: Clinical Research at the Crossroads. *The Pfizer Journal*. Vol 6:3, 2002.
3. Gene discovery shows heart failure cause, suggests treatments and screening potential [news release]. Rochester, MN: Mayo Clinic Rochester; Jan 28, 2002. Available at: www.mayo.edu/comm/mcr/news_1942.html. Accessed 3/5/02.
4. Colonoscopy more effective than barium enema for detection of colon polyps: implication for change in screening guidelines [press release]. New York, NY: memorial Sloan-Kettering Cancer Center; Jun 14, 2000.
5. UKPDS Group. Intensive blood-glucose control with sulphonylureas or insulin compared with conventional treatment and risk of complica-

tions in patients with type 2 diabetes (UKPDS 33). *Lancet.* 1998; 352:837-853.

6. Household changes can reduce asthma in children. Cincinnati, OH: CNN; Mar 5, 2001.

7. Landmark study shows behavioral interventions reduce HIV-related sexual risk behavior [news release]. Research Triangle Park, NC: Research Triangle Institute; Jun 19, 1998.

8. New Research documents success of drug abuse treatments [news release]. Bethesda, MD: NIH; Dec 15, 1997.

9. Anderson CA, Hammen CL. Psychosocial outcomes of children of unipolar depressed, bipolar, medically ill, and normal women: a longitudinal study. *J Consult Clin Psychol.* 1993; 61: 448-454.

10. Schechter AN. The crisis in clinical research: endangering the half-century National Institutes of Health Consensus. *JAMA.* 1998; 280: 1440-1442.

11. The NIH Director's Panel on Clinical Research Report to the Advisory Committee to the NIH Director. Dec 1997.

12. Report of the NIH Committee on the Recruitment and Career Development of Clinical Investigators. Mar 31, 1997.

13. US FDA. Information Sheets: Guidance for Institutional Review Boards and Clinical Investigators, 1998.

14. Getz K. Patient experiences in industry-sponsored clinical trials. In: Kalfoglou AI, Boenning DA, et al. IOM: Summary of the Symposium on Public Confidence and Involvement in Clinical Research: Clinical Research roundtable. Washington, DC: National Academy of Sciences; Sep 2000.

TEACHING TOOLS

Policy Premises

1. Health care's increasing reliance on evidence-based medicine places a heavy burden on clinical research.
2. Clinical research means many things to many people.
3. Public funding of clinical research has always lagged behind basic science bench research.
4. Clinical research involves unique challenges.
5. Modern clinical research is a team effort with heavy emphasis on patient safeguards.
6. Patient partnership is essential if clinical research is to reach its full potential.

Review

1. What are the nine core challenges associated with clinical research and outlined in the AMA's 2001 Clinical Research Summit Report?
2. What problems exist with public funding of clinical-based research?
3. Who is typically included on a clinical research team?
4. Why is safety oversight in clinical research a major challenge?
5. How does the patient participate in clinical research?
6. Why do patients choose or refuse to be in clinical trials?

Online Resources

Access online resources with this book's CD.

Institutional Review Board — Homepage
http://dir.niehs.nih.gov/dirosd/ocr/irb/

Objectives and Overview of the OHRP Quality Improvement Program
http://www.hhs.gov/ohrp/humansubjects/qip/qipdesc.pdf

Evidence-based Practice
http://www.ahrq.gov/clinic/epcix.htm

Research: A hard life at the bench
http://www.chicagotribune.com/technology/local/chi-010729p4stem,0,3962073.story

Guidelines for the Conduct of Research Involving Human Subjects at the National Institutes of Health
http://www.nihtraining.com/ohsrsite/guidelines/graybook.html

Changing Composition of Federal Funding for Research and Development and R&D Plant Since 1990
http://www.nsf.gov/sbe/srs/infbrief/nsf02315/start.htm

Health Politics Online

For Original Health Politics Programs and Slides:

Clinical Research at a Critical Juncture
http://www.healthpolitics.com/program_info.asp?p=prog_16
Slide Briefing
http://www.healthpolitics.com/media/prog_16/brief_prog_16.pdf

Patient Involvement in Research Studies

OPPORTUNITIES AND OBSTACLES

While clinical research in the new millennium holds great promise and tremendous opportunities, the realization of this potential is not without significant obstacles and barriers. Chief among them is patient participation. It is the critical ingredient for a successful clinical research study. But the reality is, most patients are unaware or uninformed.

In a recent poll of 6,000 cancer patients, 84 percent were unaware, at the time of their diagnosis, that participation in a clinical trial was an option.[1] Less than 5 percent of those surveyed participated in trials despite the fact that most experts believe there should be at least a 10 percent to15 percent participation rate.[2] In contrast, 80 percent to 90 percent of cancer-afflicted children are enrolled in clinical trials. Many believe this is a reflection of the hands-on advocacy practiced by pediatric oncology teams, and the resultant trust and confidence of parents and children in the clinical trial process.[2]

Physician advocacy and communication are critically important to ensuring patient participation. Nearly 50 percent of all patients involved in trials first learn of them through their physicians. Mass media and the Internet add another 35 percent and 9 percent, respectively, to that awareness. Friends and family contribute an additional 8 percent.

An enormous outreach is required to deliver a few active individuals willing to participate over the life of a clinical study. In 2000, a panel of experts determined that of the 6.5 million people asked to participate in clinical studies, only 675,000 people participated, for a response rate of approximately 10 percent.[1] In a second study involving 1,500 initial responders to requests for participation in a clinical trial, only 320 passed the preliminary eligibility screening. Of those, ultimately 110 enrolled in the study and only 80 completed it.[3]

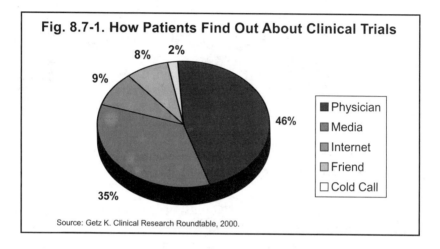

Fig. 8.7-1. How Patients Find Out About Clinical Trials

- Physician
- Media
- Internet
- Friend
- Cold Call

Source: Getz K. Clinical Research Roundtable, 2000.

In reality, the challenges of patient recruitment delay most clinical research studies. Only 18 percent of all clinical trials start on or ahead of schedule. Conversely, 82 percent are delayed by recruitment problems. Of those, 22 percent are delayed by one month, 47 percent are delayed by one to six months, and 13 percent are delayed for more than six months.[3] Despite these recruitment issues, 83 percent of the respondents to one Harris Interactive survey said that they would consider participating in a clinical research study.[4]

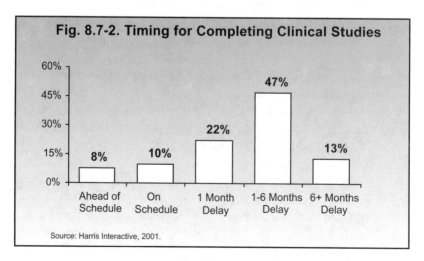

Fig. 8.7-2. Timing for Completing Clinical Studies

Source: Harris Interactive, 2001.

The pros and cons of participation in a clinical research study are well-known to patients and physicians alike. On the positive side, 58 percent chose to participate to benefit themselves or others, 48 percent believed participation would result in a fuller disclosure of all risks, 35 percent chose to enroll when it was clear that the potential benefits outweighed the reasonable risks, and 35 percent believed that the trial might yield a cure. Fully 35 percent acted based on the recommendation of their physician, while 23 percent saw participation as a way to advance science.[3,4]

On the negative side, there remains fear and caution. A full 48 percent believed that they might receive a placebo rather than active treatment. Many do not understand that most studies, and certainly those dealing with serious medical conditions like cancer, test new therapies against standard therapies, not against placebos. Patients also fail to appreciate that the clinical researcher constantly monitors results, and that the protocol defines circumstances that lead to halting a study or removing a patient from the study, if safety becomes an issue. Nonetheless, safety is an issue for patients, with 39 percent citing fear of bad side effects as a reason not to participate. Finally, 29 percent were concerned that, once the study was completed, they would lose access to a treatment that was working, and be back where they started.

The good news is that, in spite of these concerns, when patients participate, they respond favorably to the experience. In one large study, 93 percent agreed that the research team acted professionally; 97 percent said they'd experienced a thorough discussion of risks and benefits, and felt they were fully informed; and 91 percent felt the quality of care was as good as, or better than, that provided by their regular doctor.

Partnering with a clinical research team is not easy. It demands time, energy, and focus for the patient and his or her family. It means being engaged and alert, and sometimes re-asking questions and confronting the unknown. But the record shows that when patients get involved, science succeeds and we all benefit.

REFERENCES

1. Kalfoglou AI, Boenning DA, et al. IOM: Summary of the Symposium on Public Confidence and Involvement in Clinical Research: Clinical Research Roundtable. Washington, DC: National Academy of Sciences; Sep 2000.

2. Lichter, A. Bench, Bedside, and Beyond: Clinical Research at the Crossroads. *The Pfizer Journal*. Vol 6:3, 2002. p. 10-12.

3. Getz K. Patient experiences in industry-sponsored clinical trials. In: Kalfoglou AI, Boenning DA, et al. IOM: Summary of the Symposium on Public Confidence and Involvement in Clinical Research: Clinical Research Roundtable. Washington, DC: National Academy of Sciences; Sep 2000.

4. Nationwide survey reveals public support of clinical research studies on the rise [news release]. Denver, CO: Harris Interactive; Jun 27, 2001.

TEACHING TOOLS

Policy Premises

1. Patient participation is the critical ingredient for a successful clinical research study, but most patients are unaware.
2. Physician advocacy and communication are critically important to ensure patient participation.
3. An enormous outreach is required to deliver a few active participants for the life of a clinical study.
4. Challenges in patient recruitment delay most clinical studies.
5. The pros and cons for participation are well known to patients and physicians alike.
6. Most patients involved in clinical research rate the experience positively.

Review

1. In a recent poll of cancer patients, what percentage was unaware that participation in a clinical trial was an option?
2. How do patients learn about clinical trials?
3. What percent of clinical trials actually start on schedule?
4. What are the pros and cons of participation in clinical research studies?
5. Approximately what percentage of patients who were approached actually participated in clinical research trials?

Online Resources

Access online resources with this book's CD.

NIH - Clinical Trials
http://clinicaltrials.gov/ct/info/whatis#why

National Cancer Institute
http://www.cancer.gov/clinicaltrials

United States General Accounting Office Report to
Congressional Requesters. NIH Clinical trials: Various Factors
Affect Patient Participation
http://www.gao.gov/archive/1999/he99182.pdf

Lymphoma
http://www.lymphomation.org/clinical-trials-about.htm

Health Politics Online

For Original Health Politics Programs and Slides:

Patient Involvement in Research Studies
http://www.healthpolitics.com/program_info.asp?p=prog_17
Slide Briefing
http://www.healthpolitics.com/media/prog_17/brief_prog_17.pdf

CHAPTER 8.8

Patents

PROTECTING THE PUBLIC'S INTEREST

The battle between science and disease has been constant throughout human history. Just when science seems to be gaining the upper hand, microbes adapt and evolve, become immune to medicines that used to be effective, take on whole new forms and appear "brand new" as if coming out of nowhere. The SARS crisis is a prime example. For all the success we have witnessed in the 20th century, only one-third of the 30,000 known diseases currently have an effective treatment.[1]

Science will always have to think on its feet because there will always be a new threat or a brand-new challenge. Our forefathers understood that and provided a unique incentive. The word "right" is used only once in the 4,000-word United States Constitution. It's in Article 1, Section 8, Clause 8 and says that Congress shall have the power:

"To promote the progress of science and useful arts by securing for limited times to authors and inventors the exclusive right to their respective writings and discoveries."[2]

This is the basis for patent law in the United States, the provision of exclusive right to sell a product for a limited time to incentivize inventions and discovery. Abraham Lincoln shared the founding fathers' enthusiasm, commenting that patents "added the fuel of interest to the fire of genius in the discovery and production of new and useful things."[3] In spite of the numbers, there remains, even today, great confusion over what patents are and what they are not.

There are several ways to protect trade secrets. One way is to not tell anyone. Take Coca-Cola for instance. Its recipe has been a well-guarded secret since 1886. But, this doesn't work very well for medicines where scientific sharing of knowledge is central to societal well-being. Another approach is our copyright law for books, which is for the life of the author plus 50 years — way too restrictive for science, which is advancing at a gallop, and requires both protection and transparency if one's discoveries today are to lead to another's discoveries tomorrow.

For medicines, patent protection lasts for 20 years, with drug development consuming about 14 years from the time a new chemical entity is first registered.[4] So generally, more than half the patent protection is shaved away on the front end. At this point, the patented medicine is able to be sold and hopefully begin to recoup its investment. However, few do. Only one in 5,000 new chemicals registered survive. Of those that do receive FDA approval, only three in 10 ever recoup their investment — some 800 million developmental dollars per product.[5,6]

Another point of confusion is what patents actually protect. They protect the exact chemical entity, atom for atom. Change one atom and you have a brand-new chemical and a brand-new competitor. On the average, a new drug will encounter its first competitor in a class like SSRI depression drugs in just two years, and will have a second competitor in 3.1 years.

It is not a coincidence that the United States, the country with the strongest commitment to patent protection and free trade, also has the most successful research and generic pharmaceutical business in the world. This success is the result of a favorable discovery cycle built on the twin pillars of patent protection and free trade.[7]

The cycle begins with innovation, an idea worthy of investment. Given a patent, ensuring the exclusive right to the product for a limited time creates the reasonable expectation of a positive return on this investment. Investment leads to a discovery, which, if it survives the many pitfalls of rigorous testing — and that's a big "if" — can only reach its full potential if open markets exist that allow free trade. This is because free trade provides the ability to compete on level ground, based solely on the merits of the product. A good product in an open market generates profit. Profit, in turn, creates investment in future research and development leading to a new innovation and renewal of the cycle.

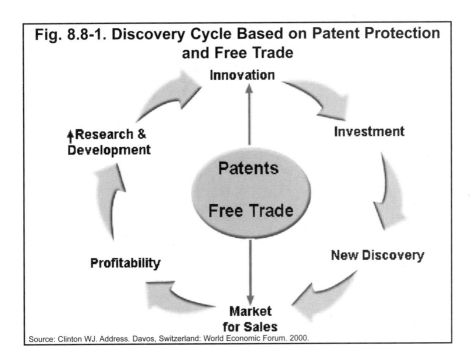

Fig. 8.8-1. Discovery Cycle Based on Patent Protection and Free Trade

Innovation

↑Research & Development

Investment

Patents

Free Trade

New Discovery

Profitability

Market for Sales

Source: Clinton WJ. Address. Davos, Switzerland: World Economic Forum. 2000.

This favorable cycle delivers concrete results in two important ways.

First, it creates a climate that will deliver more discoveries in the United States in the next 10 years than were uncovered in the past 100 years. This will not only expand availability but also affordability through price competition within individual classes of drugs. This means more hope, less surgery and hospitalization, and more years of productive life.

Second, as patent protection runs out, generic companies are free to copy the product atom for atom and sell it. Costs plunge by 90 percent, and that's great for patients. Generic companies keep trusted old standards on the market at low cost, while research companies concentrate on uncovering the next scientific breakthrough.

Though not perfect, on the whole patents not only protect products, and their discoveries, they also protect the public's interest.

REFERENCES

1. Rozek RP, Tully N. TRIPS Agreement and Access to Healthcare. *Journal World Intellectual Property*. 1999: 2(5;293-319).
2. Constitution of the United States. Article I; Section 8; Clause 8.
3. Bale HE. Pharmaceutical access and innovation; challenges and issues. Geneva: International Roundtable on Responses to Globalization; July 12-14, 1999.
4. Tufts Center for the Study of Drug Development (TCSDD). Tufts Center for the Study of Drug Development Pegs Cost of a New Prescription Medicine at $802 Million [news release]. November 30, 2001.
5. TCSDD. A Methodology for Counting Costs for Pharmaceutical R&D [backgrounder]. November 30, 2001.
6. Most Drugs Do Not Recoup R&D Investment. Source: Grabowski H, Vernon J. Returns to R&D on new drug introductions in the 1980s. *J Health Econ*. 1994; 13:383-406.
7. Clinton WJ. Address. Davos, Switzerland: World Economic Forum, January 29, 2000. Available at: http://www.weform.org. Accessed 3/14/00.

TEACHING TOOLS

Policy Premises

1. Protection of one's ideas is central to the American success story.
2. Research in pharmaceuticals can be an extraodinarily high-risk business.
3. Patents protect the exact chemical, atom for atom. Change one atom and you create a new competitor.
4. A favorable discovery cycle is built upon enlightened patent protection and free trade.
5. U.S. patent legislation will continue to deliver economic progress and improved health.

Review

1. What legal document provides the basis for patent law in the United States?
2. How long does patent protection last for medicines?
3. What percentage of FDA-approved medicines actually recoups their research investment?
4. What do patents actually protect?
5. What happens when patent protection for a medicine runs out?

Online Resources

Access online resources with this book's CD.

Progress In The Pharmaceutical Industry
http://usinfo.state.gov/products/pubs/intelprp/progress.htm

Intellectual Property
http://www.pfizer.com/are/about_public/mn_about_intellectual-propfrm.html

Intellectual Property: Overview
http://www.phrma.org/issues/intprop/

Health Politics Online

For Original Health Politics Programs and Slides:

Patents
http://www.healthpolitics.com/program_info.asp?p=prog_05
Slide Briefing
http://www.healthpolitics.com/media/prog_05/brief_prog_05.pdf

CHAPTER 9

Improving Health Care Value

"We are currently in a 'need-to-know' era in terms of health information. But tomorrow will bring the start of a 'need-to-act' era."

— ANDREA PENNINGTON
Medical Director
Discovery Health

"I do not know if the public truly understands that prevention
needs to start very early in a woman's life. Osteoporosis is a good
example. It is really a disease for which preventative steps need to
start in childhood."

— DONNA DEAN
National Institute of Health

"If a substantial part of the financing of care received by the
uninsured is already in the public sector, then some share of these
funds is potentially available for transfer to new government
efforts to extend coverage to those currently uninsured."

— KAISER COMMISSION
2003

"Cost sharing markedly decreases the use of all types of services among all types of people (with) little or no net adverse effect on health for the average person."

— THE RAND HEALTH
INSURANCE EXPERIMENT
1993

Health Care Cost and Value

WHAT WE'VE GOTTEN FOR OUR MONEY

The debate around health care over the past two decades has been fundamentally unbalanced. We never pass up a chance to raise the red flag of cost, but rarely raise the legitimate question, "What have we gotten for our money?"

First, the cost. The cost of health care in the United States has increased some 102 percent over the past two decades. Corrected for inflation, health care spending per person in 1980 was $2,207. Per capita expenditure increased by 60 percent to $3,541 in 1990 and increased by an additional 26 percent to $4,461 by 2000.[1]

While clearly this is a significant investment, America's health advanced markedly as a result during this same period. Death rates between 1980 and

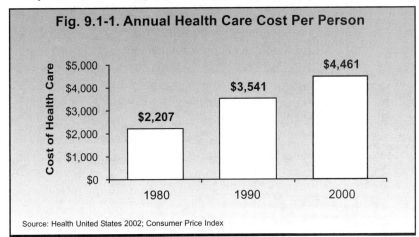

Fig. 9.1-1. Annual Health Care Cost Per Person

Cost of Health Care

$5,000
$4,000
$3,000
$2,000
$1,000
$0

1980: $2,207
1990: $3,541
2000: $4,461

Source: Health United States 2002; Consumer Price Index

2000 declined 16 percent. Average life expectancy in women rose 3 percent to 79.5 years and in men rose 6 percent to 74.1 years. Rates of disability in Americans over 65 decreased by 25 percent and days in the hospital fell from 130 to 57 per 100 persons, a 56 percent drop.[1,2,3] Stated somewhat differently, the investment in health care over the past two decades was associated with 470,000 fewer deaths, 2.3 million fewer seniors with disabilities, and 206 million fewer hospital days.[1]

Where has the most progress been made and where do challenges remain? Let's begin with heart attacks. Some 2.6 percent of the U.S. population is affected by heart attacks. The death rate from heart attacks between 1980 and 2000 declined by 46 percent, from 345 per 100,000 to 187 per 100,000. Every dollar spent on the treatment of heart attacks has generated $1.10 in heath care value.[2,4,5] What have been the major advances that provided value? The use of "clot-busting" drugs on arrival in emergency rooms has been a major advance. This advance not only resulted from the discovery and creation of this new medicine, but also from a radical change in the standard of practice across emergency departments nationwide. New technology in the form of CAT scans and Magnetic Resonance Imaging, or MRIs, allowed clinicians to better predict the most vulnerable populations earlier in the course of disease. The use of angioplasty has provided a non-invasive alternative to open heart surgery for coronary artery obstruction. New medications to control cholesterol, eliminate platelet clotting, and control the damaging effects of high blood pressure have all made a mark. And use of implantable defibrillators has lessened the chance of dying from an arrhythmia after a heart attack.[4]

The story with type 2 diabetes, by comparison, is mixed. Six percent of the U.S. population was affected by type 2 diabetes in 2003. Every dollar spent on treatment over the past two decades has generated $1.49 in health care value.[4] But during this same period of time the nation has begun to face an epidemic of obesity, which has contributed to a significant increase in the incidence — and, in turn, deaths — from diabetes.[2] That said, science and self-empowerment are responding to the challenge. Patients and families have benefited from self-monitoring glucose kits, and inhalable insulin is in the later stages of development. We have learned that high cholesterol and high blood pressure are especially lethal in diabetic patients. And the Centers for Disease Control and Prevention is now fully focused on a public health campaign to address the epidemic of obesity in the United States.[2,4]

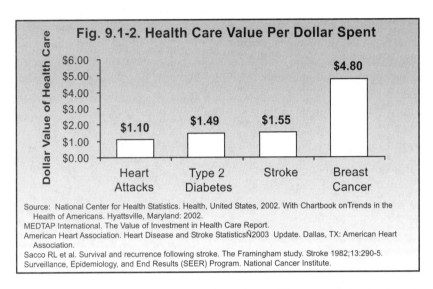

Fig. 9.1-2. Health Care Value Per Dollar Spent

Source: National Center for Health Statistics. Health, United States, 2002. With Chartbook onTrends in the Health of Americans. Hyattsville, Maryland: 2002.
MEDTAP International. The Value of Investment in Health Care Report.
American Heart Association. Heart Disease and Stroke StatisticsÑ2003 Update. Dallas, TX: American Heart Association.
Sacco RL et al. Survival and recurrence following stroke. The Framingham study. Stroke 1982;13:290-5.
Surveillance, Epidemiology, and End Results (SEER) Program. National Cancer Institute.

Stroke remains one of the most feared conditions, with its double threat to cognitive function as well as mobility. Nearly 2 percent of the American population was affected by stroke in 2003.[2,5] Our success with stroke has been significant, with $1.55 of value resulting from each dollar invested. Death rates from stroke have declined 37 percent over the past two decades, from 96 per 100,000 to 61 per 100,000.[2] Major advances have included a change in practice to encourage utilization of "clot-busting" drugs in select cases. Improvement of diagnostic imaging with CAT scans and MRIs have led to more proactive approaches to therapy. Surgical therapies improved. Anticoagulants used appropriately contributed to prevention. Finally, in cases where stroke occurred, early aggressive post-stroke rehabilitation has lessened disability.[4,7]

Success in the treatment of breast cancer has been especially significant. In 2003, 0.7 percent of the U.S. population suffered from breast cancer. Economic investment of each dollar yielded $4.80 in health care value.[4] The death rate over the past two decades has declined 21 percent, from 32 per 100,000 to 25 per 100,000.[2] That success has resulted from better screening with mammography; less invasive diagnostic procedures, like needle biopsy; breast-conserving surgery, which allowed women to more aggressively pursue early diagnosis; and improved hormonal therapy and chemotherapy. The five-year survival rate in 1980 was 77 percent; in 1995, it was 87 percent.[2,8]

Has every dollar America spent on health care been maximally benefi-cial? Certainly not. Are there opportunities to invest these dollars more wisely and efficiently, or apply our investment more equitably? Undoubtedly. That said, the value over the past two decades in individual, family and societal health is equally apparent, and far outweighs increases in health care spending. We should not lose sight of the fact that cost should always be balanced against benefit.

REFERENCES

1. Health United States 2002; Consumer Price Index.
2. National Center for Health Statistics. Health, United States, 2002. With Chartbook on Trends in the Health of Americans. Hyattsville, Maryland: 2002.
3. Manton KG, Corder LS, and Stallard E. Monitoring changes in the health of the U.S. elderly population: correlates with biomedical research and clinical innovations. *FASEB J.* 1997 (12):923-30.
4. MEDTAP International. The Value of Investment in Health Care Report. Available at http://www.medtap.com/Products/HP_FullReport.pdf.
5. American Heart Association. Heart Disease and Stroke Statistics-2003 Update. Dallas, TX: American Heart Association.
6. Mokdad AH, Bowman BA, Ford ES, et al. The continuing epidemics of obesity and diabetes in the United States. *JAMA.* 2001;286(10):1195-1200.
7. Sacco RL, Wolf PA, Kannel WB, McNamura, PM. Survival and recurrence following stroke. The Framingham study. *Stroke* 1982;13:290-5.
8. Surveillance, Epidemiology, and End Results (SEER) Program. National Cancer Institute. Available at http://www.seer.cancer.gov.

TEACHING TOOLS

Policy Premises

1. The cost of health care has increased 102 percent over the past 20 years.
2. Investments in health care have been worth the cost — Americans' health has markedly improved.
3. The death rate from heart attacks has significantly declined with the use of new drugs and a change in emergency room practice.
4. Cost should always be balanced against benefit.

Review

1. How much has health care spending increased in the past two decades?
2. What are some recent advances in the treatment of heart attacks?
3. Why, despite advances in treatment, has the diabetes death rate increased?
4. What is the relationship between the cost and value of spending on cancer care?
5. How much did the five-year survival rate for breast cancer patients change between 1980 and 1995?

Online Resources

Access online resources with this book's CD.

Follow the Money
http://www.statehealthfacts.kff.org/cgi-
bin/healthfacts.cgi?action=profile&area=United+States&catego-
ry=Health+Costs+%26+Budgets&subcategory=Personal+Health+
Care+Expenditures

Healthcare Cost and Quality
http://www.ahrq.gov/data/

Health Expenditures
http://www.cdc.gov/nchs/fastats/hexpense.htm

2003 Health Care Spending Up 7.8%
http://www.cbsnews.com/stories/2004/02/11/health/main599691.sh
tml

Cost-Value Analysis in Health Care
http://www.cambridge.org/uk/catalogue/catalogue.asp?isbn=05216
44348

Health Politics Online

For Original Health Politics Programs and Slides:

Health Care Cost: What We've Gotten For Our Money
http://www.healthpolitics.com/program_info.asp?p=prog_41
Slide Briefing
http://www.healthpolitics.com/media/prog_41/brief_prog_41.pdf

CHAPTER 9.2

The Information Highway

ALL ABOARD FOR HEALTH'S SAKE

The critical need for a better health information support system has been well recognized for more than two decades.[1] But until now, we have not been able to get our act together. Evolving technology, lack of money, no national standards, complexity, incompatibility, and overall lack of readiness to deal with the policy issues that would be triggered have all contributed to a frustratingly slow process.

But times are changing. Dr. Daniel Masys, director of biomedical informatics at the University of California, San Diego, spoke at the Institute of Medicine's (IOM's) annual meeting in 2001 and noted that the current practice of medicine "depends upon the decision-making capacity and reliability of autonomous individual practitioners for classes of problems that routinely exceed the bounds of unaided human cognition."[2] Translation — we need help. This was originally recognized in 1991 by the IOM, a non-profit organization focused on health and science policy, when the group noted that computer-based medical records are "an essential technology for patient care."[3] Eight years later the IOM report "To Err Is Human" exposed the connection between process weaknesses, the absence of information systems in health care, human error, and injuries to patients.[4] By 2003, the IOM left no doubt where it stood — it termed health information system infrastructure development "the highest priority for all health care stakeholders."[5]

Current conditions are ripe for action and are approaching a tipping point. Why now? To begin with, computer systems have advanced and are able to manage performance at a reasonable price. The Internet has become ubiquitous, no longer just a tool for elite academics, but now in the hands of the people. Software sophistication and end-point usability make its use by patients and physicians both feasible and realistic. Governments, businesses, academics, and nonprofits seem newly focused and engaged. And finally, successful local demonstration projects in Indiana and California have made it clear that health information exchange systems can work.[1,6,7]

The federal government has also weighed in. In 2001, an advisory committee to the Department of Health and Human Services put together a vision and planning report for a National Health Information Infrastructure (NHII).[8] In 2003, the Department of Health and Human Services organized a national consensus meeting to gather the opinions of 580 expert participants. All the key health care system stakeholders were represented. And, in 2004, the results from this conference were reported.[1]

Where did they find agreement? First, in the deliverables. A national health information superhighway would need to improve patient care, triggering and enabling not only modern information management, but also process re-engineering to reduce errors and variability and increase safety. Beyond acute care, the information highway would improve management of chronic diseases by promoting consistently high standards of care and allowing home monitoring with facilitated patient-clinician communications. Patient education would be expanded and individualized, and would support behavioral change. Databases, secured for privacy, would allow population research as well as public health surveillance for conditions like SARS.[1]

Obstacles remain that must be addressed. Funding for the initial investment and incentives to ensure sustainability must be provided. Linking rewards to appropriate use of technology and national standards is critical. A universal identifier number for all Americans remains critical but controversial. Dealing with legitimate privacy issues is required to place this critical piece of the puzzle. That done, legal barriers that prevent hospitals, care institutions, and doctors from working cooperatively — like the Stark statutes — need adjusting. And finally there is a list of potential, unintended consequences that must be placed on the table and addressed. These include the fear that information systems will make processes so routine that individualization of care will suffer; the fear that new technologies will become a barrier rather than a bridge between doctor and patient; and the fear that limitations on access and choice may silently find their way into information-system coding as a back door to cost control without enhancing quality.[1]

National leadership, cross-sector resourcing, and community-based participation must coalesce and tackle these manageable challenges. The consensus committee has recommended 40 to 50 demonstration projects, centered on key principles, including maintenance of confidentiality, non-proprietary status, national scalability, easy-to-use technology, low barriers to entry, standardization that ensures compatibility and connectivity, and support of the patient-physician relationship.[1]

The opportunity is here for significant improvement in quality and efficiency, but information alone is not enough. It must be friendly, real-time and usable. Community-based evolution, reflecting the grassroots reality of relationship-based care, is critical — as is the protection of patient privacy and assurances of transparency in design, execution, and ongoing management.

While the challenges are real, the benefits of a national health information highway system are increasingly indisputable.

REFERENCES

1. Yasnoff WA, Humphreys BL, Overhage JM, et al. A consensus action agenda for achieving the national health information infrastructure. *J Am Med Inform Assoc*. 2004;11:332-338.
2. Masys DR. Knowledge Management: Keeping Up with the Growing Knowledge. Presented at: 2001 IOM Annual Meeting; October 15, 2001; Washington, DC. Cited in Yasnoff WA, Humphreys BL, Overhage JM, et al.
3. Dick RS, Steen EB, Detmer DE, eds. The Computer-Based Patient Record: An Essential Technology for Health Care. Rev ed. Washington, DC: *National Academy Press*, 1997. Cited in Yasnoff WA, Humphreys BL, Overhage JM, et al.
4. Kohn LT, Corrigan JM, Donaldson MS (eds). To Err Is Human: Building a Safer Health System. Washington, DC: *National Academy Press*; 2000. Cited in Yasnoff WA, Humphreys BL, Overhage JM, et al.
5. Aspden P, Corrigan JM, Wolcott J, Erickson SM, eds. Patient Safety: Achieving a New Standard for Care. Washington, DC: *The National Academies Press*; 2004. Cited in Yasnoff WA, Humphreys BL, Overhage JM, et al.
6. Overhage JM, Dexter PR, Perkins SM, et al. A randomized controlled trial of clinical information shared from another institution. *Ann*

Emerg Med. 2002;39:14-23. Cited in Yasnoff WA, Humphreys BL, Overhage JM, et al.

7. Brailer DJ, Augustinos N, Evans LM, Karp S. Moving Toward Electronic Health Information Exchange: Interim Report on the Santa Barbara County Data Exchange. July 2003. Available at: http://www.chcf.org/documents/ihealth/sbccdeinterimreport.pdf. Accessed January 19, 2004. Cited in Yasnoff WA, Humphreys BL, Overhage JM, et al.

8. National Committee on Vital and Health Statistics. Information for Health: A Strategy for Building the National Health Information Infrastructure. November 15, 2001. Available at: http://www.Ncvhs.hhs.gov/nhiilayo.pdf. Accessed January 19, 2004. Cited in Yasnoff WA, Humphreys BL, Overhage JM, et al.

TEACHING TOOLS

Policy Premises

1. The critical need for better information system support in health has been well recognized for two decades.
2. Current conditions are ripe for action as we approach a 'tipping point.'
3. The federal government has weighed in over the past three years.
4. There is general agreement on the deliverables of a national health information systems infrastructure.
5. Remaining obstacles must be addressed.
6. National leadership, cross-sector resourcing and community participation must now coalesce to avoid further inaction.

Review

1. Why has the process to develop a health information infrastructure system been slow?
2. How have conditions changed?
3. What role has the Department of Health and Human Services played?
4. What are the benefits of having a health information infrastructure system?
5. Which obstacles still need to be addressed?

Online Resources

 Access online resources with this book's CD.

What is NHII?
http://aspe.hhs.gov/sp/nhii/FAQ.html

Executive Order
http://www.whitehouse.gov/news/releases/2004/04/20040427-4.html

Recommendations from the Institute of Medicine
http://www4.nationalacademies.org/news.nsf/isbn/0309090776?Op
enDocument

Building the National Health Information Infrastructure
http://library.ahima.org/xpedio/groups/public/documents/ahima/pub
_bok1_022849.html

Medicine Must Lead the Way
http://www.acponline.org/journals/news/apr04/washington.htm

Wondering About EHR Trends and Usage
http://www.medrecinst.com/pages/latestNews.asp?id=115

HHS Pushes Electronic Health Records
http://www.computerworld.com/governmenttopics/government/poli
cy/story/0,10801,94665,00.html

Health Politics Online

For Original Health Politics Program and Slides:

The Health Information Highway: All Aboard
http://www.healthpolitics.com/program_info.asp?p=prog_62
Slide Briefing
http://www.healthpolitics.com/media/prog_62/brief_prog_62.pdf

Health Insurance Reform

WHERE ARE WE NOW?

The U.S. health insurance system is marked by unequal distribution, a historic emphasis on intervention over prevention based on single-year budgeting rather than multi-year budgeting, limited resources, and unlimited demand.[1]

Approximately $500 billion per year is spent on health care in the United States. About $279 billion of that is contributed by employers for private employee health insurance. On average, the employer pays about three-quarters of the employee's premium, and the employee pays the balance. But not all employers offer health insurance and not all employees accept it. In 2002, 77 percent of employers offered health insurance as part of a compensation package to employees. Of those employees, 82 percent accepted it, so 63 percent of employees received employer-based insurance.[2,3]

The plans that reach employees at work are the result of a double sale. The first sale is from the health insurer to the employer and generally involves a menu of options for employees to choose from. The cost of the overall package to the employer is a function of the company it is purchased from, the various options purchased, and the degree of involvement or risk taken by the employer in managing elements of the program, like processing claims.[1]

The second sale is between the employer and employee, as various options are offered. Subsidies, educational support, and employer empathy vary widely. The insurer's primary focus is providing a quality product priced accurately to ensure profitability. The employer's primary focus is worker productivity and quality within the confines of affordability. The employee's primary focus is acquiring, at low cost, a comprehensive health-benefits package.

The factors influencing the cost of insurance are complex. They include consumer demand, scientific progress, a decrease in competition in some markets due to consolidation of the health insurance industry, variations in income from investments, fluctuating costs of reinsurance, and rising profit expectations of investors.[1] Between 1998 and 2002, the percentage of growth in health insurance premiums was four times greater than the percentage of growth in consumer prices overall.[3]

To say that health insurance, or lack thereof, is controversial in the United States would be a major understatement. In the past two decades, we have moved through three significant transformations. Until the 1980s, we were dominated by indemnity insurance, whose major cost-control strategy was to pool risk in large heterogeneous populations. Care panels were wide, with almost all doctors and hospitals participating and accessible to patients. Providers were generally paid what they billed. Benefits were narrow, covering primarily expensive in-hospital care. Limitations included steady cost inflation and a benefit package increasingly out of step with the emergence of health consumerism and prevention.[1]

Table 9.3-1. Health Insurance: Controversy & Change

	Indemnity	HMO	Consumer-Directed Health Care
Time Period:	Until 1980s	1980s-2000	2000-Present
Cost-Control Strategy:	Pool risk	Limit supply of services	Limit demand
Care Panels:	Wide	Narrow	Variable
Benefits:	Narrow	Wide	Variable
Limitations:	• Cost inflation • Outdated benefits	• No real economy of scale • Patient & Physician dissatisfaction	• Complexity • Employer cost concerns • Consumers' expectations

Source: Robinson JC. Reinvention of health insurance in the consumer era. *JAMA.* 2004;291:1880-1886.
Robinson JC. The end of managed care. *JAMA.* 2001;285:2622-2628.
Robinson JC. From managed care to consumer health insurance: the fall and rise of Aetna. *Health Aff* (Millwood). 2004;23:43-55.

From the mid-80s through 2000, Health Maintenance Organizations, or HMOs, led the way. Their cost-control strategy was to control the supply of costly services by rewarding cost-conscious behavior in doctors and hospitals.

Access to care was limited by narrowing the number of doctors and hospitals authorized to treat insured patients. In return, patients were offered comprehensive services, including outpatient, inpatient, and preventive services, as well as some pharmaceuticals at a very reasonable cost. Insurers focused on rapidly expanding market share in hopes of achieving economy of scale, an outcome that never materialized. Rather, the HMO movement came crashing down as doctors and patients revolted in a backlash of dissatisfaction over limitations on choice and access.[4]

In place of the HMO, a third approach quietly emerged, called Consumer-Directed Health Care. Its cost-control strategy is not to limit supply, but to limit demand by making patients responsible for their own choices and decisions. Care panels and benefits vary based on employee elections and their willingness to pay for various packages and tiers of service. The limitations of this approach are its inherent complexity, continued cost concerns of employers, and rising expectations of health consumers.[5]

Variable pricing and a menu of employee choices are central elements of this new health insurance strategy. The use of expansive options and choices reflects the diverse ability of employees to pay for coverage. By packaging in cost-sharing tiered networks of care, and by stratifying and targeting careful medical management of complex and expensive cases, insurers and employers hope to accurately price services, place responsibility for choice clearly on the shoulders of consumers, and carefully manage their risk. This represents a major shift from the indemnity days, when the healthy insured majority cross-subsidized the unhealthy insured minority.[1]

Success of the Consumer-Directed Health Care strategy is heavily dependent on a renewed emphasis on expert medical underwriting, predicting both health statistics and likely consumption rates of insured individuals. Not all individuals are equal in the risky business of insurance. In the privately insured, non-elderly, U.S. population, more than 60 percent are healthy, approximately 20 percent have acute diseases, 15 percent have chronic diseases, and 1 percent suffer a complex or catastrophic event in a premium year. As for cost, 56 percent is created by 5 percent of the population, and 69 percent is tied to 10 percent of the population.[1] Medical management's goal is to tailor interventions to these stratified populations. The emphasis for the healthy is prevention — keep them well; for the acutely ill — manage the care continuum with clinical protocols and utilization review; and for the chronically ill — careful case management.

Table 9.3-2. Consumer-Directed System	
Strengths	**Weaknesses**
• Consumer choice & responsibility • Priority setting on front end • Cost-conscious behavior • Accurate pricing and prevention	• Complex for diverse employee base • Limits (even self-imposed) may lead to backlash • Does not address the uninsured

So what's wrong with this picture? On the one hand, it stresses consumer choice and responsibility, priority setting on the front end, cost-conscious behavior, and accurate pricing and prevention — all good things. But on the other hand, it is remarkably complex for an employee base that is unevenly supported with education and emotional encouragement. And it is likely that limited coverage — even self-imposed by consumer choice — and economically disastrous events occurring in a small portion of the population will eventually lead to patient and physician backlash. Finally, and most significantly, it ignores the fact that a large segment of our population remains uninsured. Left unaddressed — as we have seen in the past — uninsured populations will undermine our well-intentioned but highly segmented efforts.

REFERENCES

1. Robinson JC. Reinvention of health insurance in the consumer era. *JAMA*. 2004;291:1880-1886.
2. Magee M. The safety net and caring for the uninsured. October 29, 2003. Available at: www.healthpolitics.com. Accessed June 9, 2004.
3. American Medical Association Trends Report. Health Insurance Costs and Coverage. August 2003. Available at: www.ama-assn.org/go/healthpolicy. Accessed June 9, 2004.
4. Robinson JC. The end of managed care. *JAMA*. 2001;285:2622-2628.
5. Robinson JC. From managed care to consumer health insurance: the fall and rise of Aetna. *Health Aff* (Millwood). 2004;23:43-55.

TEACHING TOOLS

Policy Premises

1. The U.S. health insurance system is marked by unequal distribution, a historic emphasis on intervention over prevention, limited resources, and unlimited demand.
2. The health insurance industry has moved into its third major transformation in two decades.
3. The cost of health insurance is rising as a result of multiple factors.
4. Not all employers provide health insurance and not all employees accept it.
5. Variable pricing and consumer choice are the central elements of the new private health insurance strategy.
6. The strengths and weaknesses of this new approach are already evident and require real-time adjustments.

Review

1. How much do U.S. employers spend on private employee health insurance each year?
2. What factors influence the cost of health insurance?
3. What type of insurance emerged after the HMO movement?
4. What are the central elements of the current health insurance strategy in the United States?
5. Which group of people is still overlooked in the U.S. health care system?

Online Resources

Access online resources with this book's CD.

Health Insurance
http://familydoctor.org/688.xml

Elderly and Uninsured
http://www.aafp.org/x26875.xml

Choosing a Plan
http://www.ahrq.gov/consumer/hlthpln1.htm#choosing

Health Insurance Coverage
http://www.cdc.gov/nchs/fastats/hinsure.htm

Estimation of Expenditures and Enrollments for Employer-Sponsored Health Insurance
http://www.meps.ahrq.gov/PAPERS/mr14_03-0009/mr14.pdf

Panel Calls for Universal Health Insurance
http://msnbc.msn.com/id/3956057/

Choosing Health Insurance That Best Meets Your Needs
http://www.ama-assn.org/ama/upload/mm/363/choosing.pdf

Implications of Health Market Trends for Consumers and the Safety Net
http://www.kff.org/insurance/7031/loader.cfm?url=/commonspot/security/getfile.cfm&PageID=36097

Health Politics Online

For Original Health Politics Programs and Slides:

Health Insurance Reform
http://www.healthpolitics.com/program_info.asp?p=prog_53
Slide Briefing
http://www.healthpolitics.com/media/prog_53/brief_prog_53.pdf

CHAPTER 9.4

The Safety Net and Care for the Uninsured

UNDERSTANDING THE NEED

A health care safety net in the United States is not a luxury, but rather a necessity. It has become necessary because we chronically possess large numbers of uninsured as a result of our employee-based health insurance system. If you're out of work in America, it's a double hit. You lose your pay and your health insurance, and that's if you were lucky enough to be in a job that provided benefits.

What we call a safety net may not reliably catch you if you're uninsured.[1] It all depends on where you live, your ability to communicate and your capacity to advocate for yourself or your family. Many participate in this loose network, including hospitals, clinics, physicians, health professionals, homecare providers and suppliers of pharmaceuticals and medical devices. The funding for these efforts is also a patchwork. It includes the patient's out-of-pocket fees, as well as payments from private insurance, public insurance through Medicare, Medicaid, veterans funds, CHAMPUS government funds and disability payments. Additionally, there are free product donations and in-kind charity care from doctors and nurses.

The bulk of the nation's expenditures for health care, about $500 billion in all, come from the private arena, where employers underwrote some $279 billion in health insurance expenditures; compared with $54 billion spent by Medicare and Medicaid for public health insurance. Not all of the care provided to the uninsured is uncompensated. In 2001, 17 percent, or $83 billion of the roughly $500 billion spent on U.S. health care, was provided for services directed at the uninsured.[2] The uninsured, themselves, paid $26 billion, private payers contributed $24 billion, Medicare and Medicaid put in almost $14 billion, and other public sources, like the Veterans Administration, accounted for nearly $19 billion.[3]

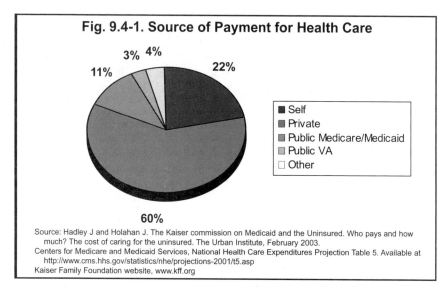

Fig. 9.4-1. Source of Payment for Health Care

Source: Hadley J and Holahan J. The Kaiser commission on Medicaid and the Uninsured. Who pays and how much? The cost of caring for the uninsured. The Urban Institute, February 2003.
Centers for Medicare and Medicaid Services, National Health Care Expenditures Projection Table 5. Available at http://www.cms.hhs.gov/statistics/nhe/projections-2001/t5.asp
Kaiser Family Foundation website, www.kff.org

What, then, is uncompensated care? The Kaiser Commission on Medicaid and the Uninsured defines uncompensated care as "care received that is not paid for, either out of pocket by the uninsured patient or by an identifiable third party or private source."[4]

A significant amount of care for the uninsured is provided each year by hospitals, clinics and physicians. In total, this care for 2001 was valued at nearly $99 billion: $40.6 billion for those uninsured the entire year and $58.3 billion for those uninsured for a portion of the year. Of that $99 billion, approximately 62 percent was compensated directly, and 38 percent was uncompensated.[4]

So what does all of this mean? It means that money is flowing into the system to care for the uninsured; it's just not going to help them buy insurance. As the Kaiser Commission stated, "In 2001, governments spent $30.6 billion covering, perhaps, 85 percent of the cost of uncompensated care. Although this is a substantial public expenditure, it represents less than 6 percent of total government spending for personal healthcare in 2001." For example, in 2001, government spending on Medicare was $247 billion, on Medicaid, $226 billion, on tax code subsidies to buy insurance, $138 billion, and on uncompensated care, $31 billion.[5] Or, viewed another way, uninsured patients in need got less care as reflected in per capita costs. The per capita cost for a privately insured patient in the United States was $2,484; for a publicly insured patient it was $2,435; and for an uninsured patient it was $1,335.[2]

The majority of public and private funds paid reactively, for uncompensated care, go to hospitals. In 2001, hospitals received $2.3 billion to $4.6 billion from private sources, $14.2 billion from federal sources and $9.4 billion from state and local sources. Up to $28.2 billion of the $40.4 billion expended (including $5.1 billion in physician charity care) went to hospitals. This is as it should be, since hospitals currently carry the greatest burden of care for the uninsured. Their contribution to the safety net includes a 24/7 community presence and responsiveness through emergency rooms, trauma units, surgical suites, hospital beds, skilled staff, equipment and supplies.[6]

Table 9.4-1. Investment in Uncompensated Care in 2001
(in billions)

	Private	Federal	State/Local	Total
Hospital	$4.6	$14.2	$9.4	$28.2
Clinics	$.13	$5.7	$1.3	$7.1
Physicians	$5.1	0	0	$5.1

Source: Davison D. Is Philanthropy Dying at the Hospital? *Philanthropy* August/September 2001.

Extending coverage to the uninsured, then, is not as impossible as it sounds. That's because we are not starting from scratch. In fact, we are providing considerable tax funds, albeit in a highly reactive, after-the-fact way. Rather than providing insurance more broadly to those in need, and incentivizing prevention, we reactively reimburse those who assume the responsibility of caring for a population of the disadvantaged and disempowered.

Extending coverage to those currently uninsured could be accomplished without new government funding. Once again, from the Kaiser Commission, "If a substantial part of the financing of care received by the uninsured is already in the public sector, then some share of these funds is potentially available for transfer to new government efforts to extend coverage to those currently uninsured. Much of the $23.6 billion in payments to hospitals…would be a reasonable candidate for reallocation…since hospitals would be the primary beneficiaries."[2]

How much medical care do uninsured patients use? Roughly half of what the insured use, but at the expense of later entry into the health care system and poorer outcomes. Who pays for the care? We do, after the fact, through tax supported public funds. How much uncompensated care do people receive now? Best estimates for 2001 were approximately $35 billion. How much did federal, state and local governments expend to cover the care of the uninsured in 2001? Best estimates are $30.6 billion, with an additional $7 to $10 billion paid to hospitals and other private sources.

The best way to create a real safety net for the uninsured is to redirect funding to provide to them what the rest of us have — and that's health insurance.

REFERENCES

1. Lewin ME and Altman S. America's Health Care Safety Net: Intact but Endangered. Washington DC. National Academy Press.
2. Hadley J and Holahan J. The Kaiser commission on Medicaid and the Uninsured. Who pays and how much? The cost of caring for the uninsured. The Urban Institute. February 2003.
3. Centers for Medicare and Medicaid Services, National Health Care Expenditures Projection Table 5. Available at: http://www.cms.hhs.gov/statistics/nhe/projections-2001/+5.asp.
4. The Kaiser Family Foundation Website. http://www.kff.org.
5. Barman LE, Uceello C and Kobes D. Tax Incentives for Health Insurance. Tax Policy Discussion paper. The Urban Institute, Washington DC.
6. Davison D. Is Philanthropy Dying at the Hospital? *Philanthropy* August/September 2001.

TEACHING TOOLS

Policy Premises

1. A health care safety net has by necessity evolved in the United States to care for a larger percentage of uninsured Americans.
2. Not all care provided to the uninsured is uncompensated.
3. A significant amount of uncompensated care is provided each year by hospitals, clinics and physicians.
4. A large amount of resources is currently expended to maintain the safety net and indirectly compensate for uncompensated care.
5. The majority of funds for uncompensated care goes to hospitals.
6. Extending coverage to those currently uninsured could be accomplished without new government funding.

Review

1. Do the bulk of the nation's expenditures for health care come from the public or private arena?
2. What is uncompensated care?
3. Where do most of the public and private funds — paid reactively, for uncompensated care — go?
4. In 2001, how much did federal, state and local governments spend to cover the care of the uninsured?
5. What is the best way to create a real safety net for the uninsured?

Online Resources

Access online resources with this book's CD.

Caring for the Nation's Uninsured - Jennifer Proctor AAMC Reporter May 2000
http://www.aamc.org/newsroom/reporter/may2000/caring.htm

The Free Care Safety Net Fact Sheet - Provided by the Access Project (Funded by the Robert Wood Foundation of Brandeis University)
http://www.accessproject.org/downloads/products/freec.pdf

Improving Access to Health Care for the Uninsured - August 2003
http://www.naph.org/Content/NavigationMenu/Issues_Advocacy/Access_to_Care_for_the_Uninsured/Improving_Access_to_Health_Care_for_the_Uninsured.htm

The Health Care Safety Net - Issue Brief January 2001
http://www.nihp.org/Issue%20Briefs/Health%20Care%20Safety%20Net%20PB.htm

Health Politics Online

For Original Health Politics Programs and Slides:

The Safety Net and Caring for the Uninsured
http://www.healthpolitics.com/program_info.asp?p=prog_28
Slide Briefing
http://www.healthpolitics.com/media/prog_28/brief_prog_28.pdf

Tiered Hospital Costs

A WORKABLE SOLUTION?

The cost of health care in the United States is once again on the rise. Between 2001 and 2002, approximately $1.6 trillion was spent on health care, a 9.3 percent rise over the prior year. This equates to $5,440 per person. Hospital spending accounted for a third of these costs and increased by 9.5 percent. This increase can be attributed to several things, including the aging of the population, new diagnostics and therapeutics, the cost of labor, and rising consumer expectations.[1]

When health care spending increases, the cost of health insurance tends to follow. Between 2002 and 2003, monthly premiums for employer-sponsored health insurance, the most dominant form, increased by 13.9 percent. The average employer paid 85 percent of the cost of premiums for individual coverage in 2003 and 73 percent of the cost of family coverage.[1,2]

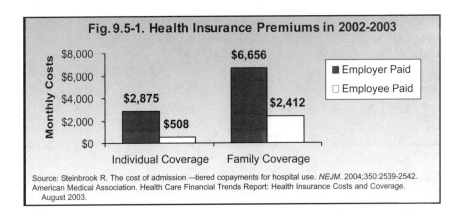

Fig. 9.5-1. Health Insurance Premiums in 2002-2003

Source: Steinbrook R. The cost of admission —tiered copayments for hospital use. *NEJM.* 2004;350:2539-2542. American Medical Association. Health Care Financial Trends Report: Health Insurance Costs and Coverage. August 2003.

As health care costs rise, insurers and employers are shifting financial responsibility for health care choices to employees. Studies have found that as employees shoulder more of this financial responsibility, they are likely to use health care services more sparingly. One study, performed between 1971 and 1982, gathered results that are still pertinent to today's health insurance situation. The RAND Health Insurance Experiment assigned about 2,000 families to insurance plans that varied, or tiered, the cost of services. The study found that "cost sharing markedly decreases the use of all types of services among all types of people." It also noted that reduced use had "little or no net adverse effect on health for the average person." But the same study also found that if people are vulnerable — either sick and poor or chronically ill — placing them at financial risk could encourage choices that hurt them.[3]

Financial risk comes in many shapes and sizes in the world of insurance. In conventional insurance plans and preferred provider organizations, employees share costs through deductibles and co-pays, and now they sometimes pay tiered costs. With this method, payments for care and treatment are based on which column their choice falls under — A, B, or C. The most common example of tiered cost sharing is in pharmaceuticals, where an older, generic drug chosen from column A may have no co-pay; an older, brand-name drug from column B may have a moderate co-pay; and a new, brand-name drug from column C may have a significant co-pay.

This latest approach of tiering choices is now being tried out for physician and hospital services as well. Insurers in several regions are experimenting with what they call "value" networks. By analyzing financial data and medical data, the insurer attempts to identify the lowest-cost, highest-quality doctors and hospitals, assign them to tiers, and steer patients to them by creating a financial incentive, such as low co-pays.

In 2003, 86 percent of employer-based insurance plans offered tiered pharmaceutical benefits, and only 6 percent offered tiers for hospital and physician networks.[4] But this approach is getting more and more attention. One example of a participating insurer is Blue Shield of California, with more than 300 hospitals in its tiered network. Eighty-five percent have been included in its "choice" tier, which doesn't require a co-pay. Patients who go to one of its other hospitals will pay a premium. A second example is Tufts Health Plan in Massachusetts. If a hospital is designated a "better quality and efficiency" hospital, patients have a $200 co-pay on the front end. But attending one of the "good quality and efficiency" institutions will cost patients $400 up front.[1]

These "value" networks are unlikely to be a workable solution in the short term. Here's why. First, measuring the quality of hospitals in order to assign them to tiers remains an inexact science. Second, studies of quality outcomes in tiered systems will be difficult to design and execute, and will take several years. Third, tiered systems will only impact costs for insured patients. The large number of uninsured people remains beyond the reach of this strategy. Furthermore, large numbers of areas in the United States have only single points of service for specialists or complex procedures. Fourth, hospitals and physicians are fundamentally uncomfortable with this approach, partly because they mistrust the accuracy of the quality measures, and partially because our complex teaching hospitals attract our sickest and most vulnerable patients, increasing the cost and at times decreasing the quality outcomes in these institutions. Finally, additional tiering of choices further magnifies health care complexity for consumers and risks undermining both patient-physician and patient-physician-hospital relations.

REFERENCES

1. Steinbrook R. The cost of admission - tiered copayments for hospital use. *NEJM*. 2004;350:2539-2542.
2. American Medical Association. Health Care Financial Trends Report: Health Insurance Costs and Coverage. August 2003.
3. Newhouse JP and the Insurance Experiment Group. Free for all? Lessons from the RAND Health Insurance Experiment. Cambridge, Mass: Harvard University Press; 1993.
4. Gabel J, Claxton G, Holve E, et al. Health benefits in 2003: premiums reach thirteen-year high as employers adopt new forms of cost sharing. *Health Aff* (Millwood). 2003:22;117-126. Cited in Steinbrook R.

TEACHING TOOLS

Policy Premises

1. The cost of health care is once again on the rise.
2. The dominant form of health care in the United States is employer sponsored.
3. Increasingly, insurers and employers are shifting financial responsibility for health care choices to employees.
4. Financial risk comes in many shapes and sizes, the latest being tiered benefits.
5. Several regions have now attempted to package physician and hospital services into tiered "value" networks.
6. "Value" networks are unlikely to be a workable solution to a fundamental problem.

Review

1. Why has hospital spending increased over the last few years?
2. What are employers and insurers doing in response to rising health care costs?
3. What is tiered cost sharing?
4. What is a "value" network?
5. Will the tiering strategy simplify health care for consumers?

Online Resources

 Access online resources with this book's CD.

Health Consumerism
http://www.benefitnews.com/detail.cfm?id=6162&terms=|hospitals||tiered|

Tiered Hospital Plans
http://www.bls.gov/opub/cwc/cm20030715ar01p1.htm

New Era of Benefits
http://content.healthaffairs.org/cgi/content/full/hlthaff.w4.210v1/DC1

Tiers Keep Costs in Tow
http://www.managedhealthcareexecutive.com/mhe/article/articleDe
tail.jsp?id=94793

Health Politics Online

For Original Health Politics Programs and Slides:

Tiered Cost Sharing: What Does It Mean for Hospital Use?
http://www.healthpolitics.com/program_info.asp?p=prog_58
Slide Briefing
http://www.healthpolitics.com/media/prog_58/brief_prog_58.pdf

Financing Home Health Care

WHO'S PAYING?

Home health care covers an increasingly important constellation of health services being delivered in a patient's home setting. Under this banner exists a complex array of professional, diagnostic, and equipment-support entities that together have, with some success, kept the frail and disabled out of hospitals and out of nursing homes.[1]

Professional services include those of doctors, nurses, dentists, dieticians, rehabilitation therapists, social workers, psychologists, podiatrists and home health aides. Diagnostic services include phlebotomy, ECG, Holter monitors, Doppler testing, oximetry, radiographic studies and a variety of point-of-care tests. Equipment support includes IV infusion sets, ventilators and oxygen, dialysis, medical alert devices, hospital beds, wheelchairs, commodes and lifts.

Table 9.6-1. Comprehensive Home Health Care Services

Professional	Diagnostic	Equipment
• Physician	• Phlebotomy	• IV infusion
• Nurse	• ECG	• Ventilator, oxygen
• Dentist	• Holter monitor	• Dialysis
• Rehab Therapist	• Doppler testing	• Medical alert devices
• Social Worker	• Oximetry	• Hospital beds
• Psychologist	• Radiographic studies	• Wheelchairs
• Podiatrist	• Point-of-care tests	• Commodes
• Home Health Aide		• Lifts

Source: Levine SA, Barry PP. Geriatric Medicine: An Evidence-Based Approach. 2003.

The size and complexity of the investment reflects the enormity of the challenge and the multiple benefits that accrue to home-based health solutions. Many older Americans are confined to their homes, and the numbers are rising. In America, four- and five-generation families are now commonplace; and third-generation Americans, voluntarily or involuntarily, have become the backbone of the unpaid family caregiver movement.[2]

Nineteen percent of the U.S. population over 5 years of age has a disability.[3] Forty-two percent of those over 65 have a disability. Of those 14 million disabled Americans 65 and older, only 1.6 million are in nursing homes, leaving 12.4 million as home-based.[2] Nine and one-half million people over the age of 50 need assistance with at least one daily living activity.[4]

Coverage of home health services comes from a variety of sources. More than 28 percent is funded through Medicare; 18.5 percent from Medicaid; 23.5 percent from private insurance; 24 percent from patient out-of-pocket; and 5.2 percent from other sources.[5] Private insurers generally dedicate approximately one percent of their budgets to home care coverage.[6]

Medicare coverage has fluctuated wildly in the past 10 to 15 years. To place the numbers in perspective, let's look at total home health care expenditures in the United States for the year 2000. About $30 billion was paid to home health agencies; $3.5 billion expended on respiratory therapy; $4.5 billion spent on home infusions; and $3 billion invested in home medical equipment.[5]

Now let's look at Medicare's contribution. In 1990, Medicare expended a total of $3.9 billion on home care.[7] At the time, it covered primarily acute and post-acute hospital care. But a variety of forces — including aging demo-

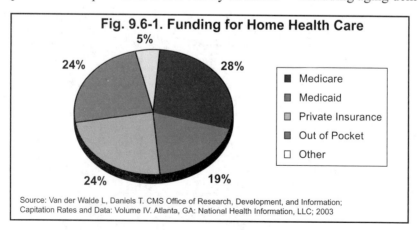

Fig. 9.6-1. Funding for Home Health Care

- Medicare — 28%
- Medicaid — 19%
- Private Insurance — 5%
- Out of Pocket — 24%
- Other — 24%

Source: Van der Walde L, Daniels T. CMS Office of Research, Development, and Information; Capitation Rates and Data: Volume IV. Atlanta, GA: National Health Information, LLC; 2003

graphics, early discharge, cost-based home care financing, and declining nursing home beds — helped support a large expansion of services, with more than half of the total resources going to patients who had not been hospitalized.[8]

By 1997, Medicare expenditures for home health services had risen to $17.2 billion, or 9 percent of the total Medicare budget. The 1997 Balanced Budget Act provided a financial push back, moving away from non-post-acute care and support for items like blood testing and home aids. As a result, by 1999, Medicare expenditure for home health care had declined to $9.7 billion, or just 4 percent of the Medicare budget. In human terms, Medicare, in 1997, served 3.5 million home-based patients with 256 million visits. By 2001, it served 2.4 million patients with 73 million visits.[9]

Yet home-based care continues to grow. It is clearly favored by patients and families, and has well-defined benefits. They include improved patient satisfaction compared to nursing homes or hospitals; more accurate information transfer, including medical diagnosis, social assessments, and medication lists; 5 to 7 percent fewer medication errors; and a 22 to 26 percent decline in acute hospitalization.[10,11,12]

Who's paying for home care, since the largest portion of the care is largely unfunded? The short-term answer is America's families — contributing not only their money, but also blood, sweat, and tears. Fully 25 percent of all U.S. citizens are unpaid home care providers. Their contributions are critical to maintaining frail and disabled patients in home settings. In fact, their contributions, translated into dollars, exceed real dollars spent by 600 percent. And for their good works, they are repaid in poorer personal health outcomes, depression and social isolation.[13,14,15]

What's the good news? People are living longer and happier, largely in home-based settings. But they are managing on the backs of, primarily, third-generation female family members who are stretched thin in every imaginable way.

Home-based caregivers need inclusion and support within care teams. If we wish to use this approach long term, support for family caregivers must include financial, logistical, and emotional expenditures to stabilize what is currently, at best, a rapidly over-stressed and over-burdened voluntary work force.

REFERENCES

1. Levine SA, Barry PP. Home Care. In: Cassel CK, Leipzig RM, Cohen HJ, Larson EB, Meier DE, Capello CF, eds. *Geriatric Medicine: An Evidence-Based Approach*. 4th ed. New York, NY: Springer-Verlag New York; 2003.
2. Census 2000 Brief. The 65 years and over population: 2000. Available at: http://www.census.gov/prod/200/pubs/c2kbr01-10pdf. Accessed 2003.
3. Census 2000 Brief. Disability status: 2000. Available at: http://www.census.gov/hhes/www/disable/disabstat2k/table1.html. Accessed July 24, 2003.
4. Kassner E, Bectel RW. Mid-life and Older Americans With Disabilities: Who Gets Help? A Chartbook. Washington, DC: Public Policy Institute, American Association of Retired Persons; 1998.
5. Van der Walde L, Daniels T. CMS Office of Research, Development, and Information. Health care industry market update: home health. Available at: http://www.cms.hhs.gov/reports/hcimu/hcimu_06282002.pdf. Accessed August 18, 2003.
6. *Capitation Rates and Data: Volume IV*. Atlanta, GA: National Health Information, LLC; 2003.
7. Cotterill PG, Gage BJ. Overview: Medicare Post-acute care since the Balanced Budget Act of 1997. *Health Care Finac Rev*. 2002; 24:1-6.
8. Welch HG, Wennberg DE, Welch WP. The use of Medicare home health services. *N Engl J Med*. 1996; 335:324-329.
9. Chen Q, Kane RL, Finch MD. The cost effectiveness of post-acute care for elderly Medicare beneficiaries. *Inquiry*. 2000-2001; 37: 359-375.
10. Ramsdell JW, Swart JA, Jackson JE, Renvall M. The yield of home visits in the assessment of geriatric patients. *J Am Geriatr Soc*. 1989; 37: 17-24.
11. Yang JC, Tomlinson G, Naglie G. Medication lists for elderly patients: clinic-derived versus in-home inspection and interview. *J Gen Intern Med*. 2001; 16:112-115.
12. Meredith S, Feldman P, Frey D, et al. Improving medication use in newly admitted home healthcare patients: a randomized controlled trial. *J Am Geriatr Soc*. 2002; 50:1484-1491.
13. Donelan K, Hill CA, Hoffman C, et al. Challenged to care: informal caregivers in a changing health system. *Health Aff* (Millwood). 2002; 21:222-231.

14. Arno PS, Levine C, Memmott MM. The economic value of informal caregiving. *Health Aff* (Millwood). 1999; 18:182-188.
15. Haley WE, Levine EG, Brown SL, Berry JW, Hughes GH. Psychological, social and health consequences of caring for a relative with senile dementia. *J Am Geriatr Soc*. 1987;35:405-411.

TEACHING TOOLS

Policy Premises

1. Home health care covers an increasingly important constellation of health services delivered in a patient's home setting.
2. Coverage of home health care services comes from a variety of sources.
3. Medicare coverage has fluctuated and comes with strings attached.
4. Home-based care is clearly favored by patients and has well-defined benefits.
5. The largest portion of the home care network is completely unfunded.

Review

1. What percentage of the U.S. population, above age five, has a medical disability?
2. In the year 2000, what were America's total home health care expenditures?
3. What are the primary sources of coverage for home-based health care?
4. What are the key patient benefits associated with home-based health care?
5. What support is needed to sustain home-based caregiving?

Online Resources

Access online resources with this book's CD.

Older Americans Act Appropriations - The National Family Caregiver Support Program
http://www.ncoa.org/content.cfm?sectionID=165&detail=70

Health Care Industry Market Update
http://www.cms.hhs.gov/reports/hcimu/hcimu_06282002.pdf

Health Politics Online

For Original Health Politics Programs and Slides:

Financing Home Health Care
http://www.healthpolitics.com/program_info.asp?p=prog_27
Slide Briefing
http://www.healthpolitics.com/media/prog_27/brief_prog_27.pdf

Improving Patient Adherence

A CONSUMER EMPOWERMENT CHALLENGE

The modern patient-physician relationship worldwide is increasingly becoming horizontal, not vertical. Studies show that physicians have largely embraced partnerships with their patients. The days of "doctor says" and "patient does" are steadily drifting into the past. In concert, one-on-one strategies are giving way to team approaches as doctors begin to acknowledge that managing both clinical and educational continuums in support of educationally empowered health consumers requires a supportive team and delegation. "Doctor's orders" are increasingly being supplemented by mutual decision-making. The long-term goal: prevention rather than intervention.[1,2]

But we're not there yet. Why not? Part of the answer is that the patient-physician relationship has evolved more rapidly than patients' and physicians' ability to reliably execute treatment plans. One indicator of this structural disconnect is the tension that has arisen over the language we use to describe patient execution and follow-through. Prior to the emergence of health consumerism, the Internet, and prevention-focused medicine, health care leaders spoke often of compliance: the extent to which a patient follows medical instructions. Today we look at adherence: the extent to which a person's behavior — taking medication, following a diet, or executing lifestyle changes — corresponds with agreed recommendations from a health care provider.[3,4]

Changes in language often signal the onset of process and system redesign. Recent publications by the World Health Organization and the American Medical Association have made it clear that adherence is a worldwide issue that will grow in significance with aging of our populations and coincident increases in the prevalence of chronic diseases.[4,5] The WHO report notes, "In developed countries, adherence among patients suffering chronic diseases averages only 50 percent." And the challenge is greater in the developing world. For example, studies show that adherence to treatment regimens for hypertension are 51 percent in the United States, 43 percent in China, but only 27 percent in Gambia.[4] Studies also reveal that the developing world is rapidly encountering a dual burden of disease as it confronts infectious diseases and malnutrition on the one hand, and marketing-driven behavioral changes that increase the incidence of chronic diseases and cancer on the other.[6]

The reasons for poor adherence are well-understood, but the solutions are only now taking shape. Adherence requires that a patient fully understand and comprehend the plan, be in full agreement with the course of action, and be committed to the execution of what is increasingly a multistep solution.[7] Thinking for a moment just about medication for a well-motivated, engaged patient with resources, what questions would be required to generate baseline information? Here are just a few: How much medication is needed? How often? Same time every day? Do I empty the bottle? Do I need a refill? Side effects? Will I become addicted? Any interactions with my other medicines? Do you have information I can take with me? Whom do I call if I have a problem? And that doesn't even begin to address more substantive lifestyle behavioral changes.

The reality is that ensuring adherence is complex. No single strategy has been known to be effective.[4] What we do know is that good follow-through is a local phenomenon and is most likely if interventions are tailored to the individual patients; if patients are supported rather than blamed; and if patients, families and communities are actively involved. Peer support can be critical, according to the WHO report, which says, "There is substantial evidence that peer support among patients can improve adherence to therapy while reducing the amount of time devoted by the health professionals to the care of chronic conditions."[4]

Measuring adherence remains problematic. The WHO report continues, "There is no 'gold standard' for measuring adherence behavior…measurement of adherence remains only an estimate of a patient's actual behavior."[4] But technology, in the form of future "smart" delivery systems that use the detection of chemical signals in the body to release appropriate dosages from internalized reservoirs of medicine are on the horizon.[8] Cross-sector partnerships are also beginning to attack behavioral change and chronic diseases in a more deliberate and multi-year manner with some success.[9]

Is the investment worth it? Economists would say "without a doubt." In the United States alone, the annual cost of poor adherence is estimated at $75 billion to $100 billion. The human cost is even more striking — 125,000 preventable deaths and 10 percent to 25 percent of all hospital and nursing home admissions.[7] As Dr. Eduardo Sabaté, medical officer of the WHO, has noted, "Better adherence will not threaten health care budgets. On the contrary, adherence will result in a significant decrease in the overall health budget. This is due to the reduction in the need for more costly interventions, unnecessary use of emergency room services and highly expensive intensive care services."[4]

Table 9.7-1. Medical Benefits of Patient Adherence

- Fewer medical complications
- Better quality of life
- Decreases in drug resistance
- Wiser use of health resources
- Decreases in pain and intervention
- Increases in work productivity

Source: Adherence to Long-Term Therapies: Evidence for Action. World Health Organization 2003.

In addition to financial benefits, the medical benefits are real, including fewer medical complications, better quality of life, decreases in antibiotic drug resistance, wiser use of limited health resources, decreases in pain and intervention, and increases in workforce productivity.[4,7]

U.N. Secretary-General Kofi Annan perhaps said it best: "When we are sick, working is hard and learning is harder still. Illness blunts our creativity, cuts out opportunities."[4]

REFERENCES

1. Magee M, D'Antonio M. *The Best Medicine*. New York: Spencer Books; 2001.
2. Magee M. Relationship Based Health Care in the United States, United Kingdom, Canada, Germany, South Africa, and Japan. Presented at the World Medical Association Annual Meeting. Helsinki, September

    11, 2003.
3. Haynes RB. Determinants of compliance: the disease and the mechan-
    ics of treatment. Baltimore: Johns Hopkins University Press; 1979.
4. Adherence to Long-Term Therapies: Evidence for action. World Health
    Organization 2003. Available at: http://www.who.int/chronic_condi-
    tions/adherencereport/en/.
5. American Medical Association. The Patient's Role in Improving
    Adherence. Available at: http://www.ama-assn.org/ama/pub/arti-
    cle/12202-8427.html. Accessed October 21, 2004.
6. Magee M. Attacking Chronic Diseases in Developing Countries.
    Available at:
    http://www.healthpolitics.com/program_info.asp?p=prog_55.
    Accessed October 21, 2004.
7. Family Medicine NetGuide. Patient Adherence Explained. Available
    at: http://www.fmnetguide.com/vo2iss1/feature.html. Accessed
    October 21, 2004.
8. American Medical Association. Facilitating Adherence with
    Technology. Available at: http://www.ama-assn.org/ama/pub/arti-
    cle/12202-8430.html. Accessed October 21, 2004.
9. Pfizer Clear Health Communication Initiative 2003-2004.

TEACHING TOOLS

Policy Premises

1. The modern patient-physician relationship is horizontal, not vertical, in nature.
2. The relationship has evolved more rapidly than patients' and physicians' ability to reliably execute treatment plans.
3. Adherence is a worldwide issue that will grow in significance with aging and increased chronic disease.
4. The reasons for poor adherence are well-understood; the solutions require individualization and community support.
5. Measuring adherence is problematic; technology may help.
6. Investing in adherence is a wise financial decision.

Review

1. How has the patient-physician relationship changed?
2. What is the rate of adherence among those patients with chronic diseases?
3. What types of actions have been proven to help improve patient adherence?
4. How might technology make a difference?
5. What is the annual cost of poor patient adherence?

Online Resources

Access online resources with this book's CD.

Patient Adherence Explained
http://www.fmnetguide.com/vo2iss1/feature.html

Compliance Action Program
http://www.americanheart.org/presenter.jhtml?identifier=1657

Interventions to Improve Adherence
http://www.bcbs.com/tec/vol18/18_12.html

Risky Behavior
http://www.defeatdiabetes.org/Articles/medications041006.htm

Defining the Patient-Physician Relationship for the 21st Century
http://www.patient-physician.com/docs/PatientPhysician.pdf

New Technology Facilitates Patient Adherence
http://www.eurekalert.org/pub_releases/2004-03/ama-ntf022604.php

Health Politics Online

For Original Health Politics Programs and Slides:

Improving Patient Adherence: A Consumer Empowerment Challenge
http://www.healthpolitics.com/program_info.asp?p=prog_70
Slide Briefing
http://www.healthpolitics.com/media/prog_70/brief_prog_70.pdf

Pricing of Pharmaceuticals

NO SIMPLE TASK

The pricing of pharmaceuticals has attracted a lot of attention recently.[1] On the surface, it seems the simplest of debates. Is the price too high, too low, or just right? What could be easier than comparing the price here versus the price there? But for economists, finding answers to these "simple" questions has been a major challenge.

Markets are largely determined by geographic boundaries and a wide range of intersecting social, economic and political factors. Conditions defining a market include the standard of living — or average earning power of the area's citizens, income disparities, employment rates, the form of government, the extent and nature of its social programs, the degree of regulatory restraints on competition, trade policy, currency rates and more.

Price differentials occur for all products across markets. For example, the price differentials for food and electronics across European Union markets vary from 50 percent to 100 percent.[2] Pharmaceutical markets vary widely, not only in pricing, but also in the factors contributing to pricing. These include the range of available compounds, the availability of newly discovered medicines, the percentage of generic versus brand name drugs that are purchased, the form and presentation of compounds, the number of competitors, the restrictions on free trade, and retail mark-ups.

This wide range of variables has often meant that comparing pricing of pharmaceuticals has been an apples and oranges situation. While no simple, perfect price comparisons exist, economists from the University of

Pennsylvania's Wharton School of Business have completed a careful study published in the respected health policy journal, *Health Affairs*. This study comes close to uncovering the real numbers.[3]

In constructing their study, the researchers compared the United States with eight other countries and considered price and mix of brand name, generic, and over-the-counter drugs. The comparisons included the 249 leading compounds. They considered exchange rate movement or currency conversion rates, purchasing power parities (PPP) on variations in gross domestic product (GDP), adjustments for income and standard of living, the regulatory climate, and timing of access to newer modern discoveries.[3]

One issue that warranted focus was the mix of brand name and generic drugs, which varied from country to country, affected price, and reflected complex social, political, medical and economic trade-offs. Many prior studies neglected to include generic pricing in the mix and, therefore, skewed results. Pricing policy for brand name and generic drugs impact each other, and together define pharmaceutical affordability.

In the United States, support for the development of brand name drugs has resulted in American dominance of new pharmaceutical discoveries over the past two decades.[4] This success, along with favorable pricing in the enormous U.S. market, has rewarded the focus of brand-name companies looking for the next breakthrough. This also means, however, that in the United States, brand name companies tend to abandon their products when they go off patent, allowing generic companies, free of development costs and the costs of competing with the giant pharmaceutical concerns, to provide old-standard, off-patent medicines at a very low price. The result is easily visible in the number comparisons between the United States and Germany, where support for discovery is less pronounced and brand names often stay with the original company after patents expire. In the United States, 58 percent of drug purchases are generic, accounting for only 18 percent of all dollars spent; while in Germany, 61 percent of drug purchases are generic, accounting for 34 percent of total expenditures.[3] Comparison studies like the one conducted at the Wharton School capture both sides of the product equation — newer brand name and older generic.

A second major area of concern is the appropriate adjustments necessary to reflect not only price, but also true purchasing power. Pricing comparisons, adjusted for currency valuations, must be adjusted a second time using the well-accepted purchasing power parity index, or PPP. The PPP takes into account a country's gross domestic product, along with its overall cost of medical goods and services. By making these adjustments, prices are seen within the context of their local economies, and we are better able to approach comparisons of the relative affordability of product in one market versus another. Quick comparisons of the United States and Canada make the point. Adjusting just for currency rates, we see prices 33 percent less expensive in Canada. But with correction for PPP, the affordability differential declines to 14 percent.[3]

What else do we know about pharmaceutical market comparisons in Canada and the United States? We know that Canada's gross domestic product, per citizen, is roughly two-thirds that of a U.S. citizen, or $21,306 compared to $33,038. The buying power of the average Canadian compared to the average American — or comparative GDP normalized to the United States — is 64 percent, a factor you would expect to be reflected to some extent in pricing. We know the PPP-adjusted drug-price index shows prices closer to those of the United States, or 86 percent of our levels. We also know that the total drug volume consumed, reflecting access to and purchasing of pharmaceuticals to support prevention and health and fight disease, is 93 percent of U.S. per capita consumption. So part of the social trade-off, on first glance, is somewhat lower Canadian pricing, 86 percent to our 100 percent, for somewhat lower access to medicines, 93 percent to our 100 percent.[3]

But one other issue emerges in the breakout comparisons of drug consumption. If you compare the use of compounds more than five years old, per capita consumption in the United States and Canada is nearly identical. But when you compare products two to five years old, Canadian access is two-thirds that of the United States. And when you look at new discoveries less than two years old, access in Canada is one-quarter of that in the United States.[3]

Pricing comparisons seem simple, but they are not. Each market, each country, balances a wide range of competing issues and interests, and then creates policy that defines its social tradeoffs. In the United States, when adjusted properly, there remains a 14 percent differential in affordability with Canada. In return, we have created the world's most successful pharmaceutical-discovery enterprise, and a large portion of our citizens receive up to a five-year jump on access to new discoveries.[4,5]

REFERENCES

1. Danzon PM and Chao LW. Cross-National Price Differences for Pharmaceuticals: How Large and Why? *Journal of Health Economics.* 2000;2:159-195.
2. European Commission. "Price Differences between EU Member States— Results of Commission Surveys," May 2001. Accessed October 17, 2003.
3. Danzon PM, Furukawa MF. Prices and Availability of Pharmaceuticals: Evidence from Nine Countries. *Health Aff.* Available at: www.healthaffairs.org/WebExclusives/Danzon. Accessed October 29, 2003.
4. Danzon PM, Wang RY and Wang L. The Impact of Price Regulation on the Launch of New Drugs. NBER Working Paper no. 9874. Cambridge, Mass.: National Bureau of Economic Research, 2003.
5. Ramsey FP. A Contribution to the Theory of Taxation. *Economic Journal.* 1927;37:47-61.

TEACHING TOOLS

Policy Premises

1. Markets are largely determined by geographic boundaries and a wide range of social, economic and political conditions within those boundaries.
2. Price differentials occur for all products across markets. Pharmaceutical markets vary widely not only in pricing, but in the factors contributing to pricing.
3. Comparing pricing of pharmaceuticals is often an apples and oranges situation. While no single perfect price comparison exists, economists are making progress.
4. The mix of brand name and generic drugs and their pricing reflects an array of complex social, political, medical and economic tradeoffs.
5. Price comparisons adjusted for currency value must be further adjusted using the purchasing power parities index (PPP).
6. True market comparisons of U.S. and Canadian pharmaceuticals reflect moderate differences in standard of living and PPP adjusted prices, as well as early access to new discoveries.

Review

1. What conditions define a pharmaceutical market?
2. What factors contribute to pricing in a pharmaceutical market?
3. In the United States, generic drugs represent what percentage of drug purchases?
4. Do Canadian patients have the same access to new discoveries — those less than five years old — as patients from the United States?
5. When pricing is properly adjusted, what percentage differential is there in affordability between drugs in Canada and the United States?

Online Resources

 Access online resources with this book's CD.

Lowering Generic Drug Prices: Less Regulation Equals More Competition
http://econ.ucalgary.ca/research/anis%20generic%20pricing.pdf

Differential Pricing for Pharmaceuticals: Reconciling Access, R&D and Patents
http://hc.wharton.upenn.edu/danzon/PDF%20Files/Diff%20Pric%20Files/Diff%20Pric%2
0for%20Pharma_Recon%20Access%20RD%20Patents_Danzon&
Towse_%20IJHCFE.pdf

International Price Comparisons for Pharmaceuticals
http://hc.wharton.upenn.edu/danzon/PDF%20Files/Intl%20Price%
20Comparisons%20for%20Pharma_Mar98%20PharmacoEcon.pdf

U.S. and Canada Price Comparisons
http://www.pnwer.org/Working_Group/Health%20Care/nga13.pdf

Health Politics Online

For Original Health Politics Programs and Slides:

Pricing Pharmaceuticals
http://www.healthpolitics.com/program_info.asp?p=prog_30
Slide Briefing
http://www.healthpolitics.com/media/prog_30/brief_prog_30.pdf

Research Versus Generic Drugs

THE BENEFITS OF PARTNERSHIPS

One of the logical reactions to the emergence of new, higher-priced drugs is to promote the use of older and lower-cost copies of formerly patented drugs, commonly called generic drugs. Most often when you hear the debate over research drugs versus generic drugs, it's an either/or proposition. But the truth is that new discoveries and older generics are extraordinarily dependent on each other for success.

Let's begin at the source — a new pharmaceutical discovery. The first thing a pharmaceutical company does when it discovers a new chemical it thinks might someday be a blockbuster discovery is to patent the chemical. When it applies for and receives the patent, it is not in exclusive company. In fact, more than five million patents have been granted since 1790, for a wide variety of products that the inventors hoped would increase efficiency or productivity, improve health, make life easier or more pleasurable.[1]

The patent, a period of exclusivity intended to allow inventors a reasonable chance of recouping development costs, exists for a wide range of new discoveries, in fields as varied as telecommunications, electronics, chemicals and pharmaceuticals.

What is unusual about the pharmaceuticals industry is the cost of testing a new chemical to ensure its safety and effectiveness prior to coming to market. It takes an average of 14 years and some $800 million for each discovery that reaches the American public. In contrast, a copy may be produced in one year, for less than $1 million.[2]

Where does the $800 million go? Ten percent goes to building the original molecule — knowing its structure and then bringing it to life through chemical and biological synthesis. Once you have the chemical in hand, an additional 14 percent is used for early screening and testing, to ensure its ability to effectively correct or improve the problem for which it was designed. An additional 5 percent is spent in early safety testing and 8 percent to formulate it at the right dose in pill or injectable form. Once all that is done, the clinical studies (up to and beyond approval of the drug) occur in thousands of human volunteers and consume an additional 41 percent. If all goes well, it's on to full-scale quality manufacturing, where an additional 8 percent investment is required. Then, to present the case to government regulators in the hope of market approval, 6 percent is expended. The point is, it's a long, complex, and laborious process, but it works.[2]

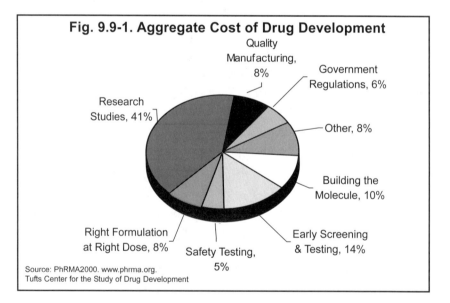

Fig. 9.9-1. Aggregate Cost of Drug Development

Quality Manufacturing, 8%

Government Regulations, 6%

Research Studies, 41%

Other, 8%

Building the Molecule, 10%

Right Formulation at Right Dose, 8%

Safety Testing, 5%

Early Screening & Testing, 14%

Source: PhRMA2000. www.phrma.org.
Tufts Center for the Study of Drug Development

Government, non-profit foundations and industry play complementary roles in the discovery process.[3] All three play a role in the first phase, basic science research to discover how the human body functions on a cellular and molecular level, and how these functions are disrupted by disease. This becomes the foundation for translational research and translating knowledge to action. This research is once again substantially supported by government, industry and foundations. Finally, those ideas that survive and have promise must now be created, tested and proven safe and useful before being blessed by the FDA. This third phase of research, called applied research, is primarily shouldered by pharmaceutical industry funding and direction. Taken as a whole, the global breakdown in investment in drug research and development is 49 percent industry, 45 percent government and 6 percent non-profit foundations.[4]

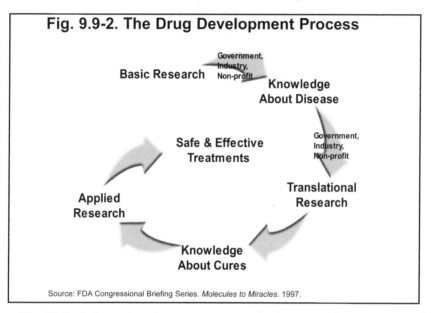

Fig. 9.9-2. The Drug Development Process

Source: FDA Congressional Briefing Series. *Molecules to Miracles*. 1997.

The United States has, by any measure, the largest and most successful pharmaceutical industry in the world. Forty-five percent of all new discoveries, between 1975 and 1994, came from U.S. companies, with the United Kingdom a distant second at 14 percent.[4] What is equally amazing is that during this same period of research industry success, the percentage of total United States prescriptions, written by doctors and filled by patients with generic drugs, increased from 18 percent to 51 percent.[5] Thus, the United States, which alone accounted for one-third of all of the world's filled prescriptions in 1999, filled roughly half of these with patented new drugs and half with the lower-cost, trusted, old standard generic drugs.[6] What led to this combined success? Most experts credit the Hatch-Waxman law, a piece of legislation passed in 1984 and formally titled the Drug Price Competition and Patent Term Registration Act of 1984. In it, legislators attempted to balance the competing interests of generic manufacturers and the prescription drug industries. The research-based industry received additional patent protection in exchange for the generic manufacturers being granted the right to use the patent holder's original research for the generic drug approval, rather than having to repeat expensive experiments on their own.

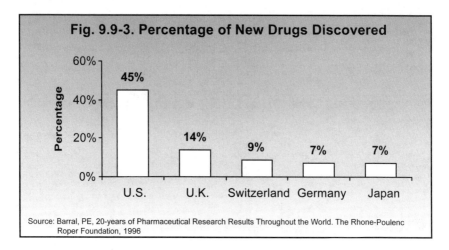

Fig. 9.9-3. Percentage of New Drugs Discovered

Source: Barral, PE, 20-years of Pharmaceutical Research Results Throughout the World. The Rhone-Poulenc Roper Foundation, 1996

This critical compromise, supported by strong patent law and free markets for competition in the United States, created a symbiotic relationship favorable to both industries. How does this favorable cycle work? It begins with the research-based industry coming up with a new discovery. The discovery becomes a product that is provided a limited period of patent protection. Once the patent expires, the generic industry creates an identical low cost copy and the market price drops, often 90 percent. The lower-cost copy is generally produced by more than one generic company, and competition increases price compression. But even at low cost, generic companies are able to make a profit since they have made no investment in the original research, development or approval, and they are not competing against the huge research companies, who chose to "let the product go" once their patent expires. Why do they choose to not compete? Because they are focused on the high-risk, high-gain world of creating the next new discovery. The net effect of the cycle, then, is to simultaneously create a viable and successful new discovery industry, while at the same time feeding and supporting a generic industry that provides low-cost and effective old standards that might otherwise disappear.[7]

The benefits of partnership, then, are obvious. Research companies provide a constant flow of new discoveries, testing the frontiers of science, providing hope and attracting private and public investment. The generic companies provide trusted old standards, expand low-cost access, help maintain confidence in the health care system and provide additional options for care. Together, working well and working in unison, they share a common goal, supporting patient care.

REFERENCES

1. Lienhard JH. The Engines of Our Ingenuity, No. 565: A Potash Patent. Available at: http://www.uh.edu/engines/epi565.htm. Accessed 4/10/00.
2. Tufts Center for the Study of Drug Development (TCSDD). Tufts Center for the Study of Drug Development Pegs Cost of a New Prescription Medicine at $802 Million [news release]. November 30, 2001.
3. PhRMA Annual Survey, 2000. Available at: www.phrma.org.
4. Discovery of New Drugs; From Basic Research to the Prescription. Source: FDA, Congressional Briefing Series, "Molecules to Miracles," 1997. As cited in: PhRMA. Pharmaceutical Industry Profile 2000. Available at: http://www.phrma.org/publications/industry/profile00.html. Accessed 5/23/00.
5. Kettler HE. Narrowing the Gap Between Provision and Need for Medicines in Developing Countries. London: Office of Health Economics; 2000. Available at: http://www.ohe.org/narrowing%5the%5Fgap.htm. Accessed 4/12/00.
6. A Global Market for Pharmaceuticals. Source: IMS Health, 2000. As cited in: PhRMA. Pharmaceutical Industry Profile 2000. Available at: http://www.phrma.org/publications/industry/profile00.html. Accessed 5/23/00.
7. U.S. International Trade Commission, Office of Industries. Review of global competitiveness in the pharmaceutical industry. USITC Staff Research Study 25. Washington, DC; April 1999. Publication 3172.

TEACHING TOOLS

Policy Premises

1. Drugs are extremely expensive to develop, yet relatively easy to copy.
2. Government and industry have complementary roles to play in new drug development.
3. The U.S. has the strongest generic industry and the strongest research pharmaceutical industry.
4. This is because strong patent protection and free markets create a symbiotic relationship favorable to both industries.
5. Both research and generic pharmaceutical industries have a role to play in developing nations.
6. It is in the public interest to have the best of both worlds — a strong research and a strong generic pharmaceutical industry.

Review

1. What is the cost of testing a new chemical to ensure its safety before it is put on the market?
2. How much does it cost and how long does it take to produce a generic drug?
3. What percentage do industry, government and non-profit foundations invest in drug research and development?
4. Generic drugs accounted for what percentage of filled prescriptions in 2002?
5. What is the Hatch-Waxman law?

Online Resources

Access online resources with this book's CD.

Tufts Center for the Study of Drug Development
http://csdd.tufts.edu/

Tufts Center for the Study of Drug Development Pegs Cost of a New Prescription Medicine at $802 Million
http://csdd.tufts.edu/NewsEvents/RecentNews.asp?newsid=6

Congressional Budget Office — How Increased Competition from Generic Drugs Has Affected Prices and Returns in the Pharmaceutical Industry
http://www.cbo.gov/showdoc.cfm?index=655&sequence=2

FDA Consumer special issue From Test Tube To Patient: New Drug Development in the United States
http://www.fda.gov/cder/about/whatwedo/testtube.pdf

PhRMA: Most Drugs Never Recoup the Average Cost of Development
http://www.phrma.org/publications/quickfacts/16.04.2003.717.cfm

Health Politics Online

For Original Health Politics Programs and Slides:

Balancing the Research and Generic Pharmaceutical Industries
http://www.healthpolitics.com/program_transcript.asp?p=prog_06
Slide Briefing
http://www.healthpolitics.com/media/prog_06/brief_prog_06.pdf

CHAPTER 9.10

Drug Importation

FROM CANADA AND BEYOND

Current price differentials between U.S. and Canadian markets have led some to support importation of drugs as a method of cost control. But is this approach wise or safe? The simple answer is no, but getting there requires laying a bit of groundwork.

The new Medicare prescription drug benefit signed into law in 2003 by President Bush puts the safety issue front and center. Congress specifically rejected a proposal that would have allowed drugs to be reimported from Canada. Under the new Medicare law, prescription medicines can be reimported from Canada only if they have a safety stamp from the Secretary of Health and Human Services.

Leaders on both sides of the aisle, along with a broad spectrum of health organizations, have opposed importation of drugs from Canada and elsewhere for good reasons. The modern legislative record goes back to the 1987 Prescription Drug Marketing Act, which allowed only pharmaceutical manufacturers to import large quantities of medicine.[1] The Medicine Equity and Drug Safety Act of 2000 declared individuals and organizations free to import medicines from developed countries as long as the Health and Human Services (HHS) department certified that the products imported were safe and effective. Previously, Democratic HHS Secretary Donna Shalala, who served under President Bill Clinton, refused to certify the practice as safe. Under the Bush administration, the department, to date, has maintained the same position, pending further study.[2]

The historic bipartisan HHS resistance to certifying the safety of imported drugs is based on realistic and well-founded concerns. It can be boiled down to three fundamental issues. First, the system of importation, most commonly facilitated by Internet and overnight delivery, bypasses the normal checks and balances built into well-established patient-physician relationships. These relationships allow for individualization of care decisions, discussion of benefits versus risks, considerations of cost and value, and generation of a meaningful accurate prescription faithfully executed by a licensed pharmacist.[3]

The second issue is that it is extremely difficult to verify the location, credentials and true identity of many of the importation-providing companies, their doctors and their pharmacists. These three entities, in a single operation, may exist on three different continents, connected only virtually, and beyond the licensing or regulatory reach of the area of residence of the patient.

The third problem is that the cost of policing and certifying safety of inflow is prohibitive, to the point that a July 22, 2003, analysis by the bipartisan Congressional Budget Office concluded that importation "would probably not produce substantial savings for the federal government."[4] Such cost would be necessary to deal with a host of product integrity issues already well known and well publicized.[5] These include product expiration, product dilution, product contamination, product replacement, wrong dosages, wrong drug, no instructions, and absence of assurances that Good Manufacturing Standards were followed in creation of the product.

Many of the worst players in this costly chain of invisible, profit-seeking middlemen are recognizable. They don't list their geographic address. They declare, "no need for prescriptions." They emphasize popular medications. They are not licensed. They extensively use spam promotion. And they demand release from liability.[5] Many are recognizable, but many are not.

Just how large are the safety problems? A recent and extensive investigation by the *Washington Post* led to a five-part series warning of "rogue medical merchants" in a multibillion-dollar shadow market. FDA Commissioner Mark McClellan, in a recent speech at the National Press Club, sounded similar concerns. He stressed that "pharmaceutical peddlers are taking advantage of regulatory gaps to move millions of prescription drugs, including controlled substances, into the United States from Mexico, Canada, and elsewhere. Rogue medical merchants who have dubious or no medical background are selling potentially dangerous drugs to people who never see the prescribing doctor in person or undergo tests."[6]

Open importation without safety verification would predictably unleash a chaotic cascade of market adjustments that, in the end, would degrade quality and deliver little long-term economic benefit. The importation roadmap looks like this: Open importation matches up the United States with Canada, an apples-to-oranges comparison. Canada possesses less than 5 percent of the revenues of its trading partner. Thus, the U.S. market has more than 20 times the buying power of Canada. What this means is that a Canadian wholesaler, faced with the prospect of easy access to such a comparatively huge opportunity, will respond and over-respond. To participate on this scale they must rapidly expand purchases from U.S. manufacturers and focus on the United States over Canada.[7]

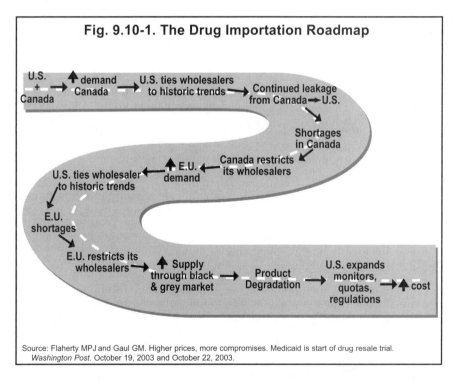

Fig. 9.10-1. The Drug Importation Roadmap

Source: Flaherty MPJ and Gaul GM. Higher prices, more compromises. Medicaid is start of drug resale trial. *Washington Post*. October 19, 2003 and October 22, 2003.

U.S. manufacturers, in turn, faced with diverting product to Canada (on its way back to the United States) and a longer supply chain, and a loss of one-third the revenue, will rapidly move (and have moved) to tie wholesaler limits to historic purchase trends.[8] Medicines will continue to leak to the United States, creating shortages of product in Canada.[9] Canadian regulators in turn will clamp down on their wholesalers, who, faced with a huge market and little product, will turn next to fixed-price European Union countries. The cycle of demand, historic trend adjustments, shortage, and local restrictions will then play out in the European Union, forcing starved wholesalers to eventually turn to counterfeiters in Asian, South American and African nations for a flow of gray and black market product. While the drugs currently taken by Canadians may be safe, dismantling our regime of safety regulations would allow bad drugs to come through Canada and flood the U.S. market.

Along the way, on this cycle, prices in Canada and the European Union may rise to lessen the margin of profit local exporting wholesalers have to gain by ignoring their own citizens.[9] And on the U.S. side, to defend against growing gray and black market products, the United States will expand monitors, quotas and regulations to manage the safety of its populace.[7]

The bottom line is that U.S. market size alone makes cost containment through importation extremely problematic. The huge U.S. market demand would rapidly overwhelm other countries' chains of supply and demand. Canada's market is just 5 percent, and Germany, the No. 1 market in the European Union, is only 30 percent the size of our market. And on the other end, without reimportation, we already receive two million medication mail packages a day, with less than one percent examined by U.S. Customs. It's literally "a BIG problem."[7,10]

Now, some states — and even local cities and counties — want to try and navigate this system on their own. Beyond the potential legal issues raised, it would be a difficult undertaking.

REFERENCES

1. Graham JR. Prescription Drug Prices in Canada and the United States-Part 4: Canadian Prescriptions for American Patients Are Not the Solution. Vancouver, Canada: The Fraser Institute; 2003. Accessed at: http://www.fraserinstitute.ca/pharmaceuticalpolicy/index.asp?snav=pa. Quoted in Calfee JE. The grim economics of pharmaceutical importation. American Enterprise Institute For Public Policy. *Health Policy Outlook*. November-December 2003.
2. Blanchard R. et al. Importing Prescription Drugs-Comparison of the Drug Import Provisions in the Medicare Reform Bills, H.R. 2427, and Current Law. Washington, DC: Congressional Research Service. 2003.

3. Nash DB. *Connecting With the New Healthcare Consumer*. Gaitherberg, MD: Aspen Publishers; 2001.
4. Congressional Budget Office. Cost Estimate of H.R:1 and S.1. Washington, DC: 2003.
5. National Association of Pharmacy Boards. Press Release. October 23, 2003.
6. McClellan M. Speech given before Fifth Annual David A. Winston Lecture National Press Club, October 20, 2003, Washington, DC.
7. Flaherty MP and Gaul GM. Higher prices, more compromises. Medicaid is start of drug resale trial. *Washington Post*. October 19, 2003 and October 22, 2003.
8. Waldie P. Ottawa fears medicine shortage. Globe and Mail. October 29, 2003.
9. Wroe, D and Colebatch, T. Deal may push up drug prices. The Age. October 23, 2003. Australia.
10. Verband Forschender Arzneimittelhersteller e.V. The Pharmaceutical industry in Germany: Statistics 2003. Available at: http://www.vfa.de/en/statistics/statoverview.html.

TEACHING TOOLS

Policy Premises

1. Current price differentials between U.S. and Canadian markets have led some to support importation of drugs as a method of cost control.
2. Historically, American leaders and health organizations have opposed importation of drugs for good reasons.
3. Bipartisan HHS resistance to certify safety has been based on real concerns.
4. Beyond safety, open importation would unleash a chaotic cascade of market adjustments that degrade quality with little cost benefit.
5. The bottom line is that the size of the United States alone makes cost containment through importation extremely problematic.
6. In the short-term, other options are available that better serve those in need. In the long-term, expansion of insurance for prescription medications is essential.

Review

1. Why has HHS consistently refused to certify the safety of imported drugs?
2. What effect would linking Canada to the huge U.S. market have on Canadian drug prices and supplies?
3. What measures might Canada take to ensure its own citizens' access to drugs?
4. How might Canada become a gateway for drugs from all over the world?
5. What alternative methods of cost control might we consider?

Online Resources

Access online resources with this book's CD.

Buyer Beware
http://www.fda.gov/cder/consumerinfo/border.htm

Imported May Equal Unapproved
http://www.fda.gov/fdac/features/2002/502_import.html

Is Reimportation Cost Effective?
http://www.aei.org/publications/pubID.19380/pub_detail.asp

Drug Reimportation Not Needed
http://www.ncpa.org/iss/hea/2003/pd072403a.html

Should the State Government Import Prescription Drugs?
http://www.jbartlett.org/pdf/policy_matters_drugs.pdf

Drug Re-Importation Bill: Cheaper Drugs Today, But Fewer Medicines Tomorrow
http://www.cei.org/gencon/003,03567.cfm

Health Politics Online

For Original Health Politics Programs and Slides:

Importing Drugs from Canada and Beyond
http://www.healthpolitics.com/program_info.asp?p=prog_32
Slide Briefing
http://www.healthpolitics.com/media/prog_32/brief_prog_32.pdf

CHAPTER 9.11

ERISA: Laws Protecting Managed Care

MAKING SENSE OF ERISA

Over the past decade or two, many people inside and outside of health care have been marginally aware of the term ERISA, but not thoroughly versed on its implications and the ideological battle it has come to represent. What is ERISA?

The Employee Retirement Income Security Act, or ERISA, was enacted in 1974 to protect employees from losing their pensions as a result of inadequate funding or mismanagement of pension plans.[1,2] A run of pension collapses and reversals at the time instigated this federal legislation. The law standardized benefit management policies, moving oversight from state to federal bodies to address state-to-state variability.[3,4,5]

Today, ERISA impacts some 140 million Americans under the age of 65 in ways that were not originally intended 30 years ago.[6] It has now become the central pillar of defining the roles and responsibilities of the health insurance industry's managed care organizations. More specifically, it's used to define the extent of their liability for both health benefits and the fallout of decisions to extend, or not to extend, coverage for a wide array of health services.

ERISA has been quite successful in providing federal protection of pension benefits but more controversial in the area of health benefits. The reasons are obvious. For pensions, the legislation ensures dollar-for-dollar replacement of pensioners' losses due to plan mismanagement. In health, however, losses extend well beyond the financial value of a denied concrete service, impacting the short- and long-term physical and mental health of the individual and the individual's family.

The core section of ERISA, at the crosshairs of intense legal battling, is Section 502 (a) (1) (B). It states the law's intent on behalf of a beneficiary "to recover benefits due to him under the terms of his plan, to enforce his rights under the terms of the plan, or to clarify his rights to future benefits under the terms of the plan."[7] The section was intended to create an "exclusive" remedy on the federal level when mistakes occurred: Underfund a pension plan, mismanage it (deliberately or not), and you will still be held responsible for delivering the dollars promised, but will not be subject to punitive or other claims that might vary state-to-state in malpractice courts.[1]

In the 1980s, when applied to a wide variety of issues flowing out of the managed care movement, ERISA created immediate controversy between doctors, patients and their insurers. The interfaces between the three have been complex from the start. They all share the effort to manage both cost and quality of health care. Their core roles, however, diverge. Managed care organizations administer health contracts that define specific benefits. They also exert judgment for a portion of their benefits by reimbursing activities that are deemed "medically necessary." An unwillingness to reimburse, at least for a portion of the population, is tantamount to eliminating access. Should their activities be proved to be in violation of their contractual promises, managed care organizations are shielded by ERISA from exposure to the full weight of state tort courts and are liable only for replacement costs for the specific item denied, such as an extra day of hospitalization or the difference in price between a drug that was denied and the one that was provided.[1]

Physicians, in contrast, carry the full weight of their medical judgments and the responsibility to provide continuity of care. Lapses expose them to the full liability of state courts, including additional medical costs and punitive damages.

The Supreme Court weighed in on the matter in the 1987 Pilot Life v. Dedeaux decision, affirming that ERISA pre-empts the remedy of punitive damages (against managed care organizations) under state law for improper processing of benefit claims, including bad faith claims.[8]

A backlash occurred during the 1990s, fueling the creation of the Bipartisan Patient Protection bills, which were passed, but not enacted, in 2001, and the belief among some consumer groups that managed care organizations were unwilling to accept accountability for their decisions.[1,9,10] During the 1990s, courts began to distinguish between the types of decisions that managed care organizations made to determine whether they should be held responsible under state malpractice law or under ERISA.[11,12]

In 2000, the Supreme Court weighed-in again in Pegram v. Herdrich, defining three types of decisions: "eligibility decisions" around contract coverage; "treatment decisions" around diagnosis and therapy; and what they called "mixed decisions" dealing with the when, where, and how of executing benefits.[13]

This third area set a legal struggle in motion, pitting state prerogatives against federal standards, and physician organizations against managed care organizations. On June 21, 2004, the Supreme Court spoke with clarity in the combined cases of Aetna Health Inc. v. Davila and CIGNA HealthCare of Texas Inc. v. Calad. The court stated that Section 502 provides the exclusive remedy for patients in ERISA plans when a managed care organization denies benefits, even if the denial is based on a decision that disputed care is not medically necessary. The Court also said that ERISA provides appropriate relief; it reinforced the principle of a comprehensive federally regulated system; and it emphasized that managed care organizations are responsible for only what the contract promises.[14]

For many, the core concerns with ERISA remain unresolved. Reacting to the June 21 decision, the president of the American Medical Association was quoted as saying, "This is a sad day for America's patients and the physicians who care for them."[15]

What are the chief concerns? First, that the Supreme Court's decision may lead to tighter managed care organization restrictions. Second, that no significant financial disincentive exists since an ERISA loss only requires them to pay what they should have paid for in the first place. Third, that a heavy burden is placed on the patient, often ill at the time, to achieve absolute clarity on the front end or rely on strong physician advocacy to achieve corrections on the back end. Finally, that this emotional vortex could adversely impact trust and confidence between patient and physician.[1]

As we look ahead, several things will likely accelerate concerns and heighten tensions, including increasing health care costs, increasing employer demands, and the shielding of managed care organizations from the fallout of some of their decisions. Is it possible to maximize the benefit of a standardized federal approach and rapid compensation for injury (even if some say it's undervalued), while at the same time providing adequate checks and balances to encourage all parties to think long term rather than short term, especially in the area of "mixed decisions"? If so, a new framework is unlikely to present itself in a reversal of federal pre-emption, but rather in an expansion of compensation or further balancing of the division of responsibility between benefits and care.

REFERENCES

1. Mariner WK. The Supreme Court's limitation of managed-care liability. *NEJM*. 2004;351:1347-1352.

2. Employee Retirement Income Security Act of 1974, 88 Stat. 829 (as amended and codified at 29 U.S.C. §§1001-1161. Cited in Mariner WK.

3. H.R. Conf. Rep. No. 93-1280 (Aug. 12. 1974). Cited in Mariner WK.

4. S. Conf. Rep. No. 93-1090 (Aug. 13, 1974). Cited in Mariner WK.

5. Mariner WK. State regulation of managed care and the Employee Retirement Income Security Act. *NEJM*. 1996;335:1986-1990. Cited in Mariner WK.

6. Fronstin P. Sources of health insurance and characteristics of the uninsured: analysis of the March 2003 current population survey. EBRI issue brief. No. 264. Washington, D.C.: Employee Benefit Research Institute, December 2003:1-34. Cited in Mariner WK.

7. ERISA §502(a)(1)(B), codified at 29 U.S.C. §1132(a)(1)(B). Cited in Mariner WK.

8. Pilot Life Ins. Co. v. Dedeaux, 481 U.S. 41 (1987). Cited in Mariner WK.

9. S. 1052, passed June 29, 2001. Cited in Mariner WK.

10. H.R. 2563, passed August 2, 2001. Cited in Mariner WK.

11. Bloche MG, Studdert DM. A quiet revolution: law as an agent of health system change. *Health Aff* (Millwood) 2004;23(2):29-42. Cited in Mariner WK.

12. Agrawal GB, Hall MA. What if you could sue your HMO? Managed care liability beyond the ERISA shield. *St. Louis Univ Law J*. 2003;47:235-298.<./a>Cited in Mariner WK.

13. Pegram v. Herdrich, 530 U.S. 211 (2000). Cited in Mariner WK.

14. Aetna Health, Inc. v. Davila; CIGNA Healthcare of Texas, Inc. v. Calad, 124 S. Ct 2488 (2004). Cited in Mariner WK.

15. Japsen B. Justices protect HMOs from big damage rewards. *Chicago Tribune*. June 22, 2004:1.Cited in Mariner WK.

TEACHING TOOLS

Policy Premises

1. The Employee Retirement Income Security Act (ERISA) was enacted in 1974 to protect employee pensions.
2. ERISA is quite good at protecting pension benefits but not as good at protecting health benefits.
3. The ERISA debate around the role of managed care organizations (MCOs) in patient care coverage and discussions was addressed by the Supreme Court in 1987.
4. A backlash through the 1990s fueled the bipartisan patient protection bills in 2001.
5. The Supreme Court weighed in firmly on June 21, 2004.
6. Concerns remain, and for many the core concerns with ERISA remain unresolved.

Review

1. When and why was ERISA first enacted?
2. Are people now being affected by ERISA in ways that were not originally intended?
3. What did the Supreme Court decide about ERISA on June 21, 2004?
4. What concerns about ERISA remain unresolved?
5. Are these concerns likely to accelerate or subside in the coming months?

Online Resources

 Access online resources with this book's CD.

What is ERISA?
http://www.dol.gov/dol/topic/health-plans/erisa.htm

The Opinion of the Court
http://a257.g.akamaitech.net/7/257/2422/21june20041210/www.su
premecourtus.gov/opinions/03pdf/02-1845.pdf

Implications of ERISA Preemption
http://www.statecoverage.net/pdf/issuebrief804.pdf

The Court Has Spoken
http://www.pbs.org/newshour/bb/law/jan-june04/scotus_6-21.html

Pegram v. Herdrich: Looking Back
http://archives.cnn.com/2000/HEALTH/02/23/scotus.hmos/

Health Consumerism
http://www.benefitnews.com/detail.cfm?id=6162&terms=|hospi-
tals||tiered|

Health Politics Online

For Original Health Politics Programs and Slides:

**The Laws that Protect Managed Care Organizations: Making
Sense of ERISA**
http://www.healthpolitics.com/program_info.asp?p=erisa
Slide Briefing
http://www.healthpolitics.com/media/erisa/brief_erisa.pdf

Medical Malpractice and Safety

YOU CAN'T GET THERE FROM HERE

Medical malpractice law was designed to accomplish certain specific social objectives. These include addressing poor quality care, fairly compensating patients for injuries resulting from negligence, and imposing justice in a manner that would make future occurrences less likely. Malpractice law is a part of the family of personal injury or tort law. For a plaintiff to succeed, she must prove that the injury suffered resulted from actions that were fundamentally inconsistent with the recognized standard of care. Whether or not such injury rises to the level of negligence is a matter of degree.[1]

In theory, it all makes sense. Courts provide oversight offering corrective action when professional oversight breaks down. Doctors and hospitals are insured and therefore assured that a claim will not lead to financial ruin. Patients show restraint, acting only when there has been an undeniable breach. And lawyers pursue only meritorious claims and discourage those that lack merit.

But in practice it doesn't come close. As three well-known scholars recently noted, the medical malpractice system "has internal logic but falls far short of its social goals of promoting safer medicine and compensating wrongfully injured patients."[1]

The medical malpractice system is fundamentally adversarial and built on a culture of blame. Doctors, hospitals, insurers and lawyers are locked into battle and patients are routinely caught in the crossfire.

This disturbing state of affairs was captured in a 1998 expert consensus editorial in the *Journal of the American Medical Association*. The editorial, which focused on improving the safety performance of our health care system, concluded that "a new understanding of accountability that moves beyond blaming individuals when they make mistakes must be established if progress is to be made."[2]

For some time prior to this statement, it had been abundantly clear that the American medical malpractice system was ineffective in managing the appropriate distribution of compensation to deserving patients. Studies in the 1970s, 1980s and 1990s drew near-identical results.[3,4] The most often-quoted study was conducted in 1984 when Harvard examined 30,000 medical records and 3,500 malpractice claims from New York hospitals. From the medical records they determined that 4 percent of patients had suffered adverse events, and that 1 percent rose to the level of negligence. But when they correlated these records with malpractice claims, they found that only 2 percent of the patients who had suffered from negligence had actually submitted claims, and only 17 percent of the malpractice claims were in any way tied to negligence.[5]

Beyond the current system's inability to connect cause to corrective action, the medical malpractice system is organizationally unstable, expensive and inefficient.[1] Three of the last four decades have witnessed major medical malpractice crises. The crisis of the 1970s involved availability of insurers. The crisis in the 1980s involved affordability, and the crisis of the 2000s involves both availability and affordability, with 18 states in critical condition and 26 states having serious difficulty.[6]

Factors contributing to our current insurer instability trace back to the 1990s and include large payouts in 1999, declining stock market investments, heavy competition leading to price compression, increased cost for reinsurance post-9/11, and wide geographic variability in awards and overhead.[1] Sixty cents of every dollar spent in the malpractice system goes to administrative costs.[7] That's twice the amount spent administering the Workers Compensation System.[8]

Attempts to correct the system have gained steam over the years, but only represent tinkering at the edges, not true reform. They include limiting access to the courts, limiting the number of claims, and limiting the size of the awards.[1] Yet even if all of these reforms were successful, they would leave America's doctors, patients, researchers and insurers very poorly served for one very critical reason: the American malpractice system, embedded in personal injury law, fundamentally undermines the patient safety movement.[2]

A head-to-head comparison tells the story. The tort system uses litigation as its lever for change. The safety movement uses quality improvement analysis. Tort law focuses on the individual. Safety focuses on the process. The tort system's punitive and adversarial style drives information down, encouraging secrecy. The safety movement uses a non-punitive and collaborative approach, which encourages openness, transparency, and continuous improvement. With tort law, exposing oneself can end one's career and harm one's mental health. In the safety movement, contributing is career-enhancing and therapeutic.[2]

Table 9.12-1. Tort System vs. Safety Movement	
Tort System	**Safety Movement**

• Litigation
• Focus on individual
• Adversarial approach
  — secrecy
• Adverse effects on clinicians' career and mental health
	• Quality improvement
	• Focus on process
	• Collaborative approach
	  — transparency
	• Career-enhancing and therapeutic for clinicians

Source: Leape LL, et. al. Promoting patient safety by preventing medical error. *JAMA* 1998;280:1444-1447.

It may seem counterintuitive, but for medical malpractice to achieve its stated social purpose it must abandon the emphasis on a tort-based approach and embrace safety. Alternate dispute resolution, no-fault systems, raising fault to the institutional level, and exploring the use of medical courts all merit consideration and could begin to break the cycle of blame and provide a level of security necessary to ensure openness and transparency.[1,2]

The resulting flow of error and risk management data would accelerate process reengineering, expose glaring disparities, expand collaborations across silos, and promote the development of common language and tools embedded in electronic information systems. It would also encourage risk-taking, which is essential for innovation, discovery and progress. All of these things are necessary if we are to reach the quality and prevention "tipping point."

We can hold on to malpractice if we like. We can battle at the edges. But until we throw off the shackles of blame, we will never have a safe system... because you just can't get there from here.

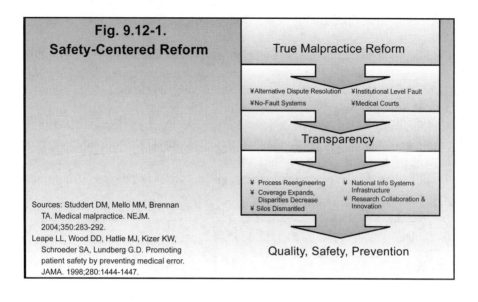

Fig. 9.12-1.
Safety-Centered Reform

True Malpractice Reform

¥ Alternative Dispute Resolution   ¥ Institutional Level Fault
¥ No-Fault Systems   ¥ Medical Courts

Transparency

¥ Process Reengineering   ¥ National Info Systems
¥ Coverage Expands,   Infrastructure
   Disparities Decrease   ¥ Research Collaboration &
¥ Silos Dismantled   Innovation

Sources: Studdert DM, Mello MM, Brennan
TA. Medical malpractice. NEJM.
2004;350:283-292.
Leape LL, Wood DD, Hatlie MJ, Kizer KW,
Schroeder SA, Lundberg G.D. Promoting
patient safety by preventing medical error.
JAMA. 1998;280:1444-1447.

Quality, Safety, Prevention

REFERENCES

1. Studdert DM, Mello MM, Brennan TA. Medical malpractice. *NEJM.* 2004;350:283-292.
2. Leape LL, Wood DD, Hatlie MJ, Kizer KW, Schroeder SA, Lundberg G.D. Promoting patient safety by preventing medical error. *JAMA.* 1998;280:1444-1447.
3. Robinson GO. The malpractice crisis of the 1970s: a retrospective. *Law Contempt. Probl* 1986;49:5-35. Quoted in Studdert et al.
4. Kinney ED. Malpractice reform in the 1990s: past disappointments, future success? *J Health Polit Policy Law.* 1995;20:99-135. Quoted in Studdert et al.
5. Localio AR, Lawthers AG, Brennan TA, et al. Relation between malpractice claims and adverse events due to negligence: results of the Harvard Medical Practice Study III. *NEJM.* 1991;324:370-6. Quoted in Studdert et al.
6. Mello MM, Studdert DM, Brennan TA. The new medical malpractice crisis. *NEJM.* 2003; 348:23, 2281-2284.
7. Kakalik JS, Pace NM. Costs and compensation paid in tort litigation. R-3391-ICJ. Santa Monica, Calif. Institute for Civil Justice, RAND, 1986. Quoted in Studdert et al.
8. Weiler PC, Hiatt HH, Newhouse JP, Johnson WG, Brennan T, Leape LL. A Measure of malpractice: medical injury, malpractice litigation

and patient compensation. Cambridge, Mass. Howard University Press; 1993. Quoted in Studdert et al.

TEACHING TOOLS

Policy Premises

1. Medical malpractice law was designed to accomplish specific social objectives.
2. The medical malpractice system is fundamentally adversarial and built on a culture of blame.
3. The current system is ineffective in the appropriate distribution of compensation.
4. The medical malpractice system is organizationally unstable, expensive, and inefficient.
5. This system also fundamentally undermines the patient safety movement.
6. To accomplish its stated social purpose, medical malpractice law must give way to safety-centered reform.

Review

1. What is medical malpractice law intended to accomplish?
2. What do studies reveal about the relationship between cases of negligence and malpractice claims?
3. Why are physicians increasingly unable to find affordable malpractice insurance?
4. How does the medical malpractice system undermine the patient safety movement?
5. How can we better prevent medical negligence and ensure patient safety?

Online Resources

Access online resources with this book's CD.

Jackpot Justice
http://www.hsph.harvard.edu/press/releases/press03012000.html

Medical Liability Reform
http://www.ama-assn.org/ama1/pub/upload/mm/-1/mlr2004.pdf

To Err Is Human: Building a Better Health System
http://books.nap.edu/html/to_err_is_human/reportbrief.pdf

Professional Liability: Tort Reform
http://www.aaos.org/wordhtml/papers/position/1118.htm

Health Politics

For Original Health Politics Programs and Slides:

The Road from Medical Malpractice to Safety: You Can't Get There from Here
http://www.healthpolitics.com/program_info.asp?p=prog_44
Slide Briefing
http://www.healthpolitics.com/media/prog_44/brief_prog_44.pdf

Epilogue

As a weekly media commentator on health care issues, I am often asked for my opinion on where our health care system is headed. I have the advantage of being able to share perspectives with a wide range of thinkers in the health care arena — and their opinions on what needs to be done about our health care system cover the entire spectrum of possibilities. Clearly, there is no single perfect set of answers.

Nor is there enough space in this book to offer all the possible scenarios for the future as they relate to the many topics we have covered — from health insurance reform to end-of-life care.

Still, I think the diverse dots that make up the current thinking in health care can be connected — and that a new vision is beginning to emerge. After 20 years of observing health care, and thinking about what's possible, some things seem undeniable. And I notice that increasingly, voices from disparate sectors and schools of thought are coalescing around these fundamental principles.

With that said, let me lay out what I believe are several general factors and trends that are defining our health care future, and what I believe is the most likely destination they are taking us — toward a new paradigm of care.

The first, and most important, factor is that we are aging as a society. We must acknowledge that this demographic change will profoundly impact health care as we know it today.

Faced with a complex health care system and the new reality of aging and chronic disease, a vast population of informal caregivers (now present in 25 percent of American families) is on the rise. They are increasingly educated, motivated and involved with health care decisions. They represent a populist force that increasingly questions the status quo.

Recognizing this rising force, and the changing dynamics of the patient-physician relationship, physicians have moved from paternalism to partnership, and are moving from individual to team-support models.

At the same time, the medical community is realizing that its infrastructure is not ideally suited for the demands this aging society will put on the health care system. There is, simply put, minimal time and space left in the doctors' offices for care. Our outpatient office-based delivery system is not ideally suited for the rigors of the future.

Combined, these forces point the system toward a logical solution: Properly supported and validated by the doctor with education, behavioral modification, early diagnosis and screening, most care decisions and care functions can take place in the home.

We can call this new paradigm home-centered health.

I believe the concept of home-centered health will grow rapidly in coming years, and it will lead to the evolution of informal caregivers into designated home health managers and their inclusion more formally into the physician-led health care team.

In this new paradigm, health care teams will coordinate both clinical and educational continuums under physician oversight. Most educational leadership will be delegated by physicians to nurses who will maintain 24/7-contact with home health managers through virtual health networks.

The virtual health networks will be here soon, thanks to incredible advances in technology. Visionary thinkers in health care technology — ranging from corporate giants such as Philips Inc. to small, entrepreneurial start-ups — are working today below the radar screen on amazing devices that will revolutionize care and make true networks possible.

The current surge of private technology investment in home health will outfit homes with pervasive motion/location sensors, intelligence analytic software, personalized prompter coaching interfaces, and internet data transfer to care networks, functionally bringing the virtual care team and its resources into the home and obviating the need for most office visits and the vast majority of hospitalizations.

As technology and demographics lead us inexorably toward this new paradigm, the health care financing system will be forced to keep pace. Health insurance will expand, be portable and involve multi-year commitments. Health insurers will reimburse physicians fairly for team management and offer incentives for home health managers by providing lower premiums to families who deliver measurably positive health outcomes and effective prevention and screening.

Pharmaceutical and device companies will invest in consumer education and behavioral modification, early diagnosis and prevention, and a new business model built around home-centered health solutions. Health information highways will be home-centric; that is, begin in the home, extend out to the caregivers and loop back to the home, rather than the other way around.

At the end of the day, caring will re-center in the home, where compassion and personalization reside. Here, caring will integrate mind, body and spirit; focus on wellness and functionality; integrate and prioritize resources along the four- or five-generation family divide; and tailor care to the unique cultural and social needs of family members.

Homes will look to their communities for value grounding, integrated social systems, and resources by exclusion if overwhelmed by complexity. Physicians and nurses will advocate for these changes because they make sense and are the only reasonable way to manage the cost and quality demands of global aging societies.

It all may sound a bit futuristic, but the elements of this new paradigm of care are either here now or at our fingertips.

And it will become a reality, thanks to the persistent demands of millions of Americans who make up a consumer empowerment movement that I believe already has built an unstoppable momentum.

We might think of the coming transition in health care as a kind of populist uprising — led by consumers who now possess the critical combination of enlightenment, empowerment, and personal motivation needed to assert control over their health care future.

Much work remains to be done before this vision of health care will be fully embraced. Some sectors of our health care system continue to cling to the silos of yesterday — in financing, in education, in technology — but if trends continue to play out as they have recently, the keepers of the silos will soon face head on the force of millions of consumers who demand change.

And we should listen to them — for after all, it's their health and their health care system. Why not strive for excellence in both?